T0321190

Controversies in the Management of Lymphomas

Cancer Treatment and Research

WILLIAM L. McGUIRE, *series editor*

R.B. Livingston, ed.: Lung Cancer 1, 1981. ISBN 90-247-2394-9

G.B. Humphrey, L.P. Dehner, G.B. Grindey, R.T. Acton, eds.: Pediatric Oncology 1, 1981. ISBN 90-247-2408-2

J.J. DeCosse, P. Sherlock, eds.: Gastrointestinal Cancer 1, 1981. ISBN 90-247-2461-9

John M. Bennett, ed.: Lymphomas 1, including Hodgkin's Disease, 1981. ISBN 90-247-2479-1

Clara D. Bloomfield, ed.: Adult Leukemias 1, 1982. ISBN 90-247-2478-3

David F. Paulson, Genitourinary Cancer 1, 1982. ISBN 90-247-2480-5

F.M. Muggia, ed.: Cancer Chemotherapy 1, 1983. ISBN 90-247-2713-8

G.B. Humphrey, G.B. Grindey, eds.: Pancreatic Tumors in Children, 1982. ISBN 90-247-2702-2

John J. Costanzi, ed.: Malignant Melanoma 1, 1983. ISBN 90-247-2706-5

C.T. Griffiths, A.F. Fuller, eds.: Gynecologic Oncology, 1983. ISBN 0-89838-555-5

F. Anthony Greco, ed.: Biology and Management of Lung Cancer, 1983. ISBN 0-89838-554-7

Michael D. Walker, ed.: Oncology of the Nervous System, 1983. ISBN 0-89838-567-9

D.J. Higby, ed.: Supportive Care in Cancer Therapy, 1983. ISBN 0-89838-569-5

Ronald B. Herberman, ed.: Basic and Clinical Immunology, 1983. ISBN 0-89838-579-2

Laurence H. Baker, ed.: Soft Tissue Sarcomas, 1983. ISBN 0-89838-584-9

CONTROVERSIES IN THE MANAGEMENT OF LYMPHOMAS

Including Hodgkin's disease

Edited by
JOHN M. BENNETT, M.D.

Head, Medical Oncology Division
Cancer Center of the University of Rochester Medical Center
Rochester, New York, U.S.A.

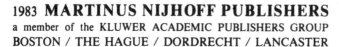

1983 **MARTINUS NIJHOFF PUBLISHERS**
a member of the KLUWER ACADEMIC PUBLISHERS GROUP
BOSTON / THE HAGUE / DORDRECHT / LANCASTER

Distributors

for the United States and Canada: Kluwer Boston, Inc., 190 Old Derby Street, Hingham, MA 02043, USA
for all other countries: Kluwer Academic Publishers Group, Distribution Center, P.O.Box 322, 3300 AH Dordrecht, The Netherlands

Library of Congress Cataloging in Publication Data

Library of Congress Cataloging in Publication Data
Main entry under title:

Controversies in the management of lymphomas.

  (Cancer treatment and research)
  Includes index.
  1. Hodgkin's disease--Treatment--Addresses, essays,
lectures. 2. Lymphoma--Treatment--Addresses, essays,
lectures. I. Bennett, John M., 1933-   . II. Series.
[DNLM: 1. Hodgkin's disease--Therapy. 2. Lymphoma--
Therapy. W1 CA693 v.16 / WH 525 C764]
RC644.C65 1983   616.99'446   83-11290
ISBN 0-89838-586-5

Copyright

© 1983 by Martinus Nijhoff Publishers, Boston.

All rights reserved. No part of this publication may be reproduced, stored in a retrieval system, or transmitted in any form or by any means, mechanical, photocopying, recording, or otherwise, without the prior written permission of the publishers,
Martinus Nijhoff Publishers, 190 Old Derby Street, Hingham, MA 02043, USA.

PRINTED IN THE NETHERLANDS

Contents

Foreword VII

Preface IX

List of contributors XIII

1. The Lukes–Butler classification of Hodgkin's disease revisited
   by James J Butler 1

2. Pitfalls in the diagnosis and classification of Hodgkin's disease:
   Surgical pathology and classification for the 1980's – Is the Lukes-
   Butler classification still relevant?
   by Thomas V. Colby. 19

3. The Reed-Sternberg cell: Biological and clinical significance
   by Marshall E. Kadin 55

4. Upon the enigma of Hodgkin's disease and the Reed-Sternberg cell
   by Clive R. Taylor. 91

5. Selection of an imaging modality for staging abdominal involvement in the malignant lymphomas – Lymphography or computed
   tomography?
   by Stephen I. Marglin and Ronald A. Castellino 111

6. The definitive management of limited and intermediate stages of
   Hodgkin's disease with radiation therapy alone
   by Richard T. Hoppe 129

7. The role of combination chemotherapy alone or as an adjuvant to
   radiation therapy in limited stages of Hodgkin's disease
   by Leonard R. Prosnitz 151

8. Chemotherapy for stage IIIA Hodgkin's disease: The proper role
   by Richard S. Stein 167

9. The Rappaport classification of the non-Hodgkin's lymphomas: Is it pertinent for the 1980's?
   by Bharat N. Nathwani 183

10. Nodular mixed cell lymphoma: Is there a potential for a prolonged disease free survival and cure?
    by Tom Anderson 225

11. Nodular mixed lymphoma: Failure to demonstrate prolonged disease free survival and cure
    by John H. Glick and Erica L. Orlow 239

12. The role of treatment deferral in the management of patients with advanced, indolent non-Hodgkin's lymphomas
    by Carol S. Portlock 257

13. Early intervention with combined modality therapy for 'favorable' non-Hodgkin's lymphomas of advanced stage
    by Timothy J. Kinsella 275

Subject index 293

Cancer Treatment and Research

Foreword

Where do you begin to look for a recent, authoritative article on the diagnosis or management of a particular malignancy? The few general oncology textbooks are generally out of date. Single papers in specialized journals are informative but seldom comprehensive; these are more often preliminary reports on a very limited number of patients. Certain general journals frequently publish good in-depth reviews of cancer topics, and published symposium lectures are often the best overviews available. Unfortunately, these reviews and supplements appear sporadically, and the reader can never be sure when a topic of special interest will be covered.

Cancer Treatment and Research is a series of authoritative volumes which aim to meet this need. It is an attempt to establish a critical mass of oncology literature covering virtually all oncology topics, revised frequently to keep the coverage up to date, easily available on a single library shelf or by a single personal subscription.

We have approached the problem in the following fashion. First, by dividing the oncology literature into specific subdivisions such as lung cancer, genitourinary cancer, pediatric oncology, etc. Second, by asking eminent authorities in each of these areas to edit a volume on the specific topic on an annual or biannual basis. Each topic and tumor type is covered in a volume appearing frequently and predictably, discussing current diagnosis, staging, markers, all forms of treatment modalities, basic biology, and more.

In Cancer Treatment and Research, we have an outstanding group of editors, each having made a major commitment to bring to this new series the very best literature in his or her field. Martinus Nijhoff Publishers has made an equally major commitment to the rapid publication of high quality books, and worldwide distribution.

Where can you go to find quickly a recent authoritative article on any major oncology problem? We hope that Cancer Treatment and Research provides an answer.

WILLIAM L. MCGUIRE
Series Editor

Preface

JOHN M. BENNETT

In the first volume in the 'Cancer Treatment and Research' series on lymphomas, the natural history, pathology, clinical staging, and therapy of these complex diseases were reviewed by a series of expert scientists. Within each modality the 'state of the art' concepts were presented and new investigational approaches elucidated.

In this second volume I have chosen an entirely different approach. Rather than provide an update of progress during the past two years in each discipline, I have focused on controversy within the broad categories that define Hodgkin's disease and the non Hodgkin's lymphomas. I have identified 8 arenas where, despite the great progress made over the past 2 decades, problems continue to exist in pathology, staging and therapeutic options. I have called upon the collective experience from those institutions where the focus has been on lymphoma management for many years.

Dr. James Butler's approach to the classification of Hodgkin's disease is a very personal one based on a large consultative referral network at the M.D. Anderson Hospital and through the South West Oncology Group. He focuses on the importance of recognizing nodularity (nodular sclerosis; nodular 'L&H'), and diffuse patterns (mixed cellularity; lymphocyte depletion). He emphasizes the misdiagnosis that can occur. A careful reading will result in the discovery of some classical gems including an awareness that only one or two Reed-Sternberg cells should be seen in lymphocyte predominance and that there is no necrosis; that solid masses of lacunar cells may mimick large cell lymphoma or metastatic carcinoma; that the use of polarized light to identify collagen and separate from reticulin fibrosis is essential for the diagnosis of nodular sclerosing Hodgkin's disease. With such attention to detail, errors in sub-classification should decrease and allow for comparisons of different treatment programs and for epidemiologic studies to be more accurate.

In the second chapter, Dr. Thomas Colby draws heavily on the extensive pathology experience of the Stanford University program. His treatise is supportive of the Lukes-Butler classification. He discusses the differences between angioimmunoblastic lymphadenopathy, 'T' cell lymphomas, malignant fibrous histiocytoma and the sub types of Hodgkin's disease. One learns that the cellular phase of nodular sclerosis has a prognosis similar to mixed cellularity Hodgkin's disease and that the number of normal appearing lymphocytes within the nodules of nodular sclerosis do not impact on prognosis.

In the next two chapters the focus narrows considerably with two excellent discussions on the origin of the Reed-Sternberg cell. Dr. Clive Taylor has mingled wit and beautiful prose with a critical dissection of the various proponents of the cell of origin. In contrast, Dr. Marshall Kadin provides an extensive analytical approach to the data. In three comprehensive tables, evidence for and against a lymphoid, macrophage/histiocyte and a dendritic/interdigitating reticulum cell is presented. Hopefully, the combined approach of cell culture, monoclonal antibodies and function studies will contribute to a final answer. The concept that the malignant cell may be related to an antigen presenting cell is intriguing because of the well-known immune defects in this disease. We still are faced with a malignant lymphoma in search of its cell of origin.

In chapter 5, Drs. Marglin and Castellino have called on their collective diagnostic experience to discuss the appropriate radiographic procedures in staging the lymphomas. Applying the Bayes theorem, relating to false positive and false negative results, we can judge for ourselves the effectiveness of computerized axial tomography (C.A.T.) versus the well established lymphangiography procedure. What becomes apparent is necessity of having local experts in lymphangiogram interpretation. It is very hard to argue against a 100% correlation with a negative study and negative laparotomy findings! Certainly one should not replace the lymphangiogram with a CAT merely because of convenience.

The next three chapters deal with a very practical consideration. How much treatment is necessary to cure the majority of patients with localized Hodgkin's disease? What is the appropriate role for combined modality therapy, i.e. combination chemotherapy, in the presence of large mediastinal masses, extranodal extensions ('E') and extensive stage IIIA disease? The results of radiotherapy for limited disease Hodgkin's disease (stages I & IIA), at Stanford University (presented by Dr. Richard Hoppe), and at Yale University (discussed by Dr. Leonard Prosnitz), are identical, with disease free survival (D.F.S.) approaching 80%.

The major differences between these two outstanding programs occurs in patients with 'B' symptoms and large mediastinums. At Stanford radiation therapy appears to be as good in I-IIB disease as it is in I-IIA. At Yale, 5 year D.F.S. is only 51%. It is hard to account for these differences on the basis of radiation equipment or planning; nevertheless the data suggests that, with the single exception of the Stanford experience, the trend is toward combined modality treatment in these 'unfavorable' localized presentations.

In chapter 8, Dr. Richard Stein defends his thesis that clinical stage $IIIA_2$ should be treated with combined modality treatment (total nodal irradiation plus 6 cycles of 'MOPP') rather than sequential treatment at relapse. Dr. Prosnitz agrees but Dr. Hoppe disagrees. A crucial consideration is the prophylactic employment of hepatic irradiation in the presence of splenic involvement (stage $IIIA_{s+}$) and the definition of massive splenic involvement. In the latter instance even the Stanford group recommends both modalities.

Lest the readers assume that this entire book is devoted to Hodgkin's disease, the remaining chapters deal exclusively with non-Hodgkin's lymphomas (NHL). Dr. Bharat Nathwani has reviewed succintly the complex classification schemas available in NHL. He presents them fairly and compares each to the National Cancer Institute's sponsored New Formulation. His support of the modified Rappaport classification for clinical trial comparisons seems very reasonable.

Drs. Tom Anderson and John Glick provide an overview of the problems of classification and the therapy of nodular (follicular) mixed cell lymphoma. The key questions relate to what cases are included by the pathologist and whether those patients who achieve a complete remission have the potential for cure. Dr. Anderson draws on his extensive experience at the National Cancer Institute, while Dr. Glick relates the large data base of the Eastern Cooperative Group. Of interest is that the referee pathologist for each program was the same. Although there are apparent differences in the outcome in the respective series, both agree that better therapy is necessary for this relatively rare NHL sub type.

The final two chapters are concerned with a most interesting and provocative discussion. At Stanford University a small group of patients with rather indolent disease (nodular histologies and diffuse well differentiated lymphocytic type) were observed without treatment treatment for months to years. The defense of this 'non treatment' until progression is eloquently stated by Dr. Carol Portlock. Dr. Timothy Kinsella takes the position that these sub types may be potentially curable and describes a new study designed to address this important issue.

In summary, this brief capsule of our table of contents is designed to provide an overview of the detailed material contained within this volume. As an editor, I believe that I have fulfilled my responsibility to solicit the best authorities in the field.

List of contributors

Tom Anderson, M.D.
Associate Professor of Medicine
Chief, Section Hematology/Oncology
Medical College of Wisconsin
Milwaukee County Medical Complex
8700 West Wisconsin Avenue
Milwaukee, WI 53226, U.S.A.

James J. Butler, M.D.
Professor of Pathology
The University of Texas System
Cancer Center
Department of Pathology
6723 Bertner Avenue
Houston, TX 77030, U.S.A.

Ronald A. Castellino, M.D.
Professor of Radiology
Stanford University Medical Center
Division of Diagnostic Radiology
Stanford, CA 94305, U.S.A.

Thomas V. Colby, M.D.
Associate Professor of Pathology
University of Utah Medical Center
Salt Lake City, UT 84132, U.S.A.

John H. Glick, M.D.
Associate Professor of Medicine
University of Pennsylvania School
of Medicine
Hematology-Oncology Section
3400 Spruce Street
Philadelphia, PA 19104, U.S.A.

Richard T. Hoppe, M.D.
Assistant Professor of Radiology
Stanford University Medical Center
Radiation Therapy Division
Stanford, CA 94305, U.S.A.

Marshall E. Kadin, M.D.
Associate Professor and Director
of Hematopathology
University of Washington
Department of Laboratory Medicine
Seattle, WA 98195, U.S.A.

Timothy J. Kinsella, M.D.
Senior Investigator
Radiation Oncology Branch
Clinical Oncology Program
Division of Cancer Treatment
National Cancer Institute
Bethesda, MD 20205, U.S.A.

Steve Marglin, M.D.
Assistant Professor of Radiology
University of Washington
Department of Radiology
Seattle, WA 98195, U.S.A.

Bharat N. Nathwani, M.D.
Department of Anatomic Pathology
City of Hope National Medical Center
Duarte, CA 91010, U.S.A.

Erica L. Orlow
Senior Research Analyst
Department of Radiation Medicine
Massachusetts General Hospital
Fruit Street
Boston, MA 02114, U.S.A.

Carol S. Portlock, M.D.
Associate Professor of Medicine
Section of Medical Oncology
Yale University School of Medicine
333 Cedar Street
New Haven, CT 06510, U.S.A.

Leonard R. Prosnitz, M.D.
Professor of Therapeutic Radiology
Division of Radiation Oncology

Box 3275, Duke University Medical Center
Durham, NC 27710, U.S.A.

Richard S. Stein, M.D.
Assistant Professor of Medicine
Vanderbilt University
Division of Hematology
1161 21st Avenue South
Nashville, TN 37232, U.S.A.

Clive Taylor, M.D.
Professor of Pathology
University of Southern California
Department of Pathology
2025 Zonal Avenue
Los Angeles, CA 90033, U.S.A.

1. The Lukes-Butler classification of Hodgkin's disease revisited

JAMES J. BUTLER

1. Introduction

The continued use of the modified Lukes-Butler classification of Hodgkin's disease (HD) since 1966 must indicate its usefulness to clinicians and pathologists. However, when one considers the number of classifications proposed for the non-Hodgkin's lymphomas in the last 10 years, its use probably also reflects the small number of pathologists with interest and experience in lymphoreticular neoplasm at the time the classification was introduced and became established. It is perhaps of interest from the historical point of view that a paper describing the nodular sclerosis type was not accepted for presentation at a national pathology meeting in 1958 [1].

Although intensive radiation therapy and combination chemotherapy have largely obliterated the differences in survival between patients with different histologic types [2, 3, 4], the incidence of non-Hodgkin's lymphomas and acute granulocytic leukemia in patients so treated indicates the need to evaluate all prognostic factors in order to individualize therapy [5]. The histologic type is one of these factors so accurate classification continues to be important. Knowledge of histologic types is also of value to the pathologist since they reflect the spectrum of histologic findings in HD and therefore help in establishing the correct diagnosis.

2. Modification of the Lukes-Butler classification

The modification [6] of the original classification made at the meeting in Rye, New York, is referred to as the Rye classification [6]. It represents a grouping of prognostically similar types in the original classification [7, 8]. The modification was said to be necessary because the six terms of the original classification were too many for clinicians to remember. This seems interesting today in view of the number of entities in the proposed classification of non-Hodgkin's lymphomas, 10 in the NCI formulation [9] and 16 in Lennert's [9]. A compari-

Bennett JM (ed), Controversies in the Management of Lymphomas. ISBN 0-89838-586-5.
© *Martinus Nijhoff Publishers, Boston. Printed in the Netherlands.*

son of the two classifications is included in Fig. 1 because young pathologists and oncologists are, in my experience, not familiar with the original classification.

While the Rye classification seems to present no problem to clinicians, its use by pathologists results in errors because the terms are not as descriptive as the original classification. Thus, I have recieved cases in which the nodular form of the L&H type of lymphocytic predominance HD had been diagnosed as nodular (follicular) lymphoma, diffuse L&H containing a large number of histocytes interpreted as mixed cellularity HD, and the reticular form of lymphocytic depletion HD called mixed cellularity HD because lymphocytic depletion was not present. The pathologist should therefore think in terms of the original classification and then translate this into the Rye classification for the clinician.

The original classification was structured so that five of the groups could be kept as pure as possible with the sixth, mixed, serving as a catchall for cases that dit not fit into the other five. Some authors [10] deplore mixed cellularity becoming a waste basket when in actuality it always has been although this was not specifically stated in the initial papers [7, 8]. Mixed cellularity is intermediate between nodular and diffuse L&H (lymphocytic predominance) and diffuse fibrosis and reticular (lymphocytic depletion); it must therefore include cases showing features, though not diagnostic changes, of these two extremes, as well as cases of nodular sclerosis with lacunar cells, sometimes in groups, without fibrosis, and those cases that do not suggest any of the other types and might be referred to as the true mixed type. A minority of the last are actually cases of nodular sclerosis that show neither fibrosis nor recognizable lacunar cells in the initial biopsy but show the characteristic findings of nodular

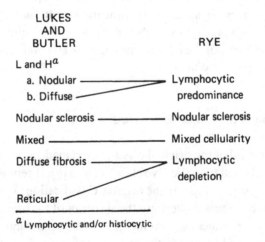

Figure 1. Comparison of Lukes–Butler and Rye classifications.

sclerosis on rebiopsy. If a pathologist has difficulty deciding whether the histology of a given case is mixed cellularity or another type, it should be placed in mixed cellularity according to the original tenets of the classification. The ultimate aim of all histological classification is to predict behavior. Use of this classification, using mixed cellularity as detailed, has done that.

3. Technical factors in diagnosis

It cannot be emphasized too strongly that the correct diagnosis of Hodgkin's disease and the determination of the histologic subtypes depends on the surgeon removing the largest lymph node possible, with its capsule intact, and the pathologist having technically excellent sections, as has been stated elsewhere [11]. Failure to satisfy either of these requirements remains the main problem in the correct diagnosis of Hodgkin's disease. Nothing is more discouraging than to receive referral slides for a difficult case in which the pathology report gives the results of flow cytometry, surface markers, and electron microscopy but in which the sections are poorly stained and two or three cells thick. It is equally disturbing to receive a lymph node 1 cm or less in diameter from a patient whose history describes 3 to 4 cm lymph nodes. No amount of experience or expertise will help to establish the correct diagnosis when the cytological features cannot be visualized or the tissue is not representative.

The emphasis in this discussion will be on features which were not emphasized in the original paper or have become apparent since then. The criteria for the different histologic types will not be repeated since they can be found in the original paper [7] and in the review by Lukes [12].

4. Definition of Hodgkin's disease

A definition of Hodgkin's disease is essential since it has become clear since the original publication that Reed–Sternberg (RS) cells are not pathognomic of Hodgkin's disease as was once thought; they have been described in both benign and malignant conditions [13, 14]. It is particularly important that pathologists remember that RS-like cells may be found in any benign or malignant proliferation of transformed lymphocytes (immunoblasts). Thus, Hodgkin's disease may be defined as a malignant process in which a diagnostic Reed–Sternberg cell is found in the background of one of the described histologic types. The patterns and cytologic features of these tumors are detailed in Table 1.

The histiocytes referred to in this discussion are monocyte related cells with

Table 1. Proper histologic background for Hodgkin's disease.

1. Nodular pattern
   a. Nodular L&H pattern with numerous L&H R–S variants in addition to lymphocytes and benign histiocytes. Rare diagnostic R–S cells.
   b. Nodular sclerosing pattern with groups of lacunar cells, partially or completely surrounded by collagen bands, and a mixture of lymphocytes, benign histiocytes, eosinophils and plasma cells. Diagnostic R–S cells often rare, but may be numerous. Large areas of necrosis common.
2. Diffuse pattern
   a. Many lymphocytes and L&H R–S variants with a varying number of benign histiocytes and possibly a few eosinophils; diagnostic R–S cells rare (Diffuse L&H).
   b. Mixture of lymphocytes, eosinophils, benign histiocytes, mononuclear R–S variants but few immunoblasts; diagnostic cells easy to find (Mixed cellularity).
   c. Cellular depletion, particularly lymphocytes, with proteinaceous material prominent; all cells noted in 'b' are present but in greatly decreased numbers; diagnostic R–S cells usually not numerous (Diffuse fibrosis).
   d. Increased number of diagnostic R–S cells, with a varying number of the cells noted in 'b'; overall cellularity usually decreased (Reticular).
   e. Increased number of bizarre multinucleated cells, some of which can be recognized as diagnostic R–S cells; the cells noted in 'b' are present but the numbers are decreased to a varying extent (Reticular).
3. Focal (interfollicular) or partial involvement
   a. Nodular sclerosing pattern with groups of lacunar cells, collagen bands, and a mixture of lymphocytes, benign histiocytes, eosinophils and plasma cells. Diagnostic R–S cells often rare, but may be numerous.
   b. Mixture of lymphocytes, eosinophils, benign histiocytes, mononuclear R–S variants but few immunoblasts; diagnostic cells easy to find (Mixed cellularity).

a large amount of cytoplasm and an elliptical or elongated nucleus with a small nucleolus. While they are thought to have the potential for phagocytosis, they rarely demonstrate this feature in HD. The nuclei of the lymphocytes in HD are frequently mildly to moderately irregular in outline; they are not as irregular as those of the cleaved or markedly irregular lymphocytes of non-Hodgkin's lymphomas. Except for occasional cases of nodular sclerosis and the reticular type of lymphocytic depletion, the process in HD rarely extends through the capsule into the pericapsular tissues. As a result, the lymph nodes of HD are classically described as discrete and not matted [15] as so frequently are those in the non-Hodgkin's lymphomas.

5. Reed–Sternberg cells and their variants

There is general agreement that RS cells are essential for the diagnosis of HD, but what constitutes an acceptable cell seems to vary judging by the photomicrographs shown by different authors [12, 16, 17]. This variation may reflect uncertainty over the significance of the RS cell variants listed in Table 2.

Table 2. Variants of Reed–Sternberg cells.

1. Diagnostic	4. Pleomorphic
2. Lacunar	5. Mononuclear
3. L&H	6. Pyknotic

While some of the cells in this list are of value in helping to identify a particular type of Hodgkin's disease and others alert one to the probability of Hodgkin's disease, as will be explained, only the diagnostic cell in the proper histologic background can establish the diagnosis. The MGP stain is of value in identifying diagnostic RS cells in those cases of HD where diagnostic RS cells are difficult to find, lymphocytic predominance and many cases of nodular sclerosis, since their nucleoli are usually strongly pyroninophilic as is their cytoplasm.

The distinction between L&H and lacunar cells remains a problem for pathologists who see HD infrequently. The problem has actually been accentuated by the use of B-5 and other modified Zenker's fixatives, which tend to make lacunar cells less easily recognized (Fig. 2). Although lacunar cells are characteristic of nodular sclerosis they may be seen in some cases of mixed cellularity that are actually cases of nodular sclerosis lacking fibrous bands. Likewise, L&H cells are characteristic of lymphocytic predominance but may be present in those cases of mixed cellularity which have too many diagnostic RS cells to be interpreted as lymphocytic predominance. The pleomorphic cell

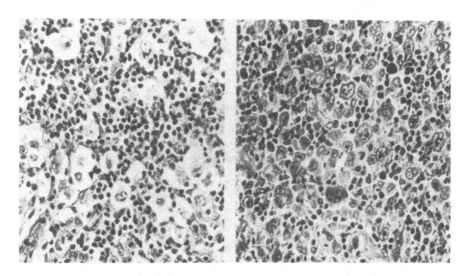

Figure 2. Lacunar cells. The sharply outlined borders, clear cytoplasm, and small nuclei with small nucleoli of the cells in tissue fixed in formalin (left) contrast with the less sharply defined borders, granular cytoplasm, larger nuclei, and more prominent nucleoli in tissue fixed in B-5 (right). × 300.

is characteristic of a minority of cases of the reticular type of lymphocytic depletion but may be seen in rare cases of nodular sclerosis (Fig. 3).

The presence of RS mononuclear variants in the correct background suggests HD and warrants a search for a diagnostic cell. This is usually the problem in cases of early or focal HD [18] where tiny foci are present in otherwise reactive lymph nodes; it is more common in lymph nodes obtained at staging laparotomy than in initial biopsies. Pyknotic or 'zombie' cells (Fig. 4) have the same significance but are more commonly seen in sections containing diagnostic RS cells. Jackson and Parker [19] first mentioned them as evidence that RS cells can undergo necrobiosis. They have subsequently been commented on only by Cross [16] and Buyssens and Bourgeois [17].

6. Rebiopsy of treated patients

In the last 10 years it has become established practice to biopsy lymph nodes that appear in previously treated patients with an established diagnosis of HD, rather than to consider them as evidence of recurrent disease. The value of this is shown by the number of biopsies that do not show evidence of HD. If HD is present in such a lymph node, one should not attempt to subclassify it if the

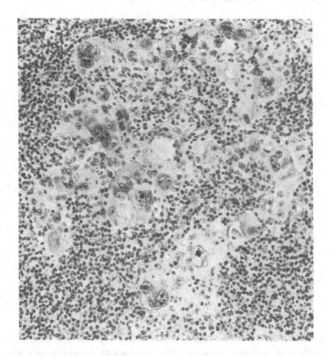

Figure 3. Pleopmorphic cells in nodular sclerosis. × 112.5.

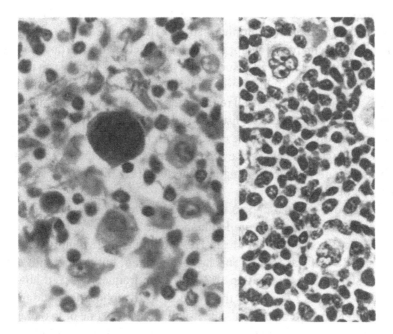

Figure 4. Right: L&H cells in formalin fixed tissue frequently show hyperlobation ('popcorn cells'); left: Pyknotic giant cell ('zombie cell'). × 450.

patient has had x-ray therapy to the area or chemotherapy; both types of therapy are lympholytic and the classification depends on the presence or absence of lymphocytes as well as the number of abnormal cells. The exception to this rule is nodular sclerosis since the pattern of fibrosis is so important for that diagnosis and is not significantly modified by the therapy given.

7. Lymphocytic predominance

The two variants of lymphocytic predominance seem to present the greatest problem in establishing the diagnosis of HD. The nodular L&H form may be misdiagnosed as follicular lymphoma, if the poorly defined nodules are recognized, or reactive hyperplasia or diffuse well differentiated lymphocytic lymphoma, if they are not. The diffuse type is often diagnosed as well-differentiated lymphocytic lymphoma because the sections are too thick and the pathologist fails to recognize the L&H cells (Fig. 4). Both are also misdiagnosed as chronic lymphadenitis or reactive hyperplasia since the clinical information is usually that the patient has a single enlarged lymph node in the high cervical or inguinal area.

In the initial study we found that both variants of lymphocytic predominance often involved only a portion of the lymph node with displacement of the uninvolved portion to the periphery so that the involved portions formed a relatively well demarcated tumor nodule with reactive follicles outside but not intermixed with the involved tissue. In the last few years I have seen rare cases in which a few reactive follicles were intermixed with the involved tissue. It is perhaps significant that these all represented stage II disease; this finding may therefore indicate progressive disease. The rim of normal lymph node around the area of involvement in some cases of both types of lymphocytic predominance is of diagnostic value since such a sharp separation between the area of involvement and the surrounding normal node (Fig. 5) is rarely seen in any other type of lymphoma.

Although our original papers stated that diagnostic RS cells were rare in both types of lymphocytic predominance, we did not state, although we implied, that the diagnosis of mixed HD should be made if more than a rare diagnostic RS cell was found. This has been stated, but perhaps not emphasized, in subsequent publications [12, 20]. I am frequently asked how many diagnostic RS cells still permit the diagnosis of lymphocytic predominance. Although it is hard to be precise, one usually finds only one or two diagnostic RS cells in several sections. If a single RS cell is found in every section examined or mononuclear variants are easily found, the pathologists must mention the likelihood that the patient has progressive disease in the report. If more than two diagnostic RS cells are present in any one section then I believe the diagnosis should be mixed cellularity with a comment regarding its origin in lymphocytic predominance. If, on the other hand, a diagnostic RS cell cannot

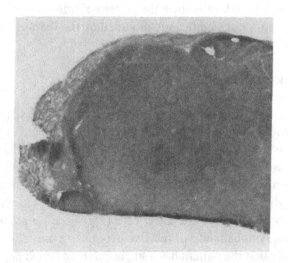

Figure 5. Lymphocytic predominance, nodular L&H type, with rim of normal lymph node (lighter zone). × 5.

be identified, then one should get step sections and look for the same cell [17] or other cells in successive sections or submit additional tissue.

8. Nodular sclerosis

It has become apparent over the years that nodular sclerosis is not limited to the supraclavicular area and mediastinum as was originally thought. It actually is the type HD most likely to present as extranodal disease on the anterior chest wall and the breast or parasternal area. Nodular sclerosis is also the type most likely to involve the lung, probably by direct spread.

Whether groups of lacunar cells without fibrous bands or with only minimal ones, the so-called cellular phase of nodular sclerosis, should be diagnosed as nodular sclerosis or mixed cellularity is controversial [10]. Studies [21, 22] have shown, however, that the overall survival of patients with this type HD is that of mixed cellularity HD.

The histologic diagnosis of nodular sclerosis is more difficult in tissues fixed in Zenker's fixatives because the sharply defined lacunar spaces present in formalin-fixed tissue are usually not seen (Fig. 2). While diagnostic RS cells were said to be usually difficult to find in the initial descriptions of nodular sclerosis [7], some have mistakenly interpreted this to mean that easily identifiable RS cells indicate mixed cellularity. As noted previously, bizarre giant cells (Fig. 3) may be seen in nodular sclerosis. In some instances the changes of nodular sclerosis will be present in only one part of the node. If the changes of nodular sclerosis are present, whether in one portion of a single node, one of many nodes, or one of several biopsies, the diagnosis of nodular sclerosis takes precedent over all other types of HD. Eosinophils are usually present and may form abscess like masses in those lymph nodes showing large areas of necrosis.

In some cases of nodular sclerosis solid masses of cells are present (Fig. 6) often with central necrosis, which may raise the possibility of large cell lymphoma or metastatic carcinoma, particularly on small biopsies [23]. In a few instances I have made the diagnosis of large cell ('histiocytic') lymphoma on adequate size biopsies from an extranodal site on the basis of a mono-morphous proliferation of large cytoplasmic cells without associated fibrosis; the true nature of the process became obvious when a subsequent lymph node biopsy for staging purposes showed classical nodular sclerosis. Only on review of the original material did the resemblance of the tumor cells to lacunar cells become obvious. This type, which I have designated as the syncytial or lacunar cell predominant variant [23], was mentioned but not emphasized in the initial papers. Its prognostic significance remains to be clearly established.

Necrosis may be seen in all types of HD except lymphocytic predominance.

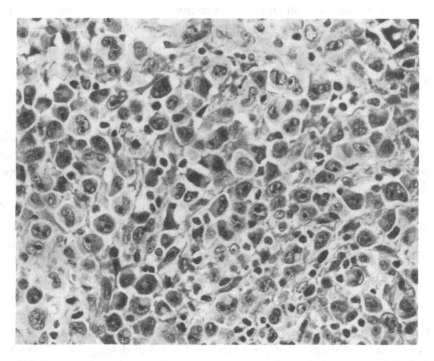

Figure 6. Lacunar cell predominant (syncytial) variant of nodular sclerosis. Areas of classical nodular sclerosis were present in another area of this biopsy. ×300.

The only type associated with large areas of necrosis prior to therapy is nodular sclerosis. Lacunar cells are usually in the viable tissues surrounding the areas of necrosis (Fig. 7). The necrotic areas often represent necrosis of masses of lacunar cells. Thus, a pathologist finding large (macroscopic) areas of necrosis in HD should be reluctant to make any diagnosis except nodular sclerosis. Microscopic areas of necrosis may be seen but are not common in mixed cellularity and both types of lymphocytic depletion.

Although it was not possible to relate the cellular composition of the nodules in nodular sclerosis to survival in our initial papers [7, 8], there was a suggestion that those nodules which were predominantly lymphocytic occurred in patients with quiescent disease while a predominance of RS cells indicated progressive disease. Recently Colby *et al.* [22] have shown a positive correlation of sclerosis, negative correlation of the number of fibroblasts, and lack of correlation of lacunar cells with relapse-free survival in patients with nodular sclerosis; the number of lymphocytes did not independently effect prognosis.

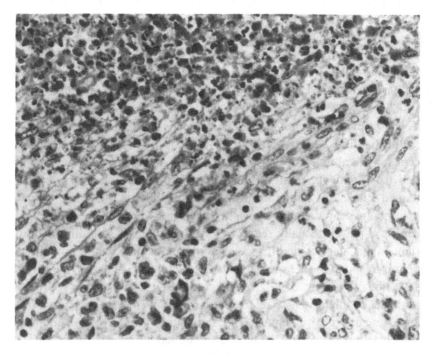

Figure 7. Nodular sclerosis with an area of necrosis surrounded by lacunar cells. × 300.

9. Mixed cellularity

A wide spectrum of histologic changes are present in mixed cellularity primarily because it encompasses such a wide variety of cases, as noted previously. Focal or interfollicular involvement should be included in mixed cellularity if the changes of nodular sclerosis are not present. Focal involvement in HD does not occur as scattered diagnostic RS cells in otherwise reactive lymphoid tissue, but as discrete foci. Though eosinophils are usually present, they are not essential for the diagnosis of mixed cellularity. Areas of necrosis are small and not commonly present.

10. Lymphocytic depletion

In 1973, Neiman *et al.* [24] described lymphocytic depletion HD as a clinicopathologic entity. Ten of their cases had the diffuse fibrosis type in which the patients had no enlarged peripheral lymph nodes. Autopsy cases with similar clinical and histologic findings were reviewed for the initial papers [7, 8] but had to be discarded since biopsy material was not available.

In all reported series the number of cases of both the diffuse fibrosis and reticular types is smaller than in our original series. This is unlikely to be due to earlier diagnosis given that our population was composed of service personnel who had to pass a physical examination prior to entry into the Armed Services. It seems more likely to reflect a change in the histologic types due to improved nutrition as suggested by the epidemiologic data of Correa and O'Connor [25].

The histologic findings of marked lymphocytic depletion, changes similar to those of the diffuse fibrosis variant of lymphocytic depletion HD, are seen, except for the absence of diagnostic RS cells, in normal or involved lymph nodes from patients treated with chemotherapy or local x-ray therapy. Enlarged spleens of patients with any histologic type HD may, following chemotherapy, show similar changes replacing scattered enlarged malpighian bodies in a pattern usually seen in Hodgkin's disease. The diffuse fibrosis variant is the most common type seen at autopsy in treated patients who appear to respond to therapy, obviously reflecting the previous therapy. The diffuse fibrosis variant continues to be confused with nodular sclerosis although the problem is now relatively uncommon since so few cases of the diffuse fibrosis type are being seen. Examination of the sections in question under polarized light is still the best means of making the distinction since the true collagen of nodular sclerosis polarizes light while the reticular fibrosis of the diffuse fibrosis type does not.

The diffuse fibrosis and reticular types frequently occur in the same lymph node, justifying the lumping of the two in the Rye classification. Whereas diffuse fibrosis is the finding at autopsy in patients who respond to therapy, the reticular type is the most common finding at autopsy in treated patients with agressive Hodgkin's disease in my experience and that of others [26, 27].

The diagnosis of the reticular type is most often an incorrect one because of the confusion with large cell lymphoma, lacunar cell predominant (syncytial) nodular sclerosis, and mixed cellularity HD [28]. The first is a problem because of the failure to realize that the untreated reticular type does not represent a monomorphic proliferation of mononuclear cells but consists of a mixture of cell types with RS cells or their variants predominating; on the other hand, it is important to remember that RS-like cells are found in all proliferations of transformed lymphocytes which large cell lymphoma represents. In the second instance, one must always think of nodular sclerosis HD when fibrosis is associated with a proliferation of large cells; when large areas of necrosis are present, the cells at the edge of the necrotic zone must be carefully evaluated since lacunar cells seem more easily identifiable there. In any case, the pathologist should make the diagnosis of the reticular type only after careful consideration of all the differential diagnostic features. If the diagnosis will affect therapy, biopsy of another lymph node, if an enlarged one is present, might be considered. The reticular variant is, my opinion, often misdiagnosed as mixed cellularity HD because, as noted previously, lymphocytic depletion may not be present in the reticular type.

10. Progression

The progression of the subtypes proposed in the original paper has been confirmed by others in treated patients [26, 29]. The exceptions to the proposed scheme of progression are almost all accounted for by those MC cases which are, as noted above, actually cases of NS without the diagnostic findings; these cases were not covered by the scheme of progression presented. As might be expected, we still have essentially no information regarding progression from one histologic type to another in untreated patients. The rare reported case usually represents a patient with unrecognized lymphocytic predominance or a patient who refuses therapy. As noted above, DF and reticular HD appear to be the common types for the majority of patients at autopsy.

11. Differential diagnosis

Only an occasional comment was made regarding differential diagnosis in the original papers since we were presenting a histologic classification of HD rather than how to establish the diagnosis. Table 3 lists the common conditions misinterpreted as Hodgkin's disease according to the histologic features likely to cause the error; it is not intended to be all inclusive. The most difficult differential diagnosis is between HD and peripheral T-cell lymphoma. In the absence of surface marker studies one must depend on the marked irregularity of the lymphocytes and the involvement of the capsule and pericapsular tissues in T-cell lymphoma. Frequently there is also a prominant vascular pattern that is unusual in HD. RS-like cells may be seen in peripheral T-cell lymphomas but are not common. The differential diagnostic features of the other conditions. mentioned are beyond the scope of this presentation but have been presented elsewhere [10, 11, 30]. The report of the Pathology Panel for Lymphoma Clinical Studies [28] details the problems in the diagnosis of HD. Their data document the problems pathologists have in differentiating HD from NHL, but from my experience understate the problem of reactive processes being misinterpreted as HD.

General guidelines for features that indicate a given lesion does not represent HD are presented in Table 4. Many of these have been referred to in the previous discussion. A prominent proliferation of immunoblasts is not seen in

Table 3. Differential diagnosis of Hodgkin's disease.

I. Focal histiocytic proliferation
    A. Toxoplasmosis
    B. Peripheral T-cell lymphoma
    C. Sarcoidosis
II. Prominence of small lymphocytes
    A. Diffuse small lymphocytic lymphoma
    B. Chronic lymphadenitis
III. Nodular pattern
    A. Reactive follicular hyperplasia
    B. Follicular lymphoma
    C. Progressive transformation of follicles
IV. Reed–Sternberg like cells present
    A. Immunoblastic proliferation
        1. Non-Hodgkin's lymphomas
        2. Immunoblastic lymphadenopathy
        3. Reactive processes
            a. Infectious mononucleosis
            b. Other viral infections
            c. Drug reactions (Dilantin)
    B. Other malignant neoplasms
        1. Metastatic
            a. Lymphoepithelioma
            b. Breast carcinoma
            c. Malignant melanoma
        2. Primary
            a. Malignant fibrous histiocytoma
V. Tissue eosinophilia
    A. Eosinophilic granuloma
    B. Tissue eosinophilia with malignant neoplasms
        1. Lymphoepithelioma
        2. Non-Hodgkin's lymphomas

HD, but is associated with RS-like cells; the histologic background is incorrect so HD should be excluded. Involvement of lymph node sinusoids is not seen in Hodgkin's disease except rarely at autopsy. What is misinterpreted as HD in sinusoids is either metastatic disease or sinusoidal large cell lymphoma [31].

The original papers reported only the findings in pretherapy lymph nodes. Only with the advent of bone marrow biopsies, more frequent liver biopsies, and staging laparotomies have criteria for involvement of extranodal sites (Table 5) become important. Though a detailed discussion of these criteria has been presented elsewhere [32] and is beyond the scope of this article, it should be emphasized that the pathologist is looking for the histologic changes of early Hodgkin's disease in all these situations. Thus, the normal size lymph node may show focal HD even though the lymphogram is negative, since histologic lesions must distort the lymph node sinuses to be seen on lympho-

Table 4. Pitfalls in the diagnosis of Hodgkin's disease.

1. Prominent immunoblastic proliferation
2. Involvement of lymph node sinuses
3. Significant irregularity of lymphocytic nuclei
4. Reed–Sternberg cell(s) in the wrong background
5. Significant involvement of lymph node capsule (and surrounding tissues)
6. Absence of L&H cells in a lymphohistiocytic proliferation

Table 5. Criteria for diagnosis of Hodgkin's disease in liver and bone marrow.

1. Initial biopsy – Diagnostic Reed–Sternberg cell in the background of one of the described histologic types
2. Biopsy in patient with established diagnosis of Hodgkin's disease
   a. Diagnostic Reed–Sternberg cell in the proper histological setting
   b. Mononuclear cell with large nucleolus (mononuclear variant) in the proper histological setting

graphy. While the spleen may be normal in size, if it is involved it will usually show macroscopic lesions; in only about 1% of spleens will a microscopic lesion be found in the absence of gross lesions. In the latter case it is important to know that the earliest location of Hodgkin's disease in the spleen is in the marginal zone of the malpighian bodies (Fig. 8). This localization is also important in helping to differentiate involvement by HD from nonspecific granulomas [33], which themselves have prognostic significance [34]; these tend to localize around the arteries and therefore are normally centrally placed in the malpighian bodies. One usually cannot subclassify HD in the spleen except when it shows, uncommonly, the characteristic changes of NS. The early foci of involvement in the liver and bone marrow are almost always microscopic areas with a background of MC; as a result, step sections are frequently necessary to satisfy the criteria for the diagnosis of HD. Skin involvement in HD always involves sites drained by involved lymph nodes [35]. The lymph nodes should be biopsied and the diagnosis of HD established from them rather than from a skin biopsy.

12. Autopsy findings

Autopsy findings in HD have been detailed by several authors [26, 27, 36] and some of their findings have already been mentioned. The most intriguing aspect of two of these reports [27, 34] has been the presence of clinically unsuspected HD in patients treated for HD who died of other causes. Why HD

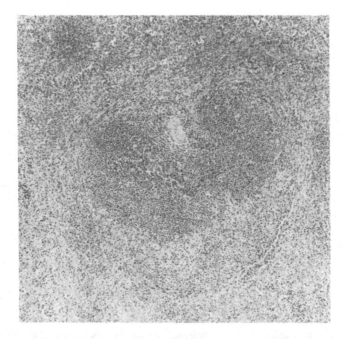

Figure 8. Involvement of the marginal zone and adjacent malpighian body in the spleen in Hodgkin's disease. × 75.

was able to exist in a symbiotic relationship with these patients is a question which we may be able to answer when we have more knowledge of the biology of this disease.

References

1. Lukes RJ, Butler JJ: Spontaneous nodular sclerosis in Hodgkin's disease. Program of the joint annual meeting of the Am Soc Clin Path and Coll of Am Path. Chicago, 1958, p 56.
2. Fuller LM, Madoc-Jones H, Gamble JF, Butler JJ, Sullivan MP, Fernandez CH, Gehan ea; New assessment of the prognostic significance of histopathology in Hodgkin's disease for laparotomy negative stage I and II patients. Cancer 39:2174–2182, 1977.
3. Fuller LM, Gamble JF, Velasquez WS, Rodgers RW, Butler JJ, North LB, Martin RG, Gehan EA, Shullenberger CC: Evaluation of the significance of prognostic factors in stage III Hodgkin's disease treated with (MOPP) and radiotherapy. Cancer 45:1352–1364, 1980.
4. Hoppe RT, Rosenberg SA, Kaplan HS, Cox RS: Prognostic factors in pathological stage III A Hodgkin's disease. Cancer 46:1240–1246, 1980.
5. Rosenberg SA: Personal communications, 1981.
6. Lukes RJ, Craver LF, Hall TC, Rappaport H, Ruben P: Report of the nomenclature committee. Cancer Res 26:1311, 1966.
7. Lukes RJ, Butler JJ: The pathology and nomenclature of Hodgkin's disease. Cancer Res 26:1063–1081, 1966.

8. Lukes RJ, Butler JJ, Hicks EB: Natural history of Hodgkin's disease as related to its pathologic picture. Cancer 19:317–344, 1966.

9. The non-Hodgkin's lymphoma pathologic classification project: National Cancer Institute sponsored study of classifications of non-Hodgkin's lymphomas: Summary and description of a working formulation for clinical usage. Cancer 49:2112–2135, 1982.

10. Dorfman RF, Colby TV: The pathologist's role in the management of patients with Hodgkin's disease. Cancer Treat Rep 66:675–580, 1982.

11. Butler JJ: Non-neoplastic lesions of lymph nodes of man to be differentiated from lymphomas. Natl Cancer Inst Monogr 32:233–255, 1969.

12. Lukes RJ: Criteria for involvement of lymph node, bone marrow, spleen, and liver in Hodgkin's disease. Cancer Res 31:1755–1767, 1971.

13. Lukes RJ, Tindle BH, Parker JW: Reed-Sternberg like cells in infectious mononucleosis. Lancet 2:1003–1004, 1969.

14. Strum SB, Park JK, Rappaport H: Observation of cells resembling Sternberg-Reed cells in conditions other than Hodgkin's disease. Cancer 26:176–190, 1970.

15. Symmers WStC: The lymphoreticular system. In: Systemic pathology vol 2, Symmers WStC (ed). Edinburgh: Churchill Livingston, 2nd ed, pp 792–793, 1978.

16. Cross RM: Hodgkin's disease: Histological classification and diagnosis. J Clin Pathol 22:165–182, 1969.

17. Buyssens N, Bourgeois N: The Sternberg-Reed cell: Mononuclear, multinucleated, or multi-lobated. Virchows Archiv A 385:335–342, 1980.

18. Strum SB, Rappaport H: Significance of focal involvement of lymph nodes for the diagnosis and staging of Hodgkin's disease. Cancer 25:1314–1319, 1970.

19. Jackson H, Parker F: Hodgkin's disease. II. Pathology. N Engl J Med 231:35–44, 1944.

20. Sullivan MP, Fuller LM, Butler JJ: Hodgkin's disease in children. In: Clinical pediatric oncology, Sutow WW, Vietti TJ, Fernbach DJ (eds). St Louis: CV Mosby Co., 2nd ed, p 413.

21. Rappaport H: Personal communications, 1980.

22. Colby TV, Hoppe RT, Warner RA: Hodgkin's disease: A clinicopathological study of 659 cases. Cancer 49:1848–1858, 1981.

23. Butler JJ: The natural history of Hodgkin's disease and its classification. In: The reticuloen-dothelial system, Bernard CW, Rebuck JW, Abell MR. Baltimore: Williams & Wilkins Co., 1975, p 184–212.

24. Neiman RS, Rosen PJ, Lukes RJ: Lymphocyte depletion Hodgkin's disease. N Engl J Med 288:751–755, 1973.

25. Correa P, O'Conor GT: Epidemiologic patterns of Hodgkin's disease. Int J Cancer 8:192–201, 1971.

26. Thomas LB, Berard CW: Hodgkin's disease: Relationship of histopathological type at diagnosis to clinical parameters and to histological progression and anatomical distribution at autopsy. Gann 15:253–273, 1973.

27. Colby TV, Hoppe RT, Warnke RA: Hodgkin's disease at autopsy: 1972–1977. Cancer 47:1852–1862, 1981.

28. Kim H, Zelman RJ, Fox MA et al.: Pathology panel for lymphoma clinical studies: A comprehensive analysis of cases accumulated since its inception. JNCI 68:43–67, 1982.

29. Strum SB, Rappaport H: Interrelations of the histological types of Hodgkin's disease. Arch Pathol 91:127–134, 1971.

30. Dorfman RF, Warnke R: Lymphadenopathy simulating the malignant lymphoma. Human Pathol 5:519–550, 1974.

31. Osborne BM, Butler JJ, Mackay B: Sinusoidal large cell 'histiocytic' lymphoma. Cancer 46:2484–2491, 1980.

32. Rappaport G, Berard CW, Butler JJ, Dorfman RF, Lukes RJ, Thomas LB: Report of the

committee on histopathological criteria contributing to staging of Hodgkin's disease. Cancer Res 31: 1862–1863, 1971.

33. Kadin ME, Donaldson SS, Dorfman RF: Isolated granulomas in Hodgkin's disease. N Engl J Med 283:859–861, 1970.
34. Sacks EL, Donaldson SS, Gordon J, Dorfman RF: Epithelioid granulomas associated with Hodgkin's disease. Cancer 41:562–567, 1978.
35. Smith JL, Butler JJ: Skin involvement in Hodgkin's disease. Cancer 45:354–361, 1980.
36. Strum SB, Rappaport H: The persistence of Hodgkin's disease in long term survivors. Am J Med 51:222–240, 1971.

2. Pitfalls in the diagnosis and classification of Hodgkin's disease: Surgical pathology and classification for the 1980's
Is the Lukes–Butler classification still relevant?

THOMAS V. COLBY

1. Introduction

Compared to the controversies surrounding the pathologic classification of the non-Hodgkin's lymphomas, the pathologic classification of Hodgkin's disease (HD) has produced barely a murmur of discontent. Perhaps the dramatically improved prognosis in patients with HD [1–3] has occasioned little need for criticism. HD is classified according to the Rye modification [4] of the histologic classification proposed by Lukes and Butler [5] (Table 1). Early series of patients classified according to this scheme showed significant and reproducible variations in survival among the different histologic subtypes [6]. However, current data show that pathologic stage is the most important prognostic factor and histologic classification per se does not have significant influence on prognosis when other parameters are held constant [7–13]. These findings have led some to question the usefulness of classification in HD.

Should classification of HD in general, and the Lukes and Butler classification in particular then be abandoned for lack of clinical usefulness? Time and energy spent by pathologists in the minutia of classification could certainly be decreased, but the importance of classification nonetheless remains. Recent improvements in the clinical management of HD relate in part to more precise criteria for histologic diagnosis which has resulted in an improvement in accuracy of the diagnosis of HD [14]. The diagnosis of HD is still the sole responsibility of the diagnostic histopathologist, and the Lukes and Butler classification ties together its varied histologic patterns. Accurate histologic diagnosis depends on familiarity with, and recognition of, all the different patterns; therefore the pathologist should primarily employ the original Lukes and Butler classification. The Rye modification may be added to the diagnosis for example in parentheses, since the clinician is usually more familar with it. The first part of this chapter will discuss recognition and diagnosis of HD with emphasis on differential diagnosis from benign and malignant lesions that can simulate HD.

The fact that pathologic stage is one of the most important prognostic

Bennett JM (ed), Controversies in the Management of Lymphomas. ISBN 0-89838-586-5.
© *Martinus Nijhoff Publishers, Boston. Printed in the Netherlands.*

variables in HD has underscored the importance of the staging laparotomy
[15]. Careful gross and microscopic evaluation is mandatory for the pathologist, and if time is limited, the patient is better served by effort in evaluation of
laparotomy specimens rather than in belaboring subtle differences in classification. The second section of this chapter will be devoted to guidelines for the
gross and microscopic evaluation of tissues removed at staging laparotomy.

The final portion of this chapter will deal with a variety of problems that
pathologists may encounter in patients with HD, including unusual morphologic patterns and post treatment changes in surgical material.

Table 1. Classification of HD.

Lukes & Butler	Rye
Nodular L&H Diffuse L&H	Lymphocyte predominance
Nodular sclerosis	Nodular sclerosis
Mixed cellularity	Mixed cellularity
Reticular Diffuse fibrosis	Lymphocyte depletion

2. Diagnosis of Hodgkin's disease

The Reed–Sternberg cell (R–S cell) continues as the cornerstone for the
histologic diagnosis of HD. This cell provides the common ground that ties
together the divergent histologic patterns of HD. The classic R–S cell is
bilobed with prominent eosinophilic nucleoli, perinucleolar clearing, thick
nuclear membrane, and relatively abundant eosinophilic to amphophilic
cytoplasm [5]. Cells with nuclei that are multilobated but otherwise identical to
R–S cells can also be considered diagnostic (Fig. 11) [14]. Except in certain
circumstances outlined below, mononuclear cells resembling R–S cells (R–S
cell variants) alone are not sufficient for a histologic diagnosis of HD.
Smudged hypereosinophilic cells with indistinct nuclei that have been termed
'mummified cells' [16] are not uncommon in HD and probably represent
degenerate R–S cells (Fig. 1). In reactive conditions transformed lymphocytes,
or immunoblasts, may mimic R–S cells, even to the point of being bilobated
[14, 17, 18]. Immunoblasts may usually be recognized by the surrounding
cellular environment (see below), their smaller amphophilic or basophilic
nucleoli with less perinucleolar clearing, and by their less voluminous
cytoplasm. In some cases the stromal background is the best (and only) key to
the identity of a cell.

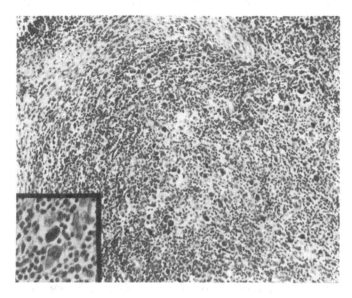

Figure 1. 'Mummified cells' appear as dark smuges in this nodule in NSHD. (H&E × 90, inset: H&E × 225).

The character of the infiltrate (stromal background or cellular milieu) amongst which R–S cells are found *is as important* for the diagnosis of HD as the R–S cell itself [5, 14, 15]. The stromal background in HD consists of a mixed population of cytologically benign cells that do not show features of transforming lymphocytes as observed in diffuse hyperplasia, the usual stromal background in which R–S-like immunoblasts are identified. The background infiltrate in HD is described as cytologically benign; however the small lymphocytes sometimes show minor degrees of nuclear atypia, particularly in lymphocyte predominant HD. The degree of nuclear atypia is significantly less than in non-HD lymphomas with the exception of some lymphocytic lymphomas whose differential diagnosis is discussed below.

Early nodal infiltrates of HD are seen as focal nodules or an interfollicular process. The location of these infiltrates is in the paracortical or 'T-zone' of the node [19, 20]. When an entire node is replaced by HD, extranodal extension is not usually a conspicuous feature in surgical material. Progressive expansion in the node is more common than early extension of the process into the perinodal soft tissue. An exception is occasionally seen with nodular sclerosing HD, which may extensively involve soft tissue even to the point of surrounding uninvolved lymph nodes. The features of nodular sclerosis are so distinctive that there is little difficulty in diagnosis of such cases.

A good histologic section, relatively free of artifacts, is the most important first step in the accurate histologic diagnosis of HD [14, 15].

2.1. Nodular lymphocyte and histiocyte (L&H) form of lymphocyte predominant Hodgkin's disease (nodular L&H LPHD)

In the nodular L&H form of LPHD large nodules partially or completely replace the lymph node. The nodules are usually two to three times the size of reactive germinal centers an have a mottled appearance at low power due to the presence of single or clustered histiocytes and/or 'L&H cells.' 'L&H cells' are characteristic of LPHD and have vesicular, lobated nuclei with less conspicuous nucleoli than in R–S cells or classic Lacunar cells and the designation 'popcorn cells' is particularly descriptive [14, 19]. R–S cells in LPHD are difficult to find and several sections often have to be examined. Acceptable Reed–Sternberg cells are often smaller than those seen in other forms of HD and they seem to 'hide' amongst a background of lymphocytes.

Despite the nodularity, the nodular L&H form of LPHD is not often confused with follicular lymphoma but cases may be misdiagnosed as atypical follicular hyperplasia. Large mottled nodules that are crowded together involving cortex and medulla of the node (thereby effacing the normal architecture) at scanning power are the initial clue that should lead one to carefully evaluate the cytology and to search for R–S and L&H cells. Nonspecific paracortical hyperplasia may produce mottled nodules but they rarely involve the entire node and although they may distort, they do not obliterate its architecture. Paracortical hyperplasia produces oval nodules that are relatively uniform, whereas the mottling in nodular L&H is more prominent at the center of the nodules. The most difficult differential diagnostic problem is the lesion termed by Lennert 'progressive transformation of germinal centers' [21]. Poppema *et al.* have postulated that progressive transformation of germinal centers may even be a precursor of nodular L&H LPHD [22]. In progressive transformation germinal centers enlarge and lose the sharp demarcation between the center and the cuff of small lymphocytes. A large vaguely mottled lymphoid nodules results. Not all germinal centers in a given lymph node show this change and they are often at various stages of progressive transformation. This feature and the lack of L&H and R–S cells in progressive transformation are helpful in differential diagnosis. Since nodular L&H LPHD may be focal and associated with reactive follicular hyperplasia, progressive transformation or both, such cases assure exceptional diagnostic difficulty. In these cases the strict criteria for the diagnosis of HD should always be adhered to and all the tissue should be extensively sampled.

Occasional cases of nodular L&H LPHD may be associated with sclerosis [13]. This is the one instance where the presence of sclerosis should not dictate placing the case in the nodular sclerosis category. Such an approach is arbitrary and is based on the observation that such lesions otherwise are typical of nodular L&H: mottled nodules with L&H cells and Reed–Sternberg cells.

2.2. Diffuse L&H LPHD

LPHD of the diffuse L&H type is less common than the nodular form [13] and it is not clear whether the two are generically related, analogous to follicular and diffuse lymphomas of follicular center cell origin. Diffuse L&H LPHD may also have clusters of histiocytes scattered through the stroma, as well as L&H cells and a paucity of R–S cells. Early cases may show only a prominence of lymphocytes and be mistaken for a benign lesion. Unless unequivocal HD can be demonstrated it is prudent to err on the side of benignancy and suggest another biopsy. In the majority of cases the node is grossly enlarged and over-run by an infiltrate predominantly composed of small lymphocytes. Chronic lymphocytic leukemia (CLL) and small lymphocytic lymphoma (well differentiated lymphocytic lymphoma-WDL) should be included in the differential diagnosis [20, 23]. We have seen a number of cases of CLL/WDL mimic the diffuse L&H form of LPHD to the extent of having L&H-like cells and R–S-like cells as well as clusters of epithelioid histiocytes. In some cases immunologic marker studies may be necessary for accurate diagnosis [23]. The pathologist must know the complete blood count of any patient in whom a diagnosis of diffuse L&H HD is under consideration, and be wary of any case of diffuse L&H in patients over the age of 40.

2.3. Nodular sclerosing HD (NSHD)

In its classic form NSHD is familiar to all pathologists. Dense lamellar relatively acellular bands of collagen surround lymphoid nodules that are composed of various numbers of lacunar cells, R–S cells, lymphocytes, histiocytes, eosinophils, neutrophils, plasma cells and fibroblasts. With the exception noted above, any case of HD that shows significant tendency to sclerosis (defined below) should be interpreted as NSHD regardless of the relative numbers of lymphocytes or atypical cells. The presence of sclerosis takes precedence in subclassification [14]. The validity of such an approach was shown in our recent comprehensive clinicopathologic study of patients with HD [13].

Some variations in the classic histology of NSHD require comment. Some cases have very few classic R–S cells depite an abundance of lacunar cells. Several sections and many levels may need to be searched before acceptable R–S cells are identified in a case that is otherwise typical of NSHD. Lacunar cells show considerable cytologic variation. Classic lacunar cells have multilobed nuclei with promonent 'penny on a plate' nucleoli and rest in a large lacuna (an artifact of formalin fixation) often visible at scanning power [5, 14]. The abundant cytoplasm of lacunar cells is best appreciated on touch prep-

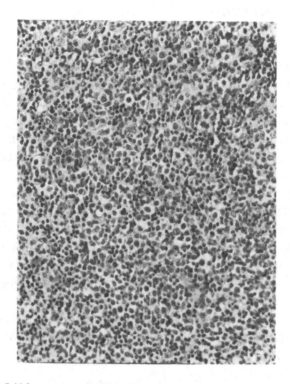

Figure 2. Selected field from a case of NSHD. Lacunae are relatively few and most of the atypical cells lack lobated nuclei. There is a strong resemblance to a non-Hodgkin's lymphoma. (H&E × 144).

arations. Some lacunar cells have single round nuclei and less prominent nucleoli but the same abundant cytoplasm as classical lacunar cells. One of the characteristic features of lacunar cells is their occurrence in sheets or clusters (Figs. 7–9). In some cases there are atypical cells that have less cytoplasm and lack the familiar multilobed nuclei and large nucleoli of classical lacunar cells (Fig. 2), but they are probably variants of lacunar cells since they show a similar tendency to cluster. When large fields of such cells are present there may be difficulty in distinguishing the lesion from large cell non-HD lymphoma (Fig. 2), or metastatic carcinoma (Fig. 9) [14]. This problem is most often encountered in mediastinal lesions and the diagnosis of HD rests on identification of fields showing the characteristic polymorphous stromal background with R–S cells and scattered lacunar cells. The occurrence of such large sheets of atypical cells in cases of Hodgkin's disease did not correlate with prognosis in our recent study [13].

When necrosis and neutrophilic infiltrate are seen in HD they are most commonly associated with NSHD [13]. Necrosis shows a significant correlation with the presence of B symptoms [13] in some instances the necrosis appears to arise in sheets of lacunar cells that are unfiltrated by neutrophils. The atypical cells that characteristically border the necrosis in HD probably represent residual viable lacunar cells. The most bizarre and gigantic atypical cells that one encounters in HD occur in NSHD; they appear to be variants of lacunar cells and individually may rival the most bizarre cells seen in tumor pathology.

Despite its characteristic histology there are several lesions that may mimic NSHD. Malignant histiocytosis (Fig. 3), metastatic nasopharyngeal carcinoma (Fig. 4) and metastatic malignant melanoma may produce histologic and cytologic features very reminiscent of NSHD, including sclerotic nodules surrounding clusters of atypical cells that may easily be mistaken for lacunar cells and/or R–S cells [15]. Careful evaluation of the entire lesion usually reveals foci that are diagnostic: monomorphous sinusoidal infiltrates in the case of malignant histiocytosis, and cohesive cell nests in metastatic carcinoma. The degree to which HD may be mimicked is surprising. The author and two colleagues considered the possibility of HD on a frozen section of a lymph node biopsy with full knowledge that the patient had a history of nasopharyngeal carcinoma six years earlier (Fig. 4). Permanent sections confirmed the presence of metastatic nasopharyngeal carcinoma. Non-Hodgkin's lymphomas may be nodular with dense sclerotic bands [24] but the resemblance to HD usually ends at scanning power: cytologic features allow ready separation. Non-Hodgkin's lymphomas may also show a more delicate intercellular fibrosis, which in the case of follicular lymphomas may be seen in the neoplastic follicles themselves. This latter type of fine sclerosis is unusual in HD.

2.4. Mixed cellularity Hodgkin's disease (MCHD)

Cases of HD that do not readily fit into one of the other five categories are arbitrarily placed into the mixed cellularity category [19, 20]. Even though MCHD has thus become a 'wastebasket' it is a sufficiently homogeneous subgroup as to have clinicopathologic characteristics distinct from the other subtypes (Table 2).

MCHD frequently contains appreciable numbers of lacunar cells [13] but it lacks the sclerosis necessary for the diagnosis of NSHD. Epithelioid histiocytes are common in MCHD [13] and give an overall eosinophilic appearance at scanning power. Differential diagnosis from lymphocyte predominant Hodgkin's disease is arbitrary and probably not of clinical significance [13]. If Reed–Sternberg cells and their variants are relatively easy to find, even if only focally, the case is designated as MCHD [5, 14, 19]. The differential diagnosis from the reticular variant of lymphocyte depleted Hodgkin's disease

26

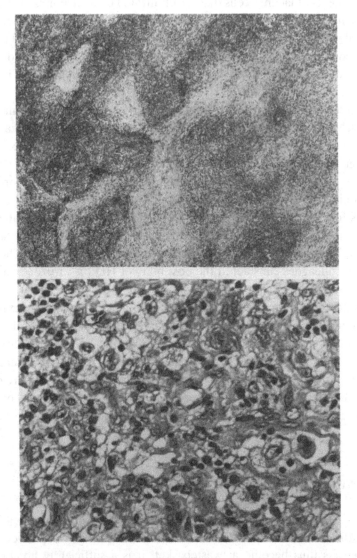

Figure 3. Malignant histiocytosis mimicking NSHD. Sclerotic bands surround polymorphous nodules in this case. The diagnosis of malignant histiocytosis was confirmed on spleen and lymph nodes taken at staging laparotomy. (H&E × 56.25).

is more a potential problem than a real one. The number of cases (in the author's experience) of lymphocyte depletion HD are few and they are sufficiently distinctive, with their large numbers of Reed–Sternberg cells, so that this differentiation can usually be accomplished.

Lymphoid hyperplasia, particularly of the diffuse type with large numbers of immunoblasts, may have R–S-like cells [14, 17]. Classic R–S cells and

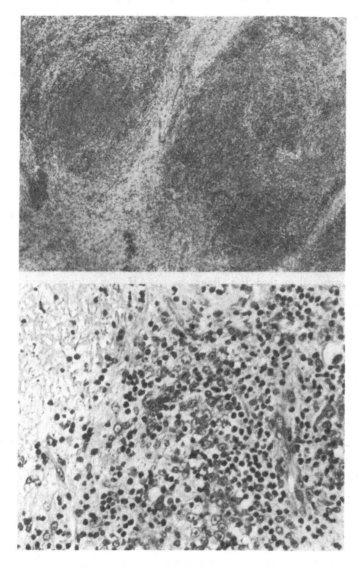

Figure 4. Metastatic nasopharyngeal carcinoma mimicking NSHD in retroperitoneal lymph nodes. Low power (top) shows polymorphous nodules surrounded by collagenous bands. Higher power (bottom) shows loosely cohesive tumor cells infiltrated by numerous eosinophils adjacent to a focus of necrosis (upper left). Characteristic cohesive nests of nasopharyngeal carcinoma were found in other foci in the node. (Top H&E × 22.5, bottom H&E × 225).

multilobed atypical cells are not a feature of lymphoid hyperplasia. The background stroma is mottled at scanning power and at higher magnification shows a broad spectrum of lymphocyte transformation rather than the polymorphous unstimulated background of MCHD. Mitotic figures and plasmacytoid cells are also often prominent in stimulated lymphoid tissue. Angioimmunoblastic lymphadenopathy with dysproteinemia (AILD) is a recently described syndrome thought to be a form of atypical lymphoid hyperplasia with predisposition to the development of lymphoma [25, 26]. It is associated with a distinctive clinical syndrome that is usually very different from that of HD. Affected lymph nodes are effaced and depleted of lymphocytes, typically with sparing of the subcapsular sinus [15] as the infiltrate extends into perinodal soft tissue. Immunoblasts and small blood vessels are prominent. Well formed germinal centers are lacking, PAS+ positive interstitial material may be found, and the infiltrate frequently includes eosinophils, plasma cells and histiocytes. Mixed cellularity Hodgkin's disease generally lacks the immunoblastic and vascular proliferation and preservation of the subcapsular sinuses, and classic R–S cells, particularly multilobed variants, are not seen in AILD.

The spectrum of T cell lymphomas has been found to include lesions which both clinically and histologically mimic AILD [27, 28] and HD and it is the author's impression that the diagnosis of AILD has decreased as T cell lymphomas have become better recognized. T cell lymphomas are particularly difficult to distinguish from MCHD and it is possible that a significant number of cases interpreted previously as MCHD might be reinterpreted today as T cell lymphomas. Another lesion that may also represent a T cell lymphoma and may be confused with MCHD is so-called Lennert's lymphoma (malignant lymphoma with high content of epithelioid histiocytes) [28, 29]. Since all of these lesions may involve the interfollicular zones like HD, differentiation from HD must be cytologic. Most cases can be separated by the identification of atypical small lymphocytes and lack of classic R–S cells (Fig. 5). Some T cell lymphomas may have bizarre cells that mimic Reed–Sternberg cells but they comprise only part of a population of large atypical cells that are much more pleomorphic and polymorphic than is typical of Hodgkin's disease. Nevertheless, some cases are nearly inseparable and may only be solved by follow-up, further tissue examination, or by immunologic studies.

2.5. Reticular variant of lymphocyte depleted Hodgkin's disease (LDHD)

The reticular variant of LDHD is characterized by the presence of numerous R–S cells and variants thereof, without any significant tendency to sclerosis. Bona fide cases are uncommon but very distinctive. The cytologic features usually allow separation from non-Hodgkin's lymphomas as many of the cells are classic R–S cells. Small numbers of lymphocytes and histiocytes are also usually present and produce an overall heterogeneity in contrast to the homogeneity that characterize most large cell non-Hodgkin's lymphomas.

2.6. Diffuse fibrosis form of LDHD

The author has seen only a few cases of the diffuse fibrosis form of LDHD. There is a background proteinaceous stroma with scattered cells interspersed in it [15, 14, 20]. Despite their paucity, the majority of the cells are atypical

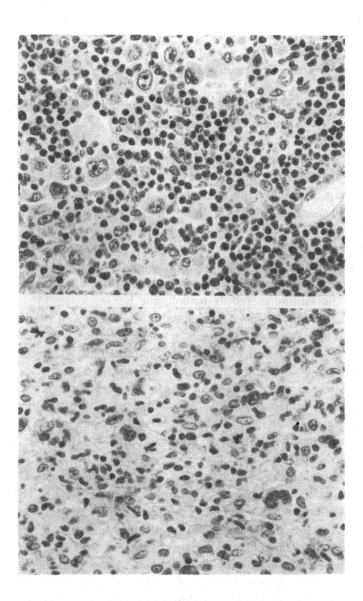

Figure 5. MCHD (top) compared with non-HD lymphoma (bottom) showing polymorphous pattern suggestive of peripheral T cell lymphoma. Both cases are Bouin's fixed. (top: H&E × 360, bottom: H&E × 260).

including some that have features of R–S cells and others that are smudged or degenerate.

Diffuse fibrosis is a rare form of HD in the U.S. and in the author's experience the majority of cases of HD that have large zones of hyaline fibrosis are nodular sclerosis [13]. These zones appear to originate from hyaline thickening of capillaries and this feature is probably analogous to the perivascular sclerosis that characterizes early sclerosis in NSHD.

2.7. Other morphologic patterns seen in Hodgkin's disease

Some cases of HD have unusual histologic features that may lead to misdiagnosis. These are summarized and described below.

1. *HD with prominent germinal centers: interfollicular HD (Fig. 6).* Reactive follicles are common in lymph nodes involved by HD [13]. In some cases the neoplastic cells are present only in the interfollicular zones overshadowed by the prominent reactive germinal centers. Such cases may be confused with reactive follicular hyperplasia and this pattern has been descriptively termed 'interfollicular HD' [30].

2. *HD mimicking toxoplasmic lymphadenitis.* HD may also be associated with clusters of epithelioid histiocytes and more rarely with infiltrate of monocytoid cells in the sinuses. When germinal centers are present, these cases may be misinterpreted as toxoplasmic lymphadenitis [31, 32]. The epithelioid cell clusters in HD are usually associated with the neoplastic components and do not encroach upon germinal centers as is characteristic of toxoplasmic lymphadenitis. Toxoplasmic lymphadenitis is associated with immunoblastic proliferation and lacks characteristic R–S cells.

3. *Syncytial sheets of lacunar cells (Figs. 7–9).* In some cases of NSHD, particularly in the mediastinum, sheets of large atypical cells with abundant cytoplasm (lacunar cells or apparent variants thereof) may be seen [13, 14, 20, 33, 34]. The designation 'syncytial' [33] is appropriately descriptive. The cells may even give the appearance of cohesion and simulate metastatic carcinoma (Fig. 9). Large sheets of noncohesive cells are reminiscent of non-Hodgkin's lymphoma. In both instances a search for characteristic foci of HD with a mixed background stroma containing scattered individual lacunar and R–S cells will lead to the correct diagnosis. Another term applied to this pattern of lacunar cells is the 'sarcomatous' variant of HD [34].

4. *HD associated with eosinophilic granuloma.* HD and eosinophilic granuloma (histiocytosis X) may coexist in the same patient and even in the same lymph node [13, 35–37]. The relationship between the two lesions is not clear. In some cases they are separate and probably coincident whereas in others they are intricately intermingled to the extent that they appear related. The

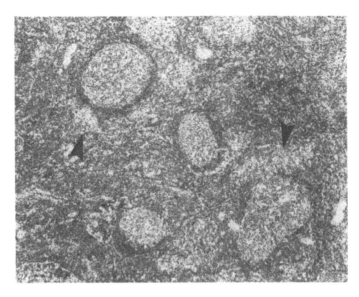

Figure 6. Interfollicular HD. The neoplastic infiltrate is between the prominent germinal centers. Clusters of atypical cells are present (arrows). (H&E × 36).

putative relationship of both R–S cells [38] and the histiocytes of eosinophilic granuloma [35] to the interdigitating reticulum cell raises interesting questions in histogenesis.

5. *HD resembling fibrous histiocytoma (Fig. 10).* Fibroblastic proliferation of HD is common, particularly in NSHD, and by itself may have prognostic significance (see below) [13]. In a small number of cases large fields mimicking malignant fibrous histiocytoma may be seen [13]. A storiform pattern may be present; however individual spindle cells do not apear malignant and the abnormal cells present appear to be R–S cell variants trapped in the proliferation of fibroblasts. Differential diagnosis of Hodgkin's disease from malignant fibrous histiocytoma is rarely a practical problem since the pathologist is usually aware that the lesion is in a lymph node and not a soft tissue tumor.

6. *Extensively necrotic HD.* A small percentage of cases of HD have large zones of geographic necrosis [13, 14] and much of it may be rimmed by a non-specific histiocytic and granulation tissue reaction. There may be a striking resemblance to granulomatous infection [39]. The necrotic debris may be infiltrated by neutrophils or eosinophils producing true eosinophilic abscesses [13]. Atypical cells, mummified cells and R–S cells are almost invariably present, at least focally, in the surrounding viable tissue. Even when one is convinced of the diagnosis of HD, if there is any question of an infection, special stains should be performed since Hodgkin's disease and infectious granulomas may certainly coexist.

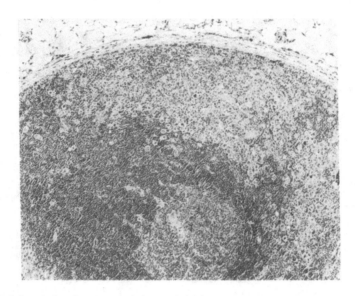

Figure 7. Subcortical and paracortical sheets of classic lacunar cells. In this focus the pattern is reminiscent of the sinusoidal infiltrates of malignant histiocytosis. (H&E × 56.25).

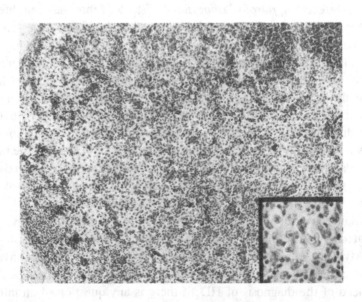

Figure 8. Sheets of lacunar cells with prominent cytoplasm imparting a histiocytic appearance at low power. (H&E × 56.25, inset × 225).

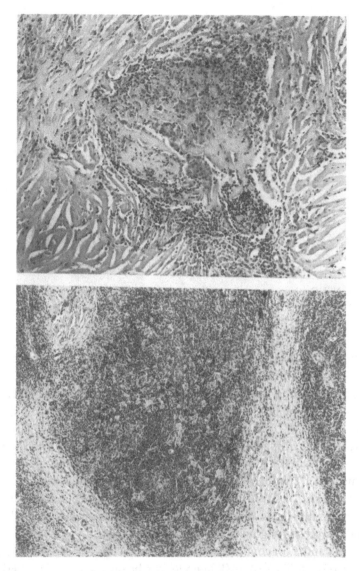

Figure 9. Top: Lacunar cells appear cohesive in the dense sclerotic collagen in this example of mediastinal NSHD. (H&E × 90). Bottom: Other fields in the same lesion show typical NSHD with non-cohesive lacunar cells scattered amongst lymphocytes and other inflammatory cells. (H&E × 56.25).

7. *HD mimicking giant lymph node hyperplasia (Fig. 11).* Lymph nodes harboring HD may occasionally have the peculiar hyalinized germinal centers identical to those seen in giant lymph nodes hyperplasia (Castleman's disease) as described by Keller *et al.* [40]. We have seen one case in which large fields resembled giant lymph node hyperplasia [41]. This case had increased vas-

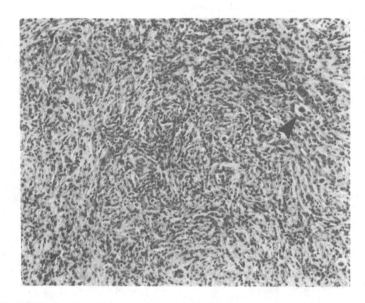

Figure 10. NSHD mimicking fibrous histiocytoma. Note storiform pattern and R–S cells (arrow). (H&E × 90).

cularity, plasma cell infiltrate, sclerosis and the distinctive germinal centers. Diagnostic fields of HD were very focal and difficult to find. The best example of this phenomenon we have seen was in a case of recurrent NSHD and it seems unlikely, at least in that instance, that there were two coincidental lesions.

8. *HD associated with other lymphoproliferative disorders.* Some of the reported occurrences of HD in patients with a history of chronic lymphocytic leukemia (CLL) probably represent nodal manifestations of CLL although bona fide cases do occur [42]. Likewise HD may rarely be found in patients with mycosis fungoides, but many such cases that have been reported probably represent mycosis fungoides in lymph nodes [43, 44]. Lymph nodes represent the earliest and most common site of extracutaneous MF [43, 45]. Despite the presence of R–S-like cells, MF in nodes can be distinguished from HD by the marked nuclear atypia present in all cells, small and large [43, 45]. CLL may either be mistaken for LPHD when small lymphocytes still comprise the majority of cells [23] or as MCHD or LDHD when the number of large and atypical R–S-like cells is prominent (Fig. 12). Dick and Maca [46] have called attention to this phenomenon, which more closely resembles a pleomorphic large cell lymphoma than HD although individual cells may be very similar to R–S cells. In any case, knowledge of skin involvement and the peripheral blood findings are invaluable in differential diagnosis [23, 45].

Composite lymphomas have two or more distinct histologic appearances in a

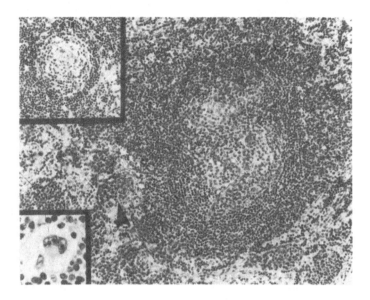

Figure 11. Relapse of NSHD in the axilla mimicking giant lymph node hyperplasia. A 3 cm diameter lymph node had extensive reactive follicles, some with prominent vessals (right), whereas others were small and hyalinized (upper inset). Sheets of plasma cells (arrows) filled interfollicular zones. Diagnostic HD was very focal (R–S cell in lower inset) and present on only one of three tissue blocks. (H&E × 90; lower inset × 360; upper inset × 90).

given specimen [47]. The majority are combinations of histologic subtypes of non-HD lymphomas, and as such, probably represent different histologic manifestations of the same neoplastic cell line [46]. A minority of composite lymphoma comprise HD and non-Hodgkin's lymphoma in the same lymph node [47]. The two lesions are usually quite distinct and readily recognized once the possibility of a composite lymphoma is considered.

Although Kaposi's sarcoma probably does not represent a lymphoproliferative disorder, its concurrence with lymphomas, including HD, is more than coincidental [49]. The association may be synchronous or metachronous, although the Kaposi's sarcoma is usually present in the skin before nodal involvement occurs. Primary nodal Kaposi's sarcoma associated with HD has been described [49].

Differential diagnosis for the histologic subtypes of HD is shown in Table 2.

36

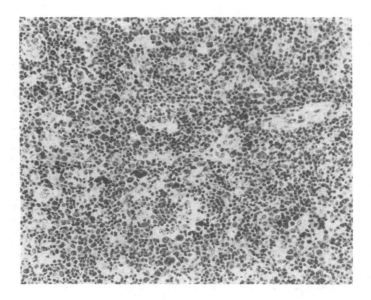

Figure 12. Pleomorphic lymph node infiltrate in a patient with a long history of CLL. Note clusters of histiocytes and bizzare R–S-like cells. In other foci the lesion was clearly a homogeneous large cell (transformed CLL) non-Hodgkin's lymphoma. (H&E × 144).

3. Further comments on subclassification and significance of histologic parameters

3.1. Cellular phase of NSHD (NSCP)

Although the definitions of the NSCP have varied, this pattern has been generally recognized as a variant of NSHD in which sclerosis is absent or poorly developed [5, 19, 50]. The relationship of NSCP to NSHD has been supported by the presence of lacunar cells and nodularity despite the relative lack of sclerosis [19, 50], the finding of NSCP in staging laparotomy tissue in cases in which the original biopsy showed characteristic NSHD [51], and by the fact that relapses in patients with NSHD showed NSCP or vice versa [52, 53]. We recently addressed the question of NSCP in diagnostic biopsy material in a large series [13]. In order for designation as NSCP, a given case had to show at least one sclerotic band extending into the lymph node parenchyma. Capsular fibrosis alone was inadequate. This definition was stricter than that used in some reports [50, 51] in which a diagnosis of NSCP was made on the basis of lacunar cells and nodularity alone. Our definition was essentially the same as that suggested by Lukes: at least one sclerotic band extending into nodal parenchyma [19]. Cases in which sclerotic bands divided a node into more than one or two nodules were designated as NSHD and the degree of sclerosis was

Table 2. HD: differential diagnosis (lymph nodes).

Type	Diagnostic considerations	
	Benign lesions	Malignant lesions
Nodular L&H	Progressive transformation of germinal centers Reactive hyperplasia (especially paracortical) Atypical follicular hyperplasia	Follicular lymphoma NSHD
Diffuse L&H	Diffuse hyperplasia	Lymphocytic proliferations (CLL, lymphocytic lymphomas) MCHD
NSHD	Reactive follicular hyperplasia (interfollicular HD) Giant lymph node hyperplasia Necrotic granulomas	Sclerotic non-HD lymphoma Malignant histiocytosis Metastatic carcinoma (especially melanoma, nasopharyngeal carcinoma) Malignant fibrous histiocytoma
MCHD	Reactive follicular hyperplasia (interfollicular HD) Diffuse hyperplasia (includes viral, drug reaction, post-vaccination) Toxoplasmic lymphadenitis Sarcoidosis AILD	Non-HD lymphomas (especially T-cell lymphomas) Chronic lymphocytic leukemia Lennert's lymphoma Malignant histiocytosis Malignant fibrous histiocytoma Atypical immune reaction
Reticular HD	Necrosis, necrotic granulomas	Non-HD lymphoma NSHD with lymphocyte depletion NSHD with sheets of atypical cells
Diffuse fibrosis	Post-treatment lymph node scarring	Non-HD lymphomas Very sclerotic NSHD

quantified. Sixty-three cases (approximately 10%) fell into the NSCP category, and as a group they showed differences from both the NS group and MCHD group: i.e. NSCP was a distinct subgroup with an overall survival similar to MCHD and significantly worse than NSHD; the relapse-free survival was more akin to NSHD [13]. The relationship between NSHD, NSCP, and MCHD for selected parameters is shown in Table 3. Among individual histologic parameters the degree of sclerosis showed a significant correlation with relapse-free survival. The presence and number of lacunar cells and/or degree of nodularity showed no such effect on relapse-free survival. Thus the relatively good prognosis associated with NSHD appeared to be related to the

Table 3. Comparison on NSHD, NSCP and MCHD.

Sub type	No. of cases	Mean age	Patho-logic stage I or II	Spleen involved	Extensive (3+) splenic disease	Lung or pleural involve-ment	Media-stinal disease
NS	397	28	57%	31%	52%	19%	78%
NSCP	63	34	62%	27%	53%	6%	50%
MCHD	146	32	44%	50%	60%	5%	33%

Sub type	Paraaortic disease	Relapsed	Relapse-free survival	Total survival
NS	26%	30%	Similar to NSCP	Significantly better than NSCP or MCHD
NSCP	25%	33%	Similar to NS	Similar to MC
MCHD	36%	24%	Slightly better than NS or NSCP (not significant)	Similar to NSCP

degree of sclerosis and not to lacunar cells or nodularity. These findings suggest that the essence of NSHD is the sclerosis itself and not the lacunar cells. The nodularity in some cases may be an epiphenomenon, secondary to the encompassing sclerosis; lacunar cells are frequent in HD, regardless of sclerosis.

3.2. 'Fibroblastic Hodgkin's disease' (Fig. 13)

In the same study [13], we found that fibroblastic proliferation (described below) was inversely related to relapse-free survival: patients with extensive fibroblastic proliferation fared significantly worse than patients lacking this feature. This finding was independent of other histologic and clinical variables. Fibroblastic proliferation was the single most significant histologic variable that influenced relapse-free survival: more than sclerosis, more than the number of lymphocytes, and more than subclassification, which by itself was not prognostically significant.

Fibroblastic proliferation is readily distinguished from sclerosis. Sclerosis is composed of relatively acellular lamellae of collagen, which in early phases are oriented around blood vessels. Sclerotic bands are birefringent. The fibroblastic proliferation produces fascicles and sheets of plump fibroblasts often infiltrated by lymphocytes and granulocytes (Fig. 13). This proliferation is a frequent finding around zones of necrosis and it may coexist with sclerosis. In

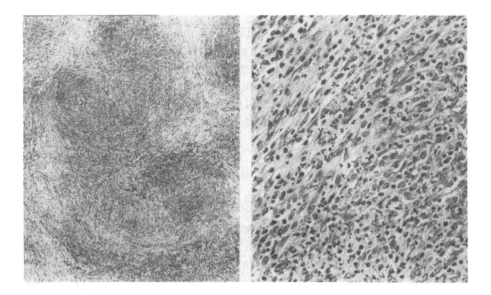

Figure 13. Fibroblastic NSHD. Fibroblast proliferation is prominent within and around nodules. The spindle cells are infiltrated by inflammatory cells. (left: H&E × 22.5; right: H&E × 225). Reprinted with the permission of J.B. Lippincott, Philadelphia, Pa., Cancer 49:1 48, 1982.

the absence of the sclerosis a case should not be designated as nodular sclerosis on the basis of nodularity and fibroblastic proliferation alone.

The mesenchymal reaction in HD has received relatively little attention in the past; most studies have concentrated on the cellular composition. The fact that sclerosis is associated with a relatively good prognosis and that a different mesenchymal response, fibroblastic proliferation, is associated with a worse prognosis is evidence that the connective tissue reaction exerts a significant role in determining prognosis and warrants further investigation [13, 54].

3.3. NSHD with lymphocyte depletion

A number of studies have shown that the number of lymphocytes influences survival in HD [2, 55–57], particularly in nodular sclerosis; however, the statistical basis for these findings and the relative effect of other parameters, such as pathologic stage has not been demonstrated in all instances. Three reported studies indicated that patients with NSHD with large numbers of lymphocytes appeared to have a better prognosis than those whose biopsy was depleted of lymphocytes [55–57]. We have shown that while increased numbers of lymphocytes, independent of other factors, were associated with a significantly better relapse-free survival in all subtypes, this was not true in the nodular sclerosing category alone [13]. Multivariate analysis indicated that fibroblastic proliferation (both in NSHD as well as all patients combined) was a better indicator of prognosis than the number of lymphocytes although both were independently predictive. The apparent influence of the number of lymphocytes, in nodular sclerosis in previously reported studies may be partially explained by the fact that in NSHD, the number of lymphocytes and fibroblasts are usually inversely related.

3.4. Histologic progression and inter-relationships of histologic subtypes of HD

Decreased numbers of lymphocytes and increased numbers of atypical cells may be seen in sequential biopsies in patients with HD and especially at autopsy [39, 53, 58]. This has often been taken as evidence of progression to a more aggressive histologic pattern; however, there is relatively little direct proof that with current therapy a lesion that looks histologically 'worse' is in fact biologically more aggressive. The evidence that supports this is circular: patients who do poorly frequently undergo repeated biopsies. Relapse biopsies in patients who have had radiation and/or chemotherapy may show a depletion of lymphocytes and less sclerosis in NSHD. This does not necessarily imply a poor response to salvage therapy [14, 58].

Lukes *et al.* [5, 19] and Butler [18] have suggested that progression among histologic subtypes usually takes place in the following manner:

LP → MC → LD

NS → Total sclerosis

The impression from such a scheme is that NS differs from the other clinical subgroups of HD. This is probably misleading. The separation of NS from other subtypes of HD is often not straightforward, as evidenced by the fact that 10% of the cases we studied were NSCP [13]. Lacunar cells are frequent in MCHD, sometimes in sheets [13], and as discussed above, the author does not consider this feature indicative of NSHD or NSCP. A number of studies have shown that relapse biopsies in patients with NSHD may show MCHD and vice versa, although in general there is a maintenance of histologic appearance, particularly when relapse occurs outside a treated site [52, 53, 58, 59]. At autopsy, lesions in patients with NSHD frequently lack sclerosis and resemble a large cell lymphoma with scattered R–S cells. Sometimes at autopsy the features of NSHD, McHD, and LDHD may all be found in different nodes at the same site [39].

4. Staging laparotomy in patients with HD

4.1. Spleen

Careful gross examination of the spleen is as important as the microscopic evaluation. The entire spleen should be sliced fresh at 2–3 mm intervals and *all* cut surfaces examined. The gross findings in the spleen are prognostically important: the presence of five or more grossly identified nodules, regardless of size, conveys a worse prognosis [12]. Suspicious foci and any obvious tumor nodules should be taken for microscopic evaluation. Four blocks are usually adequate, and overnight fixation gives best results. With careful examination, nearly all cases of splenic involvement by HD will be detected grossly. Examples in which Hodgkin's disease is identified only at microscopic examination are a rarity.

Microscopically, HD in the spleen manifests initially with atypical cells in the T zone of the white pulp [20]. The character of the lesion is usually similar to that seen in the initial lymph node biopsy. R–S cells are generally found easily, and while mononuclear variants may be indicative of a diagnosis of HD given an appropriate cellular milieu, it is more comforting to find diagnostic R–S cells. In cases in which the original node biopsy showed NSHD, sclerosis may or may not be found in the spleen.

4.2. Lymph nodes

Lymph nodes sampled at staging laparotomy should include those that were clinically suspicious on lymphangiography or other staging procedures. Though self-evident, this is not always the case. The nodes should be sliced into 2–3 mm sections and all tissue embedded for microscopic examination. If nodes are large and obviously involved grossly a single confirmatory block will suffice. Abdominal lymph nodes are especially informative in studying early lymph node involvement by HD: focal nodules and interfollicular infiltrates are relatively common. Nodules are usually highlighted by surrounding lymphangiographic reaction. In the absence of lymphangiogram effects, microscopic foci of HD are recognized as small nodules that locally distort and/or efface nodal architecture. Their composition is similar to that seen in other tissues. At scanning power small foci of HD are often paler and/or more eosinophilic than surrounding nodal tissue. R–S cells or mononuclear variants are required for a definitive diagnosis. Sectioning at multiple levels may be required to identify the smallest nodules of HD.

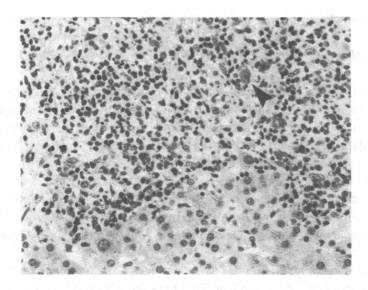

Figure 14. HD in the liver. A mixed portal infiltrate with mononuclear R–S cell variant (arrow) is present. This biopsy is from a patient who had a laparotomy and splenectomy for persistent thrombocytopenia after two cycles of MOPP chemotherapy. In addition to the apparently viable lesions in the liver, similar histologically viable nodules were present in the spleen. However, both spleen and splenic hilar nodes (Fig. 16 top) showed organizing, hemorrhagic nodules at sites of eradicated HD. (H&E × 225).

4.3. Liver and bone marrow involvement (Fig. 14)

In liver and bone marrow biopsies a diagnosis of HD can be made on the basis of finding mononuclear R–S cell variants in the appropriate cellular milieu, given a confirmed diagnosis of HD at another site [19, 50]. As shown by Weiss *et al.*, step sections, at least of bone marrow biopsies, will usually reveal characteristic R–S cells [61]. (Similar criteria can probably be applied to other small biopsies, such as transbronchial biopsies, from patients with histologically proven HD.) In our staging laparotomy material, liver or marrow involvement by HD has not occurred in the absence of splenic involvement [15], and cases in which they are involved usually have extensive splenic involvement [12].

In the liver, early infiltrates of HD are invariably portal and even with extensive involvement the infiltrates rarely spill into the lobules [62]. Individual R–S cells may rarely be seen in the sinusoids in the presence of extensive portal disease. Early portal involvement may be patchy and irregular and a suspicious infiltrate, even if only in one portal tract, should prompt the preparation of step sections.

Bone marrow involvement occurs as patchy and often extensive foci of

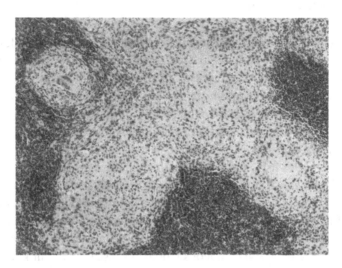

Figure 15. Granulomatous reaction in HD. Coalescent sarcoid-like granulomas are seen. Focal necrosis (lower right) was present; special stains showed no micro-organisms. (H&E × 56.25).

fibrosis with lymphoid infiltrate [61] that are relatively less cellular than the surrounding marrow tissue. Any focus of fibrosis should prompt multiple step sections and careful evaluation for R–S cells or variants thereof. Acellular scars in the bone marrow that are the result of irradiation of HD due to treatment are usually easily distinguished and discussed below.

4.4. Granulomatous reaction in HD (Fig. 15)

Epithelioid granulomas, with or without giant cells, are common in HD both in diagnostic lymph nodes and in tissues sampled at laparotomy [13, 15, 63]. In involved tissues, it is not known whether the granulomatous reaction represents an integral part of the lymphomatous process or whether it is a reaction to the neoplasm. In tissues not involved by HD the granulomas likely represent a secondary phenomenon, sometimes so extensive as to be indistinguishable from sarcoidosis. Granulomas are most commonly seen in the white pulp of the spleen but are also found in liver, bone marrow and lymph nodes. When granulomas are few and scattered they may be difficult to distinguish from lipogranulomas. One recent report has claimed that much of the granulomatous reaction seen in patients with Hodgkin's disease is, in fact, a form of lipogranuloma [64]. We think, however, that lipogranulomas and the granulomatous reaction to HD are usually distinguishable [15].

5. HD at extranodal sites

Extranodal HD is usually preceeded by involvement of lymph nodes and it is distinctly unusual for patients to present with extranodal disease alone [65], when nodal and extranodal disease are present simultaneously the former is usually biopsied for diagnosis. In our study of 659 cases, only three were diagnosed in tissue other than lymph nodes [13]. Findings such as this have led to a reluctance on the part of pathologists to diagnose extranodal HD and such a conservative approach is appropriate. Nevertheless, HD may rarely present in extranodal sites [65], and one can apply the same criteria and use a similar differential diagnosis as one uses in lymph nodes. The skin appears to be an exception since lesions occur which are morphologically identical to Hodgkin's disease but which have a clinically benign course [66]. This has led us to a *very* conservative approach in the skin in accord with Smith and Butler [67], and we are reluctant to diagnose cutaneous Hodgkin's disease without known lymph node involvement, usually in sites draining the involved skin. In any patient in which there is the slightest uncertainty about skin lesions, abnormal lymph nodes should be searched for and a biopsy performed.

6. Miscellaneous problems for the surgical pathologist

6.1. Diagnosis on frozen section

Once HD is considered and adequate tissue to confirm a diagnosis has been sampled, *there is rarely a need for definitive diagnosis at the time of frozen section.* In fact, only the exceptional frozen section is technically adequate for a confident diagnosis of Hodgkin's disease. Although by combining the architectural features seen in the frozen section with cytologic features assessed in a good touch preparation from the freshly cut node surface, one can often make a definitive diagnosis. Relatively few individuals attain enough experience with touch preparations of HD to be proficient. If touch preparations are fixed immediately in alcohol and stained with hematoxylin and eosin the cytologic features closely approximate those seen in paraffin sections. From a practical point of view frozen sections should be used to assure that adequate tissue is present for the diagnosis on permanent section. If sufficient tissue remains, this can be retained (e.g., frozen) for special diagnostic and/or experimental studies [15].

6.2. Adequacy of mediastinal biopsies

Mediastinoscopy sometimes produces tiny fragments of tissue with significant crush artifacts; however in many cases the diagnosis of HD (usually NSHD) is relatively easy. In difficult cases, which do not completely fulfill morphologic criteria, thoracotomy may be necessary. A number of mediastinal lesions, both benign and malignant including thymomas, germ cell neoplasms, non-Hodgkin's lymphomas, and giant lymph node hyperplasia among others, may have dense sclerotic bands and lymphoid infiltrates, and, in distorted tissue fragments, suggest the possibility of HD.

6.3. Histology of relapse in patients with HD

In patients with known HD, relapse is usually diagnosed without difficulty and often resembles the original lesion, especially when recurrence occurs outside treated sites [53]. Subclassification is often possible although not essential. In a minority of cases the recurrence, whether nodal or extranodal, may be pleomorphic with large numbers of atypical cells, sometimes raising the differential diagnosis of a pleomorphic non-Hodgkin's lymphoma [58, 68]. Such an appearance is in fact quite common at autopsy [37]. We have observed considerable variation in the morphologic appearance of recurrent HD and are reluctant to make a diagnosis of de novo non-Hodgkin's lymphoma without a considerable disease-free latent period and histologic features that clearly are distinct from HD. The examples of non-Hodgkin's lymphoma reported from Stanford among treated HD patients, had the appearance of diffuse undifferentiated or diffuse large cell lymphoma [69].

6.4. Treated HD (Figs. 16–18)

Nodular fibrotic residua of treated HD are common at autopsy in lymph nodes as well as spleen, liver, bone marrow and lung [39]. The changes appear to be similar regardless as to whether the patient has been treated with radiotherapy, chemotherapy, or both [70]. Such changes are also seen in surgical material. When biopsies or resections are performed during or immediately following cessation of therapy relatively acute lesions can be seen and the earliest changes we have observed in sites of treated HD are foci of recent and old hemorrhage and granulation tissue in the distribution of involvement seen in HD. Ultimately focal relatively acellular scars are all that remain and these may occasionally be associated with foam cells [39]. Interestingly, foci of recently irradiated Hodgkin's disease may be seen associated with histo-

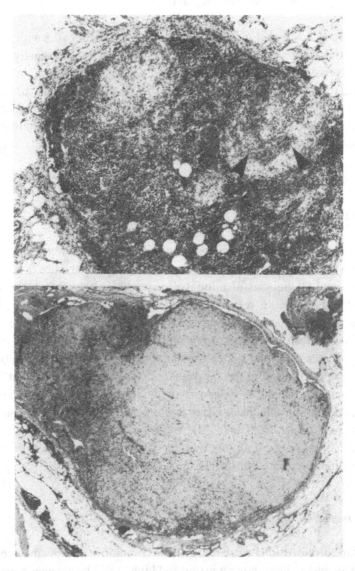

Figure 16. Effects of therapy on HD in splenic hilar lymph nodes removed at splenectomy. Top: Hemorrhagic nodules with early organization (arrows) are present. The lymph node was removed from a patient who had a splenectomy for persistent thrombocytopenia after two cycles of MOPP chemotherapy. Viable intra-abdominal HD persisted at other sites (Fig. 14). (H&E × 36). Bottom: This splenic hilar lymph node is partially replaced by nodular scars. It was removed from a patient who had completed chemotherapy 3 months previously. Laparotomy and splenectomy were performed for persistent splenomegaly. The spleen also showed the residua of treated HD, but no histologically viable HD. (H&E × 22.5).

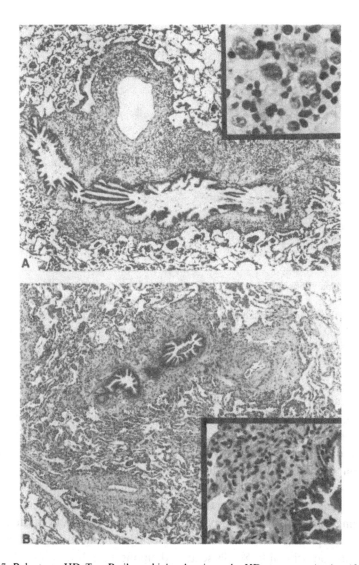

Figure 17. Pulmonary HD. Top: Peribronchial and perivascular HD at presentation in a 12-year old girl with bilateral infiltrates on chest radiograph. A mixed infiltrate including R–S variants is present (inset). (H&E × 36, inset: H&E × 360). Bottom: Histologically nonspecific peribronchial and perivascular scarring are interpreted as the residua of treated pulmonary HD. The bland cytology and fibroblastic character of the proliferation is apparent (inset). The patient was known to have HD and had had chemotherapy for clinically suspected pulmonary HD in the region of this biopsy. Lung biopsy was performed for new infiltrates, which, following biopsy evaluation, were interpreted as secondary to a nonspecific acute interstitial pneumonia. No active HD was seen. (H&E × 36; inset: H&E × 90).

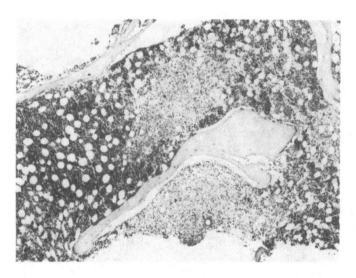

Figure 18. Two pale fibrinous foci resembling treated HD in other sites (Fig. 16). Diagnostic features of HD were absent. A staging bone marrow biopsy was not performed prior to initiation of MOPP chemotherapy. After one course a biopsy was taken. The illustrated foci are suspicious for having been sites of HD in the marrow. Definitive diagnosis, confirming or excluding this suspicion is impossible due to the mismanagement of this patient. (H&E × 36).

logically viable HD (Figs. 14, 16A) [70].

The pathologist is sometimes faced with interpretation of treated tissue from a patient who does not have a histologic diagnosis. Emergent radiotherapy for superior vena cava syndrome caused by a mediastinal mass is such a situation. Occasionally there is disease outside the treatment field that can be excised for diagnosis. Sometimes all that is available is tissue from within the treated fields. Strict criteria for the diagnosis of HD should be maintained recognizing that most of the lymphocytes will be few or absent in the treated tissue. In recognizable cases of NSHD one sees the characteristic architectural features and occasional R–S cells scattered amongst a cell-poor fibrotic background.

6.5. *The patient with HD is a compromised host*

Regardless of whether a patient with HD is on or off therapy he or she should be considered a compromised host [3, 65, 71]. As such, these patients are candidates to develop the large number of opportunistic infections that occur in this patient population. A particularly common problem for the surgical pathologist is exemplified by acute pulmonary infiltrates in a patient with a history of HD. Regardless of the histology of such lesions, a routine battery of special stains for fungi, bacteria, *Pneumocystis* and *Mycobacteria* should be performed. A similar approach should also apply to biopsies from other sites. Tissue specimens from compromised hosts may not show the histologic clues (such as granulomas in fungal infections) that the pathologist usually relies on in ordering special stains.

6.6. Cytologic diagnosis of HD

We think the initial diagnosis of HD should be by histologic and not cytologic means. In patients with a previous confirmed diagnosis of HD a cytologic diagnosis can be made with identification of the bizarre cells (lacunar cells, R–S cells) in the preparation. Most of our experience is with relapses in body fluids but fine needle aspirates will likely assume importance in the future in North Americas as in parts of Europe.

6.7. Incidental Hodgkin's disease

HD as an incidental finding is occasionally seen in tissues (usually nodes) being examined for other lesions [72]. Likewise patients with a history of HD and thought to be free of disease, who come to autopsy for an unrelated illness, may be found to be harboring occult HD at autopsy [39].

6.8. Freezing extra tissue

The pathologist is often aware of the possibility of HD when the lymph node is still fresh and in saline. In most cases of HD there is ample tissue for diagnosis and pathologists can safely freeze a portion without jeopardizing histologic diagnosis. This serves two purposes, one diagnostic and one experimental. The provision of tissue for marker studies is important if differential diagnosis of non-Hodgkin's lymphoma becomes a serious consideration and it serves as a reservoir of tissue for laboratories engaged in the research of Hodgkin's disease [15].

7. Summary

Since the vast majority of patients with HD may be cured with modern therapy and since clinical parameters (particularly pathologic stage) are the most important factors in assessing prognosis, it is not surprising that there has been little pressure to change the existing pathologic classification of HD. Even if there were reasons for change, it would probably be difficult, if not impossible, to devise a classification that significantly stratifies patients in whom the overall prognosis is so favorable. Thus classification has become relatively less important, given a confirmed diagnosis. Fine distinctions in classification and questions regarding the reproducibility of the Lukes and Butler classifications are more academic than practical considerations at this time. Nevertheless classification is still justified. The Lukes and Butler classification with its Rye Modification is familiar to pathologists and clinicians alike. It is eminently useful to the pathologist in recognizing the various patterns of HD. The primary duty of the pathologist is to make an accurate diagnosis of Hodgkin's disease and to be sure that pathologic evaluation accurately reflects the extent of involvement of tissue sampled at staging laparotomy. If there is any doubt about the initial diagnosis, surface marker studies may be helpful in some cases, consultation may be helpful in others, and in a few cases, a second lymph node biopsy may be necessary.

Acknowledgements

The author gratefully acknowledges Margaret Beers for typing the manuscript, Phil Horne for photographic assistance, and Drs. R.T. Hoppe, R.F. Dorfman, and J.S. Burke for critical review and comments.

References

1. Aisenberg AC, Linggood RM, Lew RA: The changing face of Hodgkin's disease. Am J Med 67:921–928, 1979.
2. Devita VT Jr, Simon RM, Hubbard SM, Young RC, Berard CW, Moxley JH, Frei E, Carbone PP, Canellos GP: Curability of advanced Hodgkin's disease with chemotherapy. Ann Intern Med 92:587–595, 1980.
3. Kaplan HS: Hodgkin's disease: Unfolding concepts concerning its nature, management and prognosis. Cancer 45:2439–2474, 1980.
4. Lukes RJ, Craver LF, Hall TC, Rappaport H, Rubin P: Report of the nomenclature committee. Cancer Res 26:1311, 1966.
5. Lukes RJ, Butler JJ, Hicks EB: Natural history of Hodgkin's disease as related to its pathologic picture. Cancer 19:317–344, 1966.
6. Butler JJ: Relationship of histologic findings to survival in Hodgkin's disease. Gann Monograph on Cancer Research 15:275–286, 1973.
7. Glatstein E: Hodgkin's disease and non-Hodgkin's homphomas: How important is histology? Front Radiation Ther Onc 9:203–216, 1974.
8. Fuller LM, Madoc-Jones H, Gamble JF, Butler JJ, Sullivan MP, Fernandex CH, Gehan EA: New assessment of the prognostic significance of histopathology in Hodgkin's disease for

laparotomy-negative stage I and stage II patients. Cancer 39:2174–2182, 1977.

9. Torti FM, Dorfman RF, Rosenberg SA, Kaplan HS: The changing significance of histology in Hodgkin's disease (Abstract). Proc Am Assoc Cancer Res 20:401, 1979.

10. Deforges JF, Rutherford CJ, Prio A: Hodgkin's disease. N Engl J Med 301:1212-1221, 1979.

11. Fuller LM, Gamble JF, Velasquez WS, Rodgers RW, Butler JJ, North LB, Martin RG, Gehan EA, Schultenberger CC: Evaluation of the significance of prognostic factors in stage III Hodgkin's disease treated with MOPP and radiotherapy. Cancer 45:1352–1364, 1980.

12. Hoppe RT, Rosenberg SA, Kaplan HS, Cox RS: Prognostic factors in pathological stage IIIA Hodgkin's disease. Cancer 46:1240–1246, 1980.

13. Colby TV, Hoppe RT, Warnke RA: Hodgkin's disease: A clinicopathologic study of 659 cases. Cancer 49:1848–1858, 1981.

14. Neiman RS: Current problems in the histopathologic diagnosis and classification of Hodgkin's disease. In: Pathology annual 13, part 2. Sommers SC, Rosen PP (eds) New York, Appleton-Century-Crofts, 1978, pp 289–328.

15. Dorfman RF, Colby TV: The pathologist's role in management of patients with Hodgkin's disease. Cancer Treat Rep 66:675–680, 1982.

16. Dorfman RF: Personal observations.

17. Hartsock RJ: Postvaccinial lymphadenitis. Hyperplasia of lymphoid tissue that simulated malignant lymphomas. Cancer 21:632–649, 1968.

18. Tindle BH, Parker JW, Lukes RJ: Reed-Sternberg cells in infectious mononucleosis? Am J Clin Pathol 58:607–617, 1972.

19. Lukes RJ: Criteria for involvement of lymph node, bone marrow, spleen and liver in Hodgkin's disease. Cancer Res 31:1755–1767, 1971.

20. Butler JJ: The natural history of Hodgkin's disease and its classification. In: The Reticuloendothelial System. Monographs in Pathology 16. Rebuck JW, Berard CW, Abell MR (eds). Baltimore, Williams and Wilkins, 1975, pp 184–212.

21. Lennert K: Malignant lymphomas other than Hodgkin's disease. New York, Springer-Verlag, 1978.

22. Poppema S, Kaiserling E, Lennert K: Hodgkin's disease with lymphocyte predominance, nodular type (nodular paragranuloma) and progressively transformed germinal centers – a cytohistological study. Histopathology 3:295–308, 1979.

23. Colby TV, Warnke RA, Burke JS, Dorfman RF: Differentiation of chronic lymphocytic leukemia from Hodgkin's disease using immunologic marker studies. Am J Surg Pathol 5:707–710, 1981.

24. Bennett MH: Sclerosis in non-Hodgkin's lymphoma. Br J Cancer 31:44–52, 1975.

25. Frizzera G, Moran EM, Rappaport H: Angioimmunoblastic lymphadenopathy. Diagnosis and clinical course. Am J Med 59:803–811, 1975.

26. Lukes RJ, Tindle EH: Immunoblastic lymphadenopathy. A hyperimmune entity resembling Hodgkin's disease. N Engl J Med 292:1–8, 1975.

27. Waldron JA, Leech JH, Glick AD, Flexner JM, Collins RD: Malignant lymphoma of peripheral T-lymphocyte origin: Immunologic, pathologic and clinical features in six patients. Cancer 40:1604–1617, 1977.

28. Watanabe S, Shimosato Y, Shimoyama M: Lymphoma and leukemia of T-lymphocytes. In: Pathology annual 16, part 2. Sommers SC, Rosen PP (eds), New York, Appleton-Century-Crofts, 1981, pp 155–204.

29. Kim H, Nathwani BN, Rappaport H: So-called 'Lennert's lymphoma' – Is it a clinicopathologic entity? Cancer 45:1379–1399, 1980.

30. Doggett RS, Colby TV, Dorfman RF. Interfollicular Hodgkin's disease. Am J Surg Pathol 7:145–149, 1983.

31. Dorfman RF, Remington JS: Value of lymph node biopsy in the diagnosis of acute acquired

toxoplasmosis. N Engl J Med 289:878–881, 1973.

32. Dorfman RF, Warnke R: Lymphadenopathy simulating the malignant lymphomas. Hum Pathol 5:519–550, 1974.

33. Butler JJ: Personal communication.

34. Banks PM: Sarcomatous lacunar cell Hodgkin's disease: A morphologic variant of the nodular sclerosing type. Lab Invest (Abstract) (44A), 3A, 1981.

35. Williams JW, Dorfman RF: Lymphadenopathy as the initial manifestation of histiocytosis X. Am J Surg Pathol 3:405–421, 1979.

36. Kjeldsberg CR, Kim H: Eosinophilic granuloma as an incidental finding in malignant lymphoma. Arch Pathol Lab Med 104:137–140, 1980.

37. Burns B, Colby TV, Dorfman RF: Langerkans cell granulomatosis (Histiocytosis X) associated with malignant lymphomas. Am J Surg Pathol. In press.

38. Kadin ME. Possible origin of the Reed-Sternberg cell from an interdigitating reticular cell. Cancer Treat Rep 33:601–608, 1982.

39. Colby TV, Hoppe RT, Warnke RA: Hodgkin's disease at autopsy. Cancer 47:1852–1862, 1981.

40. Keller AR, Hochholzer L, Castleman B: Hyaline-vascular and plasma cell types of giant lymph node hyperplasia of the mediastinum and other locations. Cancer 29:670–783, 1972.

41. Colby TV, Dorfman RF: Unpublished observations.

42. Choi H, Keller RH: Coexistence of chronic lymphocytic leukemia and Hodgkin's disease. Cancer 48:48–57, 1981.

43. Rappaport H, Thomas L: Mycosis fungoides. The pathology of the extracutaneous involvement. Cancer 34:1198–1229, 1974.

44. Donald D, Green JA, White M: Mycosis fungoides associates with nodular sclerosing Hodgkin's disease: A case report. Cancer 46:2505–2508, 1980.

45. Colby TV, Burke JS, Hoppe RT: Lymph node biopsy in mycosis fungoides. Cancer 47:351–359, 1981.

46. Dick FR, Maca RD: The lymph node in chronic lymphocytic leukemia. Cancer 41:283–292, 1978.

47. Kim H, Hendrickson MR, Dorfman RF: Composite lymphoma. Cancer 40:959–976, 1977.

48. van den Tweel, Lukes RJ, Taylor CR: Pathophysiology of lymphocyte transformation. A study of so-called composite lymphomas. Am J Clin Pathol 71:509–519, 1979.

49. Massarelli G, Tanda F, Denti S: Primary Kaposi's sarcoma and Hodgkin's disease in the same lymph node. Am J Clin Pathol 78:107–111, 1982.

50. Rappaport H, Berard CW, Butler JJ, Dorfman RF, Lukes RJ, Thomas LB: Report of the committee on histopathological criteria contributing to staging of Hodgkin's disease. Cancer Res 31:1864–1865, 1971.

51. Kadin ME, Glatstein E, Dorfman RF: Clinicopathologic studies of 117 untreated patients subjected to laparotomy for the staging of Hodgkin's disease. Cancer 27:1277–1294, 1971.

52. Strum SB, Rappaport H: Interrelations of the histologic types of Hodgkin's disease. Arch Pathol 91:127–134, 1971.

53. Colby TV, Warnke RA: The histology of the initial relapse of Hodgkin's disease. Cancer 45:289–292, 1980.

54. Seenmayer TA, Lagace R, Schurch W: On the pathogenesis of sclerosis and nodularity in nodular sclerosing Hodgkin's disease. Virchows Arch A Path Anat and Histol 385:283–291, 1980.

55. Keller AR, Kaplas HS, Lukes RJ, Rappaport H: Correlation of histopathology with other prognostic indicators in Hodgkin's disease. Cancer 22:487–499, 1968.

56. Coppelson LW, Rappaport H, Strum SB, Rose J: Analysis of the Rye Classification of Hodgkin's disease. The prognostic significance of cellular composition. J Natl Cancer Inst

51:379–390, 1973.

57. Patchefsky AS, Brodovsky H, Southard M, Menduke H, Gray S, Hoch WS: Hodgkin's disease: A clinical and pathologic study of 235 cases. Cancer 32:150–161, 1973.

58. Dolginow D, Colby TV: Recurrent Hodgkin's disease in treated sites. Cancer 48:1124–1126, 1981.

59. Poppema S, Lennert K: Hodgkin's disease in childhood: Histopathologic classification and relation to age and sex. Cancer 45:1443–1447, 1980.

60. Rappaport H, Berard CW, Butler JJ, Dorfman RF, Lukes RJ and Thomas LB: Report of the Committee on Histopathological Criteria Contributing to Staging of Hodgkin's Disease. Cancer Res 31:1864–1865, 1971.

61. Weiss RB, Brunning RD, Kennedy BJ: Hodgkin's disease in the bone marrow. Cancer 36:2077–2083, 1975.

62. Kim H, Dorfman RF, Rosenberg SA: Pathology of malignant lymphomas in the liver: application in staging. In: Progress in liver disease. Popper H, Schaffner F (eds), V. New York, Grune and Stratton, 1976, pp 683–698.

63. Kadin ME, Donaldson SS, Dorfman RF: Isolated granulomas in Hodgkin's disease. N Engl J Med 283:859–861, 1970.

64. Pak HY, Friedman NB: Pseudosarcoid granulomas in Hodgkin's disease. Hum Pathol 12:832–837, 1981.

65. Kaplan HS: Hodgkin's disease, 2nd ed. Cambridge Massachusetts, Harvard University Press, 1980.

66. Dorfman RF: Unpublished observations, 1981.

67. Smith JL, Butler JJ: Skin involvement in Hodgkin's disease. Cancer 45:354–361, 1980.

68. Colby TV, Carrington CB: Malignant lymphoma of the lung simulating lymphomatoid granulomatosis. Am J Surg Pathol 6:19–32, 1982.

69. Krikorian JG, Burke JS, Rosenberg SA, Kaplan HS: Occurrence of non-Hodgkin's lymphoma after therapy for Hodgkin's disease. N Engl J Med 300:452–458, 1979.

70. Colby TV: Unpublished observations, 1982.

71. Fisher RI, DeVita Jr, Bostick F, Vanhaelen C, Howser DM, hubbard SM, Young RC: Persistent immunologic abnormalities in long-term survivors of advanced Hodgkin's disease. Ann Int Med 92:595–599, 1980.

72. Miller GA Jr. Jarowski CH, Coleman M, Cibull ML, Posteraro AF, Weksler ME: Incidental discovery at radical mastectomy of inapparent Hodgkin's disease in long term survivors. Cancer 42:318–325, 1978.

3. The Reed–Sternberg cell: Biological and clinical significance

MARSHALL E. KADIN

1. Evidence for the Reed–Sternberg cell as the malignant cell in Hodgkin's disease

The nature of the malignant cell in Hodgkin's disease has remained an enigma for more than 150 years. The Reed–Sternberg cell is essential for an unequivocal diagnosis of Hodgkin's disease [1, 2] and therefore is generally accepted to represent the malignant cell of Hodgkin's disease (Table 1). The frequency of diagnostic Reed–Sternberg cells increases with advanced clinical stages of disease [3] and with progression of Hodgkin's disease over time towards more unfavorable histological types [4, 5]. Measurements of Reed–Sternberg cell DNA content and cytogenetics have demonstrated a marked degree of aneuploidy and marker chromosomes [6, 7]. The rate of synthesis of DNA seems to be slower for Reed–Sternberg cells than for mononuclear Hodgkin giant cells. Peckham and Cooper found essentially no *in vitro* tritiated thymidine (3H-TdR) labelling of Reed–Sternberg cells in cell suspensions of excised lymph nodes [7]. They proposed that the Reed–Sternberg cell is a nonproliferating cell arising from incomplete cytokinesis (cell division) during mitosis of a mononuclear Hodgkin giant cell (Fig. 1). However, a small proportion of Reed–Sternberg cells were found to incorporate DNA precursor when Hodgkin's tissues were perfused with 3H-TdR *in vivo* avoiding the cell damage that occurs in the preparation of cell suspensions [8]. Meyer and Higa found that the S-phase fraction of atypical mononuclear and multinucleated Hodgkin's cells was higher than that of lymphocytes in two of three cases of Hodgkin's disease. They studied thin slices of Hodgkin's tissue incubated

Table 1. Evidence for the Reed–Sternberg cell as the malignant cell in Hodgkin's disease.

1.	Essential for diagnosis of Hodgkin's disease [1, 2]
2.	Increased number in advanced stages of Hodgkin's disease [3, 4, 5]
3.	3H-TdR labelling, aneuploidy and marker chromosomes of Hodgkin giant cells [6, 7, 8, 9, 10]
4.	Persistence of Reed–Sternberg cells in cell lines and xenografts [10, 11, 12, 13, 14]

Bennett JM (ed), Controversies in the Management of Lymphomas. ISBN 0-89838-586-5.
© *Martinus Nijhoff Publishers, Boston. Printed in the Netherlands.*

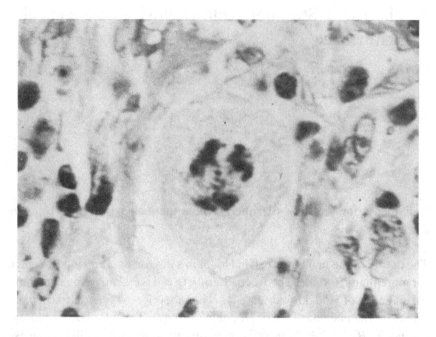

Figure 1. Multipolar mitosis of mononuclear Hodgkin's giant cell in tissue section of cervical lymph node biopsy. Abnormal mitoses and incomplete cell division are thought to give rise to R–S cells.

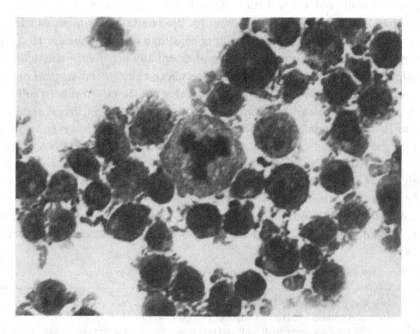

Figure 2. Tripolar mitosis in giant cell from L428 cell line of Hodgkin's disease. Note similarity to dividing cell in Fig. 1.

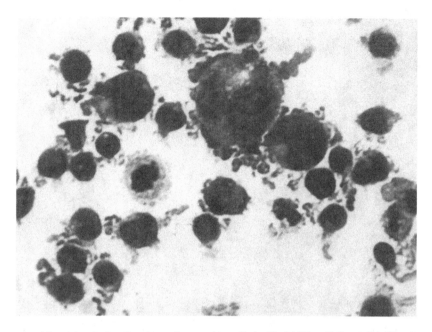

Figure 3. Binucleate R–S cell among pleomorphic cells in Hodgkin's cell line L428. Note resemblance to lymphoblastoid cell lines.

with 3H-TdR under hyperbaric conditions [9]. In studying growth of cell cultures derived from splenic lesions of Hodkin's disease, we [10, 11] and Kaplan and Gartner [12] observed 3HTdR labelling of multinucleated cells and abnormal multipolar mitoses. Schadt *et al.* also demonstrated abnormal mitoses (Fig. 2) and the persistence of multinucleated Reed–Sternberg cells (Fig 3) in neoplastic cell lines derived from pleural effusions of patients with nodular sclerosing Hodgkin's disease [13]. Reed–Sternberg cells were found when the cell lines were injected to form tumors in the brain of nude mice [13, 14]. Thus we can conclude that Reed–Sternberg cells are part of a continuum of tumor giant cells that represent the neoplastic cellular component of Hodgkin's disease.

2. Morphological variants of Reed–Sternberg cells

Lukes demonstrated distinctive morphological variants of Reed–Sternberg cells in association with specific histologic types of HD [1]. A Reed–Sternberg cell with a popcorn-like nucleus having twisted nuclear lobules, delicate chromatin and small nucleoli characterizes the lymphocyte predominance, L and H type Hodgkin's disease (Fig. 4). Poppema described special L and H

58

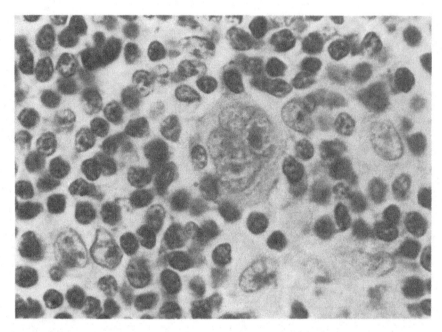

Figure 4. R–S cell variant with twisted polyploid nucleus in lymphocyte predominance, L&H type Hodgkin's disease.

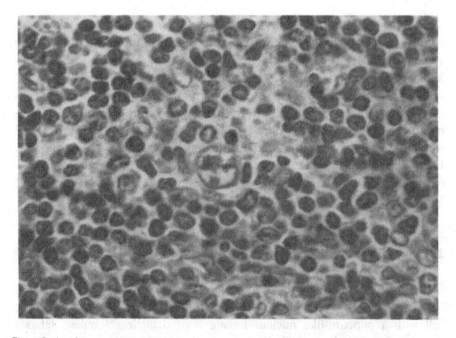

Figure 5. An abnormal blast cell with small amount of cytoplasm in the distinctive nodular para-granuloma type of Hodgkin's disease.

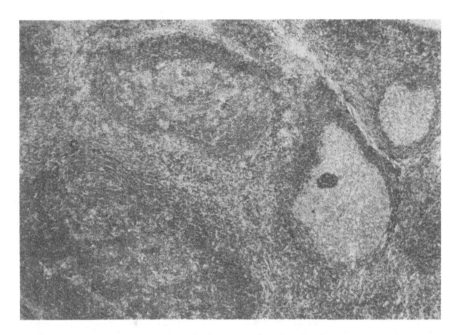

Figure 6. Progressively transformed germinal centers in lymph node of patient with nodular para-granuloma type Hodgkin's disease.

variants of Reed–Sternberg cells, resembling immunoblasts, in the unique nodular paragranuloma (lymphocyte predominance) type of Hodgkin's disease (Fig. 5). This unusual type may arise from progressively transformed germinal centers in some cases of Hodgkin's disease (Fig. 6) [15, 16].

The lacunar variant of the Reed–Sternberg cell has proven to be a highly reliable indicator of the nodular sclerosing type of Hodgkin's disease (Fig. 7) [1, 17]. In some cases, identification of lacunar cells in lesions with little or no sclerosis forecast the presence of more advanced sclerosis at other sites [17]. Thus the phrase 'cellular phase' of nodular sclerosis was coined to depict this type of Hodgkin's disease [1, 17]. Lacunar cells are best identified in formalin-fixed tissues where their pale staining cytoplasm is retracted from surrounding cells and stroma. Their nuclei may be single, multiple or hyperlobated but are generally small with inconspicuous nucleoli (Fig. 8). For accuracy and re-producibility in large series, Lukes recommends that both lacunar cells and collagen bands be required for a diagnosis of nodular sclerosing Hodgkin's disease [1].

A pleomorphic or sarcomatous variant of the Reed–Sternberg cell typifies the reticular lymphocyte depletion type of Hodgkin's disease (Fig. 9). These cells can be so bizarre in appearance that they are confused with mega-karyocytes or nonlymphoreticular tumor cells (Fig. 10).

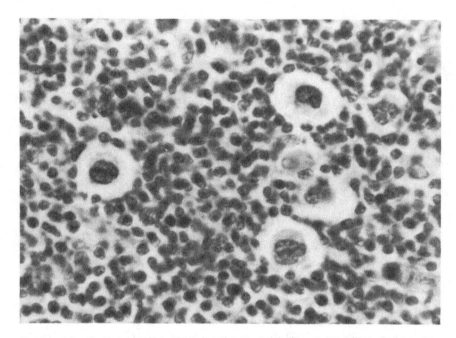

Figure 7. Lacunar type R–S cells in cellular phase of nodular sclerosing Hodgkin's disease.

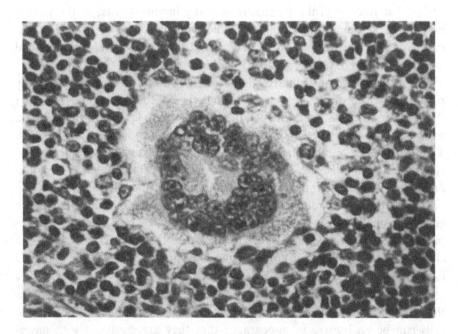

Figure 8. Many small nuclei in lacunar variant of R–S cell.

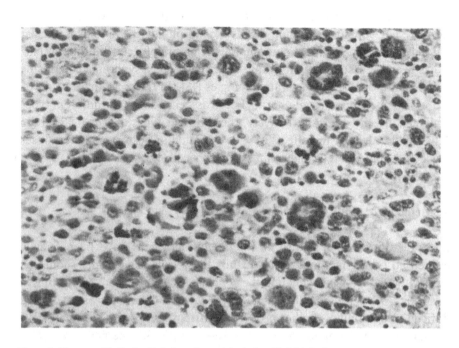

Figure 9. Pleomorphic R–S cells in lymphocyte depletion Hodgkin's disease.

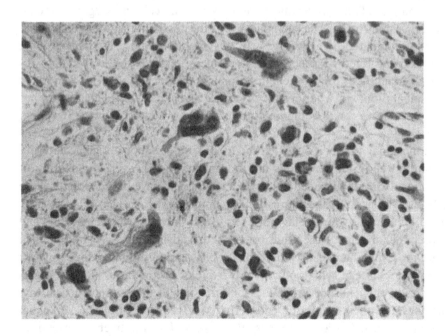

Figure 10. Sarcomatous type of R–S cells in lymphocyte depletion Hodgkin's disease.

The relationship between diagnostic Reed–Sternberg cells with huge inclusion-like nucleoli and these non-diagnostic morphological variants is unclear but may be of importance in determining the nature of Reed–Sternberg cells. It has been suggested that Hodgkin's disease may be a syndrome comprising two or more diseases of separate etiologies [18]. In that case there could be more than one kind of Reed–Sternberg cell associated with the different types of Hodgkin's disease. Alternatively, the different types of Reed–Sternberg cells could represent the effects of wide variation of host immune responses towards a single kind of malignant Hodgkin's cell [19].

3. Methods for study of Reed–Sternberg cells

Interpretations of the nature of Reed–Sternberg cells have been heavily influenced by the methods used to study these cells. The reader should be aware of this factor in evaluating the conclusions of investigators working in this area. Because of the cellular heterogeneity of Hodgkin's disease, it is often difficult to determine whether properties attributed to Reed–Sternberg cells do not actually belong to some of their adjacent look-alike neighbors. This may be true especially for morphological studies that attempt to compare the fine structural and surface characteristics of Reed–Sternberg cells with other cell types [20–24]. To overcome this difficulty some investigators have sought to develop cell lines representative of the malignant cells in Hodgkin's disease [10–14]. This effort has been complicated by the possibility that cell cultures are readily dominated by an overgrowth of lymphoblastoid cells that resemble Hodgkin and Reed–Sternberg cells in many respects. With the availability of improved methods for cytogenetics, immunodeficient animals for tumor cell transplantation, and a variety of cell surface and cytochemical markers, it has now become easier to compare cultured with noncultured Reed–Sternberg cells [12–14].

Monoclonal antibodies can be used to look for common antigenic determinants of Reed–Sternberg cells and normal cells. However, the sharing of common determinants need not imply a common lineage or function for these cells as evidenced by the expression of common ALL antigen (CALLA) on renal tubular and glomerular cells, fetal small intestine epithelial cells, and myoepithelial cells of the adult breast [25], and thymocyte-related antigen (T6) on Langerhans cells [26]. Conversely, undifferentiated immature or neoplastic cells can lack or only weakly express certain of the surface characteristics of their normal progenitors. For example, developing cortical thymocytes and their neoplastic counterparts, T cell lymphoblastic leukemia/lymphoma, usually do not express the mature T cell antigen T3 found on medullary thymocytes and the majority of functionally mature peripheral T cells [27].

Functional studies of Hodgkin's cells can contribute another dimension to our knowledge about the nature of Reed–Sternberg cells. Results of these studies may also help to explain some of the unusual clinical manifestations of Hodgkin's disease. Functional studies will be limited by the ability of investigators to selectively deplete Hodgkin's disease cell suspensions of populations of non-malignant cells, or to verify that 'Hodgkin' cell lines actually are derived from the malignant cells of Hodgkin's disease.

Since it has been proposed from epidemiologic and clinicopathologic studies that Hodgkin's disease may not represent a single disease entity, but two or more diseases of possibly separate etiologies [18, 28], a necessary step in defining the Reed–Sternberg cell will be to determine whether there are any significant differences between Reed–Sternberg cells from patients of different age, sex, race, and national origin, or from patients with different histologic types of Hodgkin's disease [16, 29–30].

4. Proposed cellular origin of the Reed–Sternberg cell

The morphologic resemblance of Reed–Sternberg cells to immunoblasts led Tindle *et al.* to suspect that Reed–Sternberg cells were transformed lymphoid cells [31]. They demonstrated immunoblasts indistinguishable from Reed–Sternberg cells in lymph nodes of patients with infectious mononucleosis. Anagnostou and co-workers traced a spectrum of lymphoid appearing cells through immunoblasts to lacunar cells and Reed–Sternberg cells in nodular sclerosing Hodgkin's disease [32]. Glick emphasized ultrastructural similarities of Reed–Sternberg cells and transformed lymphocytes noting especially their large nuclei with dispersed chromatin, large nucleoli, and great numbers of cytoplasmic polyribosomes [33]. He noted that Reed–Sternberg cells lacked the rough endoplasmic reticulum characteristic of transformed B lymphocytes. Reed–Sternberg cells, he thought, more closely resemble the large transformed cells in malignant lymphomas of peripheral T origin. In Japan, where T cell lymphomas are common, it can be difficult to distinguish Hodgkin's disease from pleomorphic T cell lymphoma [34, 35] (Fig. 11).

In tissue culture, there is even greater difficulty is distinguishing Hodgkin's cells from transformed lymphocytes. Hodgkin's cells in culture (Figs. 2 and 3) closely resemble Epstein Barr virus-transformed lymphoblastoid cell lines. Thus it is difficult to be certain of the origin of large multinucleated cells, indistinguishable from Reed–Sternberg cells, in long term cultures derived from splenic lesions of patients with Hodgkin's disease. On the basis of distinctive nuclear features, we divided cells in culture into two morphologic groups, lymphocytes and Hodgkin's cells [10]. However, a small proportion of cells, estimated at less than one percent, had morphologic features of both

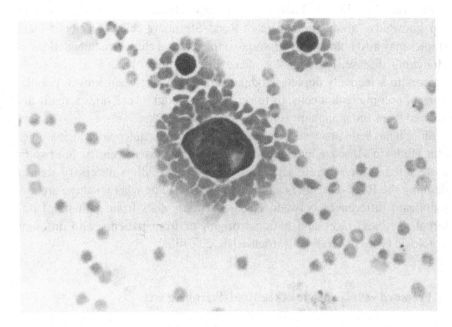

Figure 11. Sheep erythrocyte rosette formation of tumor giant cell from pleomorphic T cell lymphoma resembling Hodgkin's disease.

lymphocytes and Hodgkin's cells raising the possibility of a transition between the two apparently separate cell types. Dorfman demonstrated ultrastructural similarities between Reed–Sternberg cells and large binucleated cells in culture, while cautioning against extrapolation of *in vitro* observations to surgical biopsy material [36].

4.1. Thymic or T cell origin

Thomson suggested that Hodgkin's disease is of thymic origin. He described the appearance of Reed–Sternberg-like cells with 'owl's eye' or 'mirror image' nuclei in the histogenesis of Hassall's corpuscles of the thymus [37]. His concept did not find support in the observations of Marshall and Wood who could find gross thymic lesions in only 26 percent of 86 patients dying of Hodgkin's disease [38] or in the clinicopathological analysis of Keller and Castleman who detected no histologic evidence of Hodgkin's disease in the thymus in 50% of 54 cases initially confined to the mediastinum [39].

Nevertheless, Order and Hellman's discovery of high concentrations of Hodgkin's disease tumor-associated antigens in the neonatal thymus and other tissues rich in thymic-derived T lymphocytes prompted speculation and research on a possible T lymphocyte origin for the Reed–Sternberg cell. They

Table 2. Theories/evidence for and against derivation of the Reed–Sternberg cell from a lymphoid cell.

Authors	Year (Ref.)	Theory/Evidence
Lukes & Tindle	1972 [31]	Reed–Sternberg cells resemble immunoblasts in infectious mononucleosis
Order *et al.*	1972 [40]	Hodgkin tumor antigens in neonatal thymus and malignant thymoma
Leech	1973 [50	Reed–Sternberg cells are immunoglobulin positive
Kadin *et al.*	1974 [64]	Reed–Sternberg cells lack E rosette receptor and fetal thymic antigens
Taylor	1974 [52]	Reed–Sternberg cells contain monotypic, bitypic, or no immunoglobulin
Landaas	1977 [53]	Reed–Sternberg cells do not contain monoclonal immunoglobulin
Kadin *et al.*	1978 [54]	Immunoglobulin in Reed–Sternberg cells is exogenous in origin
Poppema *et al.*	1978 [58]	Immunoglobulin associated with other serum proteins and degenerative changes in Reed–Sternberg cells
Isaacson	1979 [57]	Absence of J chain in Reed–Sternberg cells
Poppema *et al.*	1979 [63]	L and H type Reed–Sternberg cells contain IgG and one light chain type per cell in nodular paragranuloma Hodgin's disease

proposed that a virus-altered T cell could trigger a chronic-graft verus host reaction resulting in malignant transformation of a bystander reticulum cell [40]. Alternatively a virus could transform the T cell directly into a Hodgkin tumor cell [41]. Either process would account for the early appearance of anergy [42], progressive loss of T cell function [43], and other related abnormalities often observed during the course of Hodgkin's disease [44, 45].

To examine this hypothesis directly we isolated malignant cells from involved lymph nodes and studied them for T cell surface characteristics. None were found. Reed–Sternberg cells did not form sheep erythrocyte (E)-rosettes or react with an antiserum specific for human thymocytes and peripheral T cells [46]. Subsequently, Pinkus *et al.* reported occasional Reed–Sternberg cell variants forming E-rosettes and staining focally for alpha-naphthyl acetate esterase in a T cell pattern, concluding that there was a T cell origin for part of the Hodgkin tumor cell population [47]. Recent studies with panels of monoclonal antibodies against the E-rosette receptor and other T cell differentiation antigens gave negative results, indicating that it is unlikely that Reed–Sternberg cells are closely related to T cells at either early or late stages of thymocyte differentiation [48, 49].

4.2. B cell origin

Leech found surface membrane and intracellular immunoglobulin in lymph node cell suspensions containing Reed–Sternberg cells, turning attention towards a possible B cell origin for the Reed–Sternberg cell [50]. In more comprehensive studies of fixed tissues, Garvin *et al.* and Taylor confirmed the presence of intracellular IgG in Reed–Sternberg cells [51–52], but in most cases the immunoglobulin was polyclonal or bitypic, associated with both kappa and lambda light chains [52–54], thus raising the question whether Reed–Sternberg cells were unlike malignant B cells in non-Hodgkin's lymphomas that synthesize immunoglobulin of only one light chain type [55]. Bernau *et al.* claimed to localize immunoglobulin to sites of protein synthesis in Reed–Sternberg cells, but their illustrations show only diffuse cytoplasmic staining of immunoglobulin and none localized within the cisterne of in the rough endoplasmic reticulum [56]. Against the possibility of immunoglobulin synthesis in Reed–Sternberg cells was the finding that the J chain, present in normal B-immunoblasts and B cell lymphomas synthesizing immunoglobulin, was absent in Reed–Sternberg cells [57]. Because we found that viable Reed–Sternberg cells could internalize aggregates of human IgG, we suggested that internalization of immune complexes circulating in the serum of Hodgkin's disease patients and binding to the tumor cell membrane was the mechanism whereby Reed–Sternberg cells acquired exogenous IgG [54]. Alternatively the IgG could enter Reed–Sternberg cells through a leaky cell membrane, possibly damaged by tumor directed antibodies, including IgG. This would explain the usually diffuse cytoplasmic staining of IgG in Reed–Sternberg cells, the associated degenerative changes, and the detection by some investigators of certain other low molecular weight serum proteins in Reed–Sternberg cells [58, 59]. Similar patterns of staining of IgG in the cytoplasm of tumor cells has been described in carcinomas of the ovary, lung, and liver, and in tumors of neurogenic origin [60–62].

These observations apply to RS cells from patients with the most common types of HD, mixed cellularity and nodular sclerosis. A unique RS cell variant thought to be derived from an atypical B-immunoblast in progressively transformed germinal centers has been proposed in the rare nodular paragranuloma type of Hd [15, 63]. In contrast to other types of Hodgkin's disease, immunohistology of nodular paragranuloma shows a mixture of L and H type RS cells that individually stain either for kappa or lambda light chains but no RS cells that stain for both light chains [63]. Only IgG heavy chains are found in L and H type RS cells. Because the L and H variants appear to be derived from more than one clone, one must question the neoplastic nature of RS cells in the nodular paragranuloma type of HD. Nodular paragranuloma seems to be a distinct entity since it does not progress to mixed cellularity or nodular sclerosis and has a different epidemiology than these other types of HD [16]. However, rare cases of nodular paragranuloma appear to progress to lymphocyte depletion in which the cytology of the tumor cells is compatible with immunoblastic lymphoma [15]. This is consistent with the concept that nodular paragranuloma represents a progressive proliferation of B-immunoblasts [63].

4.3. Marcophage/hostiocyte

Reed–Sternberg cells have either few or no ultrastructural and cytochemical characteristics of normal macrophages [22–24, 64–68], (Fig. 12) and rarely, if ever, show evidence of phagocytosis in vivo (Fig. 13). Immune rosetting of Reed–Sternberg cells has not been detected in frozen sections of Hodgkin's disease [69–70]. However, many investigators have reported that cells identified as Reed–Sternberg cells in vitro can bind immune complexes of erythrocytes and antibody (EA), or erythrocytes, antibody and complement (EAC) [54, 71–74] (Fig. 14), especially after enzyme removal of lymphocytes from the surface of Reed–Sternberg cells [72]. We have found some large dividing cells interpreted as Hodgkin's cells forming EA rosettes (Fig. 15). Erythrophagocytosis was also occasionally observed [54]. Additional in vitro studies testing for phagocytosis of opsonized yeast and Staphylococci have shown that Reed–Sternberg cells are not 'professional phagocytes' when compared to normal histiocytes from the same Hodgkin's disease tissues (Fig. 16) [21].

Differences between Reed–Sternberg cells and histiocytes become less clear when comparisons are made between Reed–Sternberg cells and malignant histiocytes. Using freshly isolated tumor cells from 3 patients with histiocytic medullary reticulosis (malignant histiocytosis), and a continuous tumor cell line established from one of these patients, we found that Reed–Sternberg cells and malignant histiocytes showed similar weak immune rosetting with EA and EAC [75]. Neither Reed–Sternberg cells nor malignant histiocytes from the tumor cell line MH-1 reacted with monoclonal antibodies 20.2 and 20.3 that detect surface antigens of normal monocytes and tissue macrophages [76]. These results suggest that the lack of certain normal macrophage antigens on Reed–Sternberg cells is, by itself, insufficient to distinguish then from malignant macrophages. Malignant histiocytes generally gave stronger more diffuse staining for nonspecific esterase and acid phosphatase than Reed–Sternberg cells that commonly have only small amounts of these enzymes in a focal paranuclear position (Fig. 17). These differences were smaller when Reed–Sternberg cells were placed in tissue culture (Fig. 18). Poppema found similar paranuclear staining of Reed–Sternberg cells and histiocytes for alpha-1-antitrypsin [77].

Table 3. Theories/evidence for and against a macrophage/histiocyte origin for the Reed–Sternberg cell.

Authors	Year	(Ref.)	Theory/Evidence
Dorfman	1961	[64]	Reed–Sternberg cells lack non-specific esterase and acid phosphatase enzymes characteristic of normal histiocytes
Carr	1975	[65]	Ultrastructural evidence of lysozymes, microfibrils, and complex surface projections similar to those of macrophages or reticulum cells
Kay	1975	[22]	Scanning E.M. surface lamellae of Reed–Sternberg cells similar to those of macrophages
Parmley *et al.*	1976	[67]	Reed–Sternberg cells lack ultrastructural evidence of endocytic activity
Stuart *et al.*	1977	[72]	Reed–Sternberg cells do not react with anti-monocyte serum
Kaplan & Gartner	1977	[12]	Cell lines from spleens of Hodgkin's disease contain binucleate giant cells with receptors for IgGFc and complement, phagocytosis and secretion of lysozyme
Papadimitriou *et al.*	1978	[59]	Intracytoplasmic alpha-1-antichymotrypsin and lysozyme, globules of IgG in some Reed–Sternberg cells
Kadin *et al.*	1978	[54]	Noncultured Reed–Sternberg cells can internalize aggregates of IgG, show infrequent erythrophagocytosis of IgGEA *in vitro*
Kadin *et al.*	1979	[75]	Neoplastic histiocytes of malignant histiocytosis are similar to Reed–Sternberg cells. Both have weak receptors for IgGFc, infrequent erythrophagocytosis of EA *in vitro* and absence of several normal macrophage antigens
Peiper *et al.*	1980	[20]	Ultrastructure of prominent cytoplasmic processes, well-developed Golgi, fibrillar bodies and lysozomes
Poppema	1980	[77]	Reed–Sternberg cells and histiocytes have similar paranuclear staining for alpha-1-antitrypsin

4.4. Myeloid cells

Diehl *et al.* examined the surface-membrane antigens of cultured L428 Hodgkin's cells with a panel of more than 40 monoclonal antibodies. A positive reaction was observed with most, but not all, antibodies detecting antigens on monocytes and immature myeloid cells [78]. In another study conducted by Stein and co-workers, biopsies from patients with Hodgkin's disease were examined with murine monoclonal antibodies raised against human acute myelomonocytic leukemia (AMML) cells [79]. Three of seven

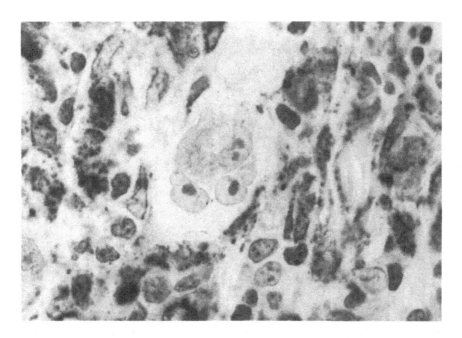

Figure 12. Dark granular acid phosphatase in normal histiocytes, but not R–S cell, from mixed cellularity Hodgkin's disease. Two micron methacrylate sections showing complex convoluted nucleus of R–S cell (center) stained according to method of Beckstead *et al.* [68]).

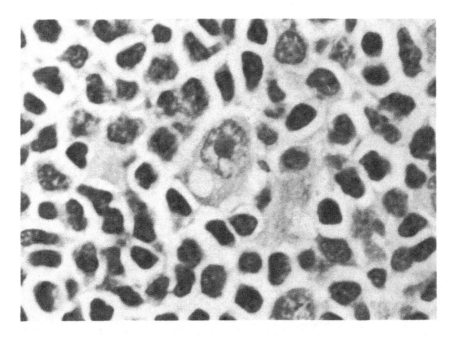

Figure 13. Cell interpreted as mononuclear Hodgkin's cell with intracytoplasmic erythrocyte in lymph node biopsy of lymphocyte predominance Hodgkin's disease.

70

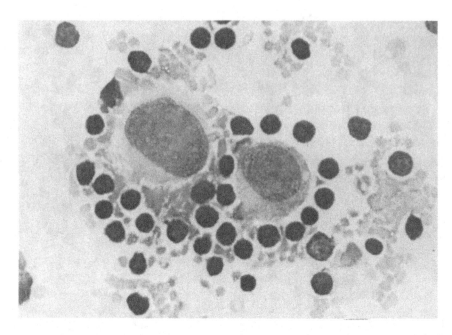

Figure 14. IgG-coated sheep erythrocytes (EA) rosetting one of two Hodgkin's giant cells *in vitro*. Surrounding T lymphocytes are not rosetted with EA.

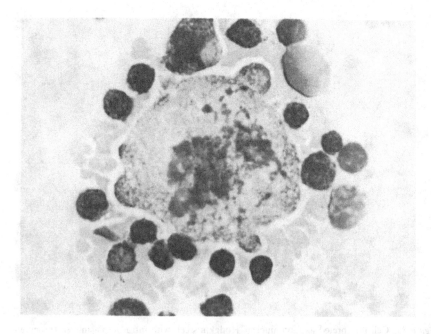

Figure 15. Large mitotic cell considered to be dividing Hodgkin's cell rosetting with EA *in vitro*.

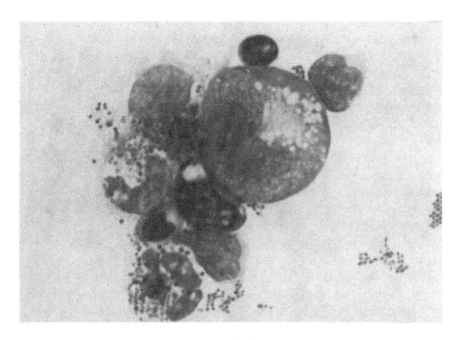

Figure 16. In vitro phagocytosis of opsonized *Staphylococci* by normal macrophages but not R–S cell which contains only numerous cytoplasmic vacuoles.

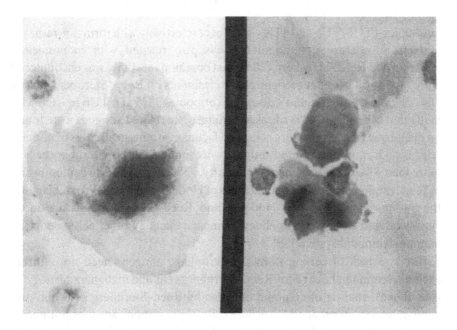

Figure 17. R–S cell (left) and interdigitating reticulum cell (right) with similar paranuclear focal staining for alpha naphthyl acetate esterase.

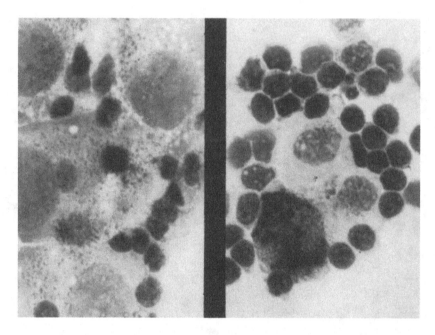

Figure 18. Increased amounts of acid phosphatase granules in R–S cell (left) after one week in tissue culture. At right for comparison, heavier staining of histiocyte but only weak staining of inter-digitating reticulum cells.

antibodies – TU5, TU6 and TU9 – that react selectively with formalin-resistant antigens of mature granulopoietic cells also reacted with mononuclear Hodgkin and Reed–Sternberg cells. Most common reactivity was encountered with antibody TU9, that recognized determinants on Reed–Sternberg cells in 76% of 75 cases of Hodgkin's disease. Antibodies TU5 and TU6 reacted with malignant cells in only 47% of cases. Granulocyte related antigens were found on diagnostic Reed–Sternberg cells, and lacunar variants in all cases of nodular sclerosis. Granulocyte-related antigens were found on Reed–Sternberg cells in more than 90% of cases of mixed cellularity, 75% of lymphocyte depletion and 38% of lymphocyte predominance types of Hodgkin's disease. From this study the authors concluded that Hodgkin and Reed–Sternberg cells are more closely related to cells of granulocytic-lineage than any other cell type in the hemato–lymphoid system [79].

Just as a lack of certain normal macrophage antigens need not entirely exclude a common lineage for Reed–Sternberg cells and malignant histiocytes (see above), sharing of common antigens by Reed–Sternberg cells and myeloid–monocytoid progenitors or late cells of granulopoiesis does not necessarily indicate a myeloid origin for Reed–Sternberg cells. Since Reed–Sternberg cells have no obvious morphological or cytochemical characteristics of myeloid cells, and the bone marrow is clinically involved in less than 10% of patients at the onset of Hodgkin's disease, the derivation of Reed–Sternberg cells from myeloid cells seems unlikely.

4.5. Dendritic reticulum cell

Using the Marshall metalophil method, Curran and Jones demonstrated large and pleomorphic dendritic cells throughout lesions of Hodgkin's disease [80]. The distribution, size and number of metalophil dendritic cells coincided with that of Hodgkin and Reed–Sternberg cells in adjacent sections stained with hematoxylin and eosin. Many dendritic cells had nuclei and nucleoli of Reed–Sternberg cells. However, some of the largest Reed–Sternberg cells seemed to lack a dendritic structure and showed no evidence of metalophilia. Normal dendritic cells occur mainly within the mantle zone and subjacent germinal center zone of lymphoid follicles. Halie *et al.* noted a close relationship of

Table 4. Theories/evidence for and against derivation of the Reed–Sternberg cell from a dendritic-/interdigitating reticulum cell.

Authors	Year [Ref.]	Theory/Evidence
Curran & Jones	1978 [80]	Population of metalophile dendritic cells in lymphoid follicles correspond in numbers, size, and distribution to Reed–Sternberg cells of Hodgkin's disease
Halie *et al.*	1978 [81]	Small Hodgkin foci in spleen corresponds to distribution of antigen trapping cells in follicles and periarteriolar lymphocyte sheath
Baldwin & Cohen	1981 [82]	Reed–Sternberg cells resemble primitive dendritic cells in spleen of *Xenopus laevis* frogs
Hansmann & Kaiserling	1981 [83]	Lacunar cells of nodular sclerosis have ultrastructure similar to interdigitating reticulum cells
Poppema *et al.*	1982 [94]	Reed–Sternberg cells have Ia-like antigens and are surrounded by helper T4 lymphocytes similar to interdigitating reticulum cells
Kadin	1982 [84]	Reed–Sternberg cells and interdigitating cells have similar cytology, cytochemistry and surface characteristics
Beckstead *et al.*	1982 [68]	Reed–Sternberg and interdigitating reticulum cells have similar focal paranuclear staining for acid phosphatase and nonspecific esterase
Schwab *et al.*	1982 [96]	Antibody against L428 Hodgkin cell line does not react with dendritic or interdigitating reticulum cells
Watanabe *et al.*	1983 [87]	Reed–Sternberg cells lack S100 protein of interdigitating cells

Reed–Sternberg cells to follicular B-cell regions in small focal lesions of Hodgkin's disease within the spleen [81].

Baldwin and Cohen found a possible analogue for Reed–Sternberg cells and human dendritic cells within the spleen of normal *Xenopus laevus* frogs [82]. In the white pulp of the spleen of these frogs are large, mitotically active cells with abundant clear cytoplasm, large hyperlobated nuclei and prominent nucleoli. These Reed–Sternberg-like cells extend long cytoplasmic processes into the red pulp trapping foreign material including IgG. This cell which most likely represents a primitive dendritic cell may be used to study the phylogenetic origin of dendritic cells and the origin and function of Reed–Sternberg cells in Hodgkin's disease.

4.6. Interdigitating reticulum cells

Hansmann and Kaiserling described lacunar cells with bizarrely shaped nuclei and cytoplasmic structures resembling the tubulovescicular system of inter-digitating cells in cases of nodular sclerosis and some cases of mixed cellularity Hodgkin's disease [83]. Similar to Reed–Sternberg cells, interdigitating cells (IDC) have weaker receptors for the Fc portion of IgG than do histiocytes [84]. The possible relationship between lacunar cells and interdigitating cells was first discussed by Lennert [85] and Kadin [21].

Interdigitating cells occur exclusively in the thymus and thymic dependent regions of human lymphoid tissue [86], where the earliest focal lesions of Hodkin's disease are found [1, 17], (Fig. 19). Here they make close contact with other IDC and neighboring T lymphocytes to which they are thought to present antigen. We compared Reed–Sternberg cells with IDC recovered from dermatopathic lymph nodes. Both Reed–Sternberg cells and IDC showed strong expression of HLA-DR (Ia-like antigens), maintained close physical contact with helper-inducer T cells *in vitro,* and lacked several normal macrophage antigens [48]. Poppema *et al.* demonstrated similar findings for Reed–Sternberg cells and IDC *in situ* in frozen sections of lymph node and spleen [49]. Other similarities between Reed–Sternberg cells and IDC are their lack of lymphoid and myeloid characteristics, smaller content of acid phosphatase and nonspecific esterase than that of histiocytes, and similar bizarre nuclear morphology with peripheral condensed heterochromatin [48, 86]. However, Reed–Sternberg cells seem to lack membrane ATPase [48] and S100 protein [87] characteristic of IDC. We postulated that some abnormalities of cell mediated immunity in Hodgkin's disease could be due to abnormal antigen presentation by Reed–Sternberg cells which had undergone malignant transformation from IDC.

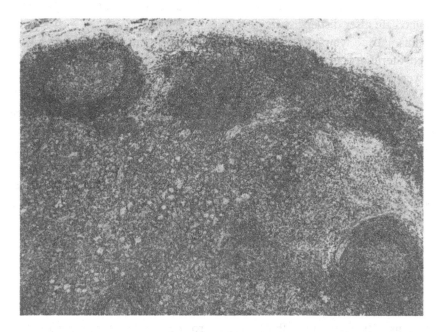

Figure 19. Early focal lesion of Hodgkin's disease in thymic dependent region of lymph node with preserved germinal centers.

4.7. Murine lymphoid dendritic cell

Steinman and Cohn described a lymphoid dendritic cell in the spleen of mice that they considered to be analogous to the human IDC [88]. This murine lymphoid dendritic cell (MLDC) is distinguished from other cells by its unusual spiny surface projections, irregular adherence to glass and a bizarre angular nucleus with marginated heterochromatin. The MLDC lacks surface immunoglobulin, T cell antigens, receptors for complement or the Fc portion of IgG, and can be further distinguished from macrophages by its lack of murine macrophage antigens Mac 1 and F4/80 [89]. MLDC appear more sensitive than macrophages to low doses of steroids and radiation [90]. They have a more rapid cell turnover than macrophages and appear to originate from nonadherent cells in the bone marrow and red pulp of the spleen [90]. Their strong expression of Ia-antigens is a constituitive trait that does not vary with the immunological state of the host, and is retained in mice raised in a pathogen-free environment [88]. Because of their high content of Ia-antigens, MLDC are potent stimulators of the mixed leukocyte culture reaction (MLC) [91]. In contrast macrophage subpopulations typically vary in their expression of Ia-antigens and are weaker stimulators of the MLC. MLDC appear to function as essential accessory cells for T cell responses *in vitro*. Close cell contact is a prerequisite and clusters of dendritic cells and T-lymphocytes reaggregate after dispersion *in vitro* [92].

Thus murine lymphoid dendritic cells share a number of properties with Reed–Sternberg cells and IDC (Table 5). There are also important differences between these cells. IDC have surface membrane Mg^{2+} dependent ATPase [93] that was not detected on Reed–Sternberg cells [48] or MLDC [88]. The Fc Receptors of IDC are weak [84], are often not detected on Reed–Sternberg cells [54, 94], and are never found on MLDC [88]. Moreover MLDC can be found in Peyer's patches of the gut [88] where Hodgkin's disease is rarely found at initial diagnosis [17, 95].

It remains to be studied whether the murine lymphoid dendritic cell corresponds to a unique unidentified cell type that should be considered as a candidate for precursor of the Reed–Sternberg cell (see below).

4.8. Unidentified cell type

Two neoplastic cell lines with unique features were established from pleural effusions of two patients with nodular sclerosing type Hodgkin's disease [13]. Both cell lines were determined to be neoplastic on the basis of structural and numerical chromosome abnormalities with a monoclonal pattern of marker

Table 5. Comparison of MLDC[a], IDC[b] and R-S cell.

Property	MLDC	IDC	R-S
T-cell region	+	+	+
Irregular nucleus	+	+	+
Cytoplasmic processes	+	+	+
NSE, Ac PHOS	weak	weak	weak
5′ nucleotidase	−	−	−
Mg^{2+} ATPase	−	+	−
FC–C_3 receptors	−	+	+
Endocytosis			
Lymphocyte Ag	−	−	−
Ig, Thy-1			
Mac antigens	−	−	−
Mac 1 (20.2)			
F4/80 (20.3)			
Ia-antigens	+ +	+ +	+
T-cell adherence	+	+	+
Bone marrow origin	+	?	?

[a] MLDC = Murine lymphoid dendritic cell.
[b] IDC = Interdigitating reticulum cell.

chromosomes; heterotransplantability to the brain of nude mice; and lack of Epstein Barr virus specific antigens that characterize most non-neoplastic B lymphoblastoid cell lines. Both Hodgkin's cell lines lacked surface and cytoplasmic Ig, T cell differentiation antigens, receptors for C_3b, C_3d, IgGFc, for mouse or sheep erythrocytes and had no detectable lysozyme, myeloperoxidase or chloracetate esterase. Each Hodgkin's cell line had Ia-like antigens, surface receptors for T cells and small amounts of staining for acid phosphatase and non-specific esterase. These latter characteristics correspond closely to those of non-cultured Reed–Sternberg cells.

A conventional rabbit antiserum was raised against the cell line L428 [62]. This antiserum seemed to show selective reactivity with at least two distinct nuclear and cytoplasmic antigens of mononuclear Hodgkin and Reed–Sternberg cells. However, the antiserum did not appear to react with any normal cells and therefore did not shed light on the origin of the malignant cell in Hodgkin's disease.

Recently a hybridoma monoclonal antibody (Ki-1) raised against cell line L428 was found to be specific for Hodgkin and Reed–Sternberg cells, and a small previously unrecognized population of cells in normal tonsils and lymph nodes [96]. A few scattered Ki-1 positive cells were also found among hematopoietic cells in the bone marrow. The detection of Ki-1 antigen on these normal cells suggests that it is a normal differentiation antigen, instead of a viral or tumor-specific antigen [96].

The small population of normal Ki-1 positive cells could be detected only with a highly sensitive three-layer immunoperoxidase labelling technique. Ki-1 positive cells were located mainly between, around and within B-cell follicles. They had a prominent single nucleolus and large amount of antibody-stained cytoplasm. Ki-1 positive cells were found to be more numerous in the parafollicular regions of lymph nodes affected by Piringers (Toxoplasma) lymphadenitis (96).

At the time of this writing, the normal cell equivalent for the Ki-1 positive cell has not been identified. However, the anti Ki-1 antibody does not appear to react with any of the other previously mentioned cell types i.e., it does not appear to react with normal T or B lymphocytes, macrophages, dendritic or interdigitating reticulum cells. The Ki-1 positive cells could represent a progenitor to one or more of these mature human cell types, and as an immature precursor cell could lack some of their mature cell surface characteristics. Ki-1 positive cells could also correspond to the previously described dendritic cells of the frog [82] or mouse [88], which appear to be necessary for normal processing or presentation of antigen to lymphocytes. Alternatively Ki-1 positive cells may be a unique-human cell type whose function remains to be determined.

5. Biologic activities of Hodgkin and Reed-Sternberg cells

The foregoing discussion devoted little attention to biological properties of Reed–Sternberg cells that might help to determine the nature of these cells and explain some of the clinical characteristics of Hodgkin's disease. The following section deals with biological assays that have been used to examine the function of Hodgkin and Reed–Sternberg cells *in vitro*.

5.1. Effect of Hodgkin's cell line conditioned media on granulopoiesis

Cell culture conditioned media of L428 cells were found to have a stimulatory effect on *in vitro* myelopoiesis [78]. Conditioned media of the original cell line L428 contained significant amounts of granulocyte colony stimulating factor (CFU-C). More potent CFU-C activity was derived from supernatants of adherent Hodgkin's cell line L428 KSA, derived by exposure of calf-serum adopted L428 cells (L428 KS) to the phorbol ester TPA. More than 85% of colonies stimulated by L428-KSA conditioned medium contained Sudan black-positive granulocytic cells. Eosinophilic CSF activity was also present, but in lower concentrations. No stimulation of erythropoiesis or macrophage colony formation was detected.

5.2. Effect of Hodgkin cell line conditioned media on spontaneous cell-mediated cytolysis

To examine the phenomenon of immune deficiency in HD, Diehl *et al.* tested L428-KSA–conditioned media for a factor that might suppress cell-mediated immune reactions [78]. They tested spontaneous cell mediated cytotoxic activity of lymphocytes from healthy donors against L428-KS and K562 target cells, with and without the addition of L428–KSA conditioned medium. In comparison to untreated cells, there was a significant ($p = 0.005$) decrease of cytolysis of both target cells after treatment of effector lymphocytes with L428-KSA conditioned medium.

5.3. Monokines–fibroblast and lymphocyte growth factors (Interleukin 1) from Hodgkin's disease cell cultures

Newcom and O'Rourke found that both serum-containing and serum-free media conditioned by short-term cell cultures from 8 lymph nodes replaced by nodular sclerosing Hodgkin's disease produced factor(s) that potentiated fibroblast growth *in vitro* [97]. Increased mitotic rate and transformation (lack of contact inhibition) of Balb/c 3T3 cells, human diploid fibroblasts and human embryonic fibroblasts were observed following stimulation with Hodgkin's disease culture supernatants. Selective removal of cells comprising the Hodgkin's disease cell suspension showed that the effect was most potent when there was enrichment for Hodgkin giant cells and the effect was not reduced by depletion of lymphocytes or fibroblasts. Removal of normal macrophages decreased but did not eliminate the proliferative activity or non-adherent growth of 3T3 cells in agar. A similar stimulation of fibroblast growth was not derived from supernates of a mixed cellularity Hodgkin's disease lymph node or a variety of non-Hodgkin's lymphomas, suggesting that this feature is relatively specific for nodular sclerosing Hodgkin's disease.

Ford *et al.* established autologous fibroblast cultures from tumor nodules of spleens removed at staging laparotomy for nodular sclerosing Hodgkin's disease. The fibroblast cultures became quiescent in serum-starved media but were restimulated to proliferation, measured quantitatively by tritiated-thymidine incorporation, following incubation with dialyzed supernatants from 24-h Hodgkin cell cultures. The fibroblast growth factor was released spontaneously but its production was enhanced by stimulation of Hodgkin's disease cells with lipopolysaccharide [98].

Hodgkin's disease adherent cell conditioned media was also measured for Interleukin 1 activity in a murine thymocyte proliferation assay. Twenty-four hour Hodgkin's disease culture supernates containing 5% fetal calf serum were dialyzed against balanced salt solution and then assayed for their effect on mouse thymocyte populations in the presence of Concanavalin A. These assays showed an IL-1-like stimulatory effect of the Hodgkin's cell culture conditioned media as measured by mouse thymocyte tritiated thymidine incorporation [98].

In other preliminary experiments, IL-1 activity appeared to be a product of non-malignant macrophages in Hodgkin's disease cell cultures [99].

5.4. In vitro studies of antigen presentation by Hodgkin cell cultures

Because of the possible derivation of the Reed–Sternberg cell from an antigen-presenting cell, it would be attractive to learn whether cultured Hodgkin's cells are capable of presenting antigen to T-cells for proliferation. Preliminary experiments conducted in my laboratory with collaborators at the Fred Hutchinson Cancer Center show that mixture of L428 cells with appropriately HLA-DR matched T-cells from peripheral blood leads to presentation of antigen poly(glutamic acid-alanine-tyrosine) (GAT) for specific proliferation in a secondary response *in vitro*; this proliferation is inhibited in the presence of a monoclonal anti-Ia antibody, indicating that the APC cell function provided by L428 operates along normal HLA-regulated pathways [100].

6. Significance of the Reed–Sternberg cell in the future control of Hodgkin's disease

Criteria used to identify and determine the nature of the Reed–Sternberg cell could also have a significant favorable impact on the future control of Hodgkin's disease. These criteria could be used for the more accurate diagnosis and staging of Hodgkin's disease, to determine whether Hodgkin's disease is one or more distinct disease entities, and to uncover the nature of the immune defect in Hodgkin's disease.

6.1. Histopathologic diagnosis and staging of Hodgkin's disease

Review of initial diagnostic material by a panel of expert hematopathologists revealed 13% of mistaken diagnoses of Hodgkin's disease among a group of 289 cases registered as Hodgkin's disease by the Southwest Oncology Group (101). Mixed cellularity and lymphocyte depletion were the most frequently mistaken histologic types and nodular sclerosis the least frequently mistaken type. Most incorrect diagnoses of Hodgkin's disease were actually large cell lymphomas with pleomorphic features. Less commonly confused with Hodgkin's disease were angioimmunoblastic lymphadenopathy and Lennert's lymphoma. Uncommon clinical presentations, especially presentation at unusual extra-nodal sites, were found to be clues to a possible mistaken diagnosis of Hodgkin's disease.

A variety of benign disorders with Reed–Sternberg-like cells commonly have been mistaken for Hodgkin's disease. Specific entities easily confused with Hodgkin's disease include infectious mononucleosis, herpes viral infections, toxoplasma and hydantoin-induced lymphadenopathies [102].

Staging of Hodgkin's disease is influenced by the morphological criteria for organ involvement. In a patient with an established diagnosis of Hodgkin's disease, atypical mononuclear cells with prominent nucleoli or other variants of Reed-Sternberg cells are often accepted as evidence of involvement of liver and bone marrow, especially in the setting of unexplained marrow fibrosis [1, 102]. Isolated sarcoid-like granulomas must not be mistaken for Hodgkin's disease in the liver, bone marrow or spleen [33, 102, 103]. Evidence that such granulomas do not indicate organ involvement by Hodgkin's disease was found by the lack of any relationship between location of granulomas and sites of subsequent relapse in 55 patients with Hodgkin's disease and associated granulomas [104]. Early focal involvement of spleen and abdominal lymph nodes are other difficult diagnostic problems in the pathologic staging of Hodgkin's disease. Immunological criteria for Reed–Sternberg cells would provide more objectivity for the histologic diagnosis of Hodgkin's disease in these difficult circumstances.

Much debate has surrounded the need for surgical staging of Hodgkin's disease [105, 107]. It would be a great advantage to have a non-invasive method to identify high risk patients with hematogenous spread of Hodgkin's disease. Blood vessel invasion has been proposed as histological evidence of hematogenous spread in unfavorable histologic types of Hodgkin's disease [108–109] (Fig. 20). However, this feature may not be detected in carefully studied patients who develop extra-nodal dissemination of their disease [110]. In addition, Reed–Sternberg cells are recognized only rarely in the blood of patients with Hodgkin's disease [111] and can be difficult to distinguish from transformed lymphocytes in patients with viral infections [112–113]. It may become possible to achieve a more accurate and sensitive detection of blood-borne malignant cells when specific immunologic criteria for the Reed–Sternberg cell are developed. Ideally patients who lack this high risk characteristic can receive more limited therapy and avoid second malignancies

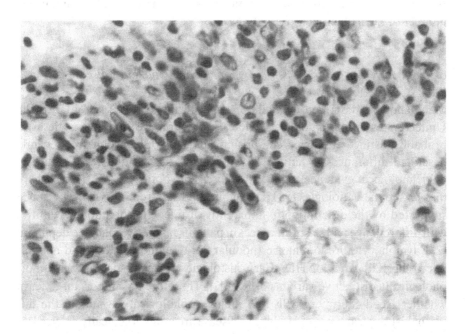

Figure 20. Hodgkin's cell with large nucleolus entering vascular lumen (center) and another in vessel wall at upper left. Vascular invasion is a possible source of hematogenous spread of Hodgkin's disease.

and other sequelae of aggressive combined drug and radiotherapy for treatment of Hodgkin's disease [114–117].

6.2. Immune defects of Hodgkin's disease

Virtually all patients with Hodgkin's disease, including those with apparent localized involvement, suffer from a selective, often subtle impairment of cell mediated immunity [118]. This defect is expressed clinically as an increased susceptibility to certain types of bacterial, fungal and viral infections [119]. Previous laboratory studies have focused on peripheral manifestations of the cellular immune defect such as cutaneous anergy [120–123], decreased lymphocyte responsiveness to mitogen or antigen [124–129], abnormal numbers and composition of peripheral T cell subsets [44, 129–131].

None of these studies have examined the possible central role of the Reed–Sternberg cell as a source of the immune defect in Hodgkin's disease. The availability of Hodgkin's disease cell lines makes it possible to test the hypothesis that Reed–Sternberg cells are abnormal antigen presenting cells. If Hodgkin's cells are shown to have this function, it will be important to learn whether impairment of cell mediated immunity in Hodgkin's disease can be related to abnormal antigen presentation by Hodgkin's cells or to a diminished number of normal antigen-presenting cells.

6.3. Single versus multiple disease hypothesis for Hodgkin's disease

MacMahon has described a bimodal age-specific incidence curve for HD in the United States as epidemiological evidence for 2 or more separate entities with probably distinct etiologies comprising HD [18]. Gutensohn has recently described differences in patient age and social class at diagnosis as further epidemiological evidence for the 'two-disease hypothesis' [28]. Hence there may be separate etiologies for HD in adults and children. This concept can be supported by the description of apparently distinct clinicopathologic entities with different age and sex preferences in patients having lymphocyte depletion [29], lymphocyte predominance (nodular paragranuloma) [16], and nodular sclerosing [30] types of HD. Each histologic type is associated with morphologically distinctive variants of RSC [1]. Therefore it is important to learn whether Reed–Sternberg cells and their morphological variants in the different histological types of Hodgkin's disease are immunologically diverse [15, 79], or identical [96]. Any differences detected can provide clues for additional studies of the epidemiology and etiology of Hodgkin's disease.

7. Conclusion

This writing takes place at a very exciting time when promising new research is being done on the nature of the Reed–Sternberg cell. The development of new cell lines, including L428, by Diehl and co-workers [13, 14] in Germany can be a great breakthrough, if the derivation of cultured cells from neoplastic cells of Hodgkin's disease can be confirmed. The immunologic identity of cultured and non-cultured Reed–Sternberg cells is supported by the specific reactivity of Ki-1 monoclonal antibody, raised against L428 cells, with Reed–Sternberg cells in tissue sections of Hodgkin's disease [96]. Since L428 cells are derived from nodular sclerosing Hodgkin's disease, a specific subtype of Hodgkin's disease, it will be important to determine whether observations made with Ki-1 antibody apply equally well to other types of Hodgkin's disease, as suggested by the initial results [96]. The Ki-1 positive cells in normal lymphoid tissues appear to be mononuclear cells located in close relationship to the follicular mantle zone of lymph nodes and tonsils. Interestingly, the tonsil is rarely a primary site of Hodgkin's disease [95].

Functional studies offer an alternative method of studying Hodgkin's cells with possible relevance to the clinical manifestations of the disease. The function of the Ki-1 positive cell is unknown. However L428 cell conditioned media supports *in vitro* granulopoiesis and suppresses spontaneous cell-mediated cytotoxicity. The secretion of lymphocyte and fibroblast growth factors by Hodgkin's cells is currently being investigated. Our own investigation links the Reed–Sternberg cell to an antigen-presenting cell, and studies are now being done to test the capacity of L428 cells to present antigen(s) to HLA-DR matched T cells *in vitro*. Evidence linking the Reed–Sternberg cell to an antigen-presenting cell could be relevant to the well known defect in cell mediated immunity in Hodgkin's disease.

8. Summary

The Reed–Sternberg cell has gained general acceptance as representing the malignant cell in Hodgkin's disease. The frequency of diagnostic Reed–Sternberg cells and morphological variants differ in the several histological types of Hodgkin's disease. Interpretations of the nature and origin of the Reed–Sternberg cell have been influenced by the methods used to identify and study these cells. Tissue culture and immunological studies offer the advantage of overcoming the cellular heterogeneity of Hodgkin's lesions. Evidence is reviewed for and against the derivation of Reed–Sternberg cells from T and B lymphocytes, macrophages, dendritic and interdigitating reticulum cells. Laboratory animal models of Reed–Sternberg cells are discussed. A previously unrecognized cell type may be the progenitor of the Reed–Sternberg cell, if recent cell lines are confirmed as being derived from neoplastic cells of Hodgkin's disease. Monoclonal antibodies against these cells can be used for more accurate diagnosis and staging of Hodgkin's disease. Functional studies of Hodgkin and Reed–Sternberg cells can provide knowledge to better understand the nature of the malignant cell and immune defect in Hodgkin's disease. Improved survival and decreased morbidity from Hodgkin's disease are expected from a better understanding of the enigma of the Reed–Sternberg cell.

References

1. Lukes RJ: Criteria for involvement of lymph node, bone marrow, spleen, and liver in Hodgkin's disease. Cancer Res 31:1755–1767, 1972.
2. Rappaport H: Tumors of the hematopoietic system. Atlas of Tumor Pathology, Section III, Fascicle 8, Armed Forces Institute of Pathology, Washington D.C., 2966.
3. Berard CW, Thomas LB, Axtell LM, Kruse M, Newell G, Kagan R: The relationship of histopathological subtype to clinical stage of Hodgkin's disease at diagnosis. Cancer Res 31:1776–1785, 1971.
4. Strum SB, Rappaport H: Interrelations of the histologic types of Hodgkin's disease. Arch Pathol 91:127–134, 1971.
5. Lukes RJ, Butler JJ, Hicks EB: Natural history of Hodgkin's disease as related to its pathologic picture. Cancer 19:317–344, 1966.
6. Seif GSF, Spriggs AI: Chromosome changes in Hodgkin's disease. J Nat Cancer Inst 39:557–570, 1967.
7. Peckham MJ, Cooper EH: Proliferation characteristics of the various classes of cells in Hodgkin's disease. Cancer 24:135–146, 1969.
8. Peckham MJ, Cooper EH: Cell proliferation in Hodgkin's disease. Nat Cancer Inst Monogr 36:179–189, 1973.
9. Meyer JS, Higa E: S-Phase fractions of cells in lymph nodes and malignant lymphomas. Arch Pathol Lab Med 103:93–97, 1979.
10. Kadin ME: *In vitro* study of multinucleated cells in Hodgkin's disease. Nat Cancer Inst Monogr 36:211–217, 1973.
11. Kadin ME, Asbury AK: Long term cultures of Hodgkin's tissue. A morphologic and radioautographic study. Lab Invest 28:181–184, 1973.
12. Kaplan HS, Gartner S: 'Sternberg-Reed' giant cells of Hodgkin's disease: cultivation *in vitro*, heterotransplantation, and characterization as neoplastic macrophages. Int J Cancer 19:511–525, 1977.
13. Schaadt M, Diehl V, Stein H, Fonatsch C, Kirchner HH: Two neoplastic cell lines with unique features derived from Hodgkin's disease. Int J Cancer 26:723–731, 1980.
14. Diehl V, Kirchner HH, Schaadt M, Fonatsch C, Stein H, Gerdes J, Boie C: Hodgkin's disease: establishment and characterization of four *in vitro* cell lines. J Cancer Res Clin Oncol 101:111–124, 1981.
15. Poppema S, Kaiserling E, Lennert K: Hodgkin's disease with lymphocytic predominance, nodular type (nodular paragranuloma) and progressively transformed germinal centres. A cytohistological study. Histopathol 3:295–308, 1979.
16. Poppema S, Kaiserling E, Lennert K: Epidemiology of nodular paragranuloma (Hodgkin's disease with lymphocytic predominance, nodular). Cancer Res Clin Oncol 95:57, 1979.

17. Kadin ME, Glatstein E, Dorfman RF: Clinicopathologic studies of 117 untreated patients subjected to laparotomy for the staging of Hodgkin's disease. Cancer 27:1277–1294, 1971.

18. MacMahon B, Cole P, Newell GR: Hodgkin's disease: One entity or two? Lancet 1:240–241, 1971.

19. Smithers DW: Hodgkin's disease: one entity or two? Lancet 2:1285–1288, 1970.

20. Peiper SC, Kahn LB, Ross DW, Reddick RL: Ultrastructural organization of the Reed–Sternberg cell: its resemblance to cells of the monocyte-macrophage system. Blood Cells 6:515, 1980.

21. Kadin ME: A reappraisal of the Reed–Sternberg cell. A commentary. Blood cells 6:525, 1980.

22. Kay MMB, Kadin M: Surface characteristics of Hodgkin's cells. Lancet 1:748, 1975.

23. Kadin ME: Surface characteristics of Hodgkin's cells. Lancet 1:1088, 1975.

24. Kay MMB: Surface characteristics of Hodgkin's cells. Lancet 2:459, 1975.

25. Metzgar RS, Borowitz MJ, Jones NH, Dowell BL: Distribution of common acute lymphoblastic leukemia antigen in nonhematopoietic tissues. J Exp Med 254:1249–54, 1981.

26. Murphy GR, Bhan AK, Sato S, Harrist TJ, Mihm MC: Characterization of Langerhans cells by use of monoclonal antibodies. Lab Invest 45:465–468, 1981.

27. Reinherz EL, Kung PC, Goldstein G, Levey RH, Schlossman SF: Discrete stages of human intrathymic differentiation: Analysis of normal thymocytes and leukemic lymphoblasts of T cell lineage. Proc Natl Acad Sci USA 77:1588–1592, 1980.

28. Gutensohn NM: Social class and age at diagnosis of Hodgkin's disease: new epidemiologic evidence for the 'two-disease' hypothesis. Cancer Treat Rep 66:689–695, 1982.

29. Neiman RS, Rosen PJ, Lukes RJ: Lymphocyte-depletion Hodgkin's disease. A clinicopathologic entity. N Engl J Med 288:751–755, 1973.

30. Hanson TAS: Histological classification and survival in Hodgkin's disease. A study of 251 cases with special reference to nodular sclerosing Hodgkin's disease. Cancer 17:1595–1603, 1964.

31. Tindle BH, Parker JW, Lukes RJ: 'Reed–Sternberg cells' in infectious mononucleosis? Am J Clin Pathol 58:607–617, 1972.

32. Anagnostou D, Parker JW, Taylor CR, Tindle BH, Lukes RJ: Lacunar cells of nodular sclerosing Hodgkin's disease. Cancer 39:1032–1043, 1977.

33. Glick AD, Leech JH, Flexner JM, Collins RD: Ultrastructural study of Reed–Sternberg cells. Comparison with transformed lymphocytes and histiocytes. Am J Pathol 85:195–208, 1976.

34. Hanaoka M: Clinical pathology of adult T cell leukemia. Acta Haematol Jpn 44:1420–1430, 1981.

35. Kikuchi M, Mitsui T, Matsui N et al.: T-cell malignancies in adults. Histopathological studies of lymph nodes in 110 patients. Jpn J Clin Oncol 9 (Suppl 1) 407–422, 1979.

36. Dorfman RF, Rice DF, Mitchell AD, Kempson RL, Levine G: Ultrastructural studies of Hodgkin's disease. Nat Cancer Inst Monogr 36:221–238, 1973.

37. Thomson AD: The thymic origin of Hodgkin's disease. Br J Cancer 9:37–50, 1955.

38. Marshall AHE, Wood C: The involvement of the thymus in Hodgkin's disease. J Path Bact 73:163–166, 1957.

39. Keller AR, Castleman B: Hodgkin's disease of the thymus gland. Cancer 33:1615–1623, 1974.

40. Order SE, Hellman S: pathogenesis of Hodgkin's disease. Lancet 1:571–573, 1972.

41. De Vita VT: Lymphocyte reactivity in Hodgkin's disease: a lymphocyte civil war. New Engl J Med 289:801–802, 1973.

42. Aisenberg AC: Studies on delayed hypersensitivity in Hodgkin's disease. J Clin Invest 41:1964–1970, 1962.

43. Levy R, Kaplan HS: Impaired lymphocyte function in untreated Hodgkin's disease. N Engl J Med 290:181–186, 1974.

44. Schulof RS, Bockman RS, Garofalo JA, Cirrincione C, Cunningham-Rundles S, Fernandes G, Day NK, Pinsky CM, Incefy GS, Thaler HT, Good RA, Gupta S: Multivariate analysis of T-cell functional defects and circulating serum factors in Hodgkin's disease. Cancer 48:964–973, 1981.

45. Twomey JJ, Laughter AH, Farrow S, Douglass CC: Hodgkin's disease. An immunodepleting and immunosuppressive disorder. J Clin Invest 56:467–475, 1975.

46. Kadin ME, Newcom SR, Gold SB, Stites DP: Origin of Hodgkin's cells. Lancet 11:167–168, 1974.

47. Pinkus GS, Hargreaves HK, McLeod JA, Nadler LM, Rosenthal DS, Said JW: Naphthyl acetate esterase activity – A cytochemical marker for T lymphocytes. Am J Pathol 97:17–42, 1979.

48. Kadin ME: Possible origin of the Reed–Sternberg cell from an interdigitating reticulum cell. Cancer Treat Rep 66:601–608, 1982.

49. Poppema S, Bhan AK, Reinherz EL, Posner MR, Schlossman SF: In situ characterization of cellular constituents in lymph nodes and spleens involved by Hodgkin's disease. Blood 59:226–232, 1982.

50. Leech J: Immunoglobulin-positive Reed–Sternberg cells in Hodgkin's disease. Lancet 1:265–266, 1973.

51. Garvin AJ, Spicer SS, Parmley RT, Munster AM: Immunohistochemical demonstration of IgG in Reed–Sternberg and other cells in Hodgkin's disease. J Exp Med 139:1077–1083, 1974.

52. Taylor CR: An immunohistological study of follicular lymphoma, reticulum cell sarcoma and Hodgkin's disease. Eur J Cancer 12:61–75, 1976.

53. Landaas TO, Godal T, Halvorsen TB: Characterization of immunoglobulins in Hodgkin cells. Int J Cancer 20:717–722, 1977.

54. Kadin ME, Stites DP, Levy R, Warnke R: Exogenous origin of immunoglobulin in Reed–Sternberg cells of Hodgkin's disease. N Engl J Med 299:1208–1214, 1978.

55. Levy R, Warnke R, Dorfman RF, Haimovich J: The monoclonality of human B cell lymphomas. J Exp Med 145:1014–1028, 1977.

56. Bernau D, Feldman G, Vorhauer W: Hodgkin's disease: ultrastructural localization of intracytoplasmic immunoglobulins within malignant cells. Br J Haemat 40:51–57, 1978.

57. Issaacson P: Immunochemical demonstration of J chain: A marker of B-cell malignancy. J Clin Path 32:802–807, 1979.

58. Poppema S, Elema JD, Halie MR: The significance of intracytoplasmic proteins in Reed–Sternberg cells. Cancer 42:1793–1803, 1978.

59. Papadimitriou CS, Stein H, Lennert K: The complexity of immunohistochemical staining pattern of Hodgkin and Sternberg–Reed cells – demonstration of immunoglobulin, albumin, -antichymotrypsin and lysozyme. Int J Cancer 21:531–541, 1978.

60. Dorsett BH, Ioachim HL, Stolbach L, Walker J, Barber HRK: Isolation of tumor-specific antibodies from effusions of ovarian carcinomas . Int J Cancer 16:779–786, 1975.

61. Gerstl B, Eng LR, Bigbee JW: Tumor-associated immunoglobulins in pulmonary carcinoma. Cancer Res 37:4449–4455, 1977.

62. Stein H, Gerdes J, Kirchner H, Diehl V, Schaadt M, Bonk A, Steffen T: Immunohistological analysis of Hodgkin's and Sternberg–Reed Cells: Detection of a new antigen and evidence for selective IgG uptake in the absence of B cell, T cell and histiocytic markers. J Cancer Res Clin Oncol 101:125–134, 1981.

63. Poppema S, Kaiserling E, Lennert K: Nodular paragranuloma and progressively transformed germinal centers. Ultrastructural and immunohistologic findings. Virchows Arch [Cell Pathol] 31:211–225, 1979.

64. Dorfman RF: Enzyme histochemistry of the cells in Hodgkin's disease and allied disorders. Nature 207:606–608, 1961.
65. Carr I: The ultrastructure of the abnormal reticulum cells in Hodgkin's disease. J Pathol 115:45–50, 1975.
66. Peiper SC, Kahn LB, Ross DW, Reddick RR: Ultrastructural characterization of Reed–Sternberg cell as a monocyte-macrophage. Blood Cells 6:515–523, 1980.
67. Parmley RT, Spicer SS, Morgan SK, Grush OC: Hodgkin's disease and myelomonocytic leukemia. An ultrastructural and immunocytochemical study. Cancer 38:1188–1198, 1976.
68. Beckstead JH, Warnke R, Bainton DF: Histochemistry of Hodgkin's disease. Cancer Treat Rep 66:609–613, 1982.
69. Poppema S, Elema JD, Halie MR: The localization of Hodgkin's disease in lymph nodes. A study with immunohistological, enzyme histochemical and rosetting techniques on frozen sections. Int J Cancer 24:532–540, 1979.
70. Cossman J, Deegan M, Schnitzer B: Complement receptor B lymphocytes in nodular sclerosing Hodgkin's disease. Cancer 39:2166–2173, 1977.
71. Payne SV, Jones DB, Haegert DG, Smith JL, Wright DH: T and B lymphocytes and Reed–Sternberg cells in Hodgkin's disease lymph nodes and spleens. Clin Exp Immunol 24:280–286, 1976.
72. Stuart AE, Williams ARW, Habeshaw JA: Rosetting and ther reactions of the Reed–Sternberg cell. J Pathol 122:81–90, 1977.
73. Jaffe ES, Shevach E, Frank M, Berard C, Green I: The immunological identification of malignant lymphoreticular cells, J Reticuloendothel Soc 15:76a–77a, 1974.
74. Hayhoe FG, Burns F, Cawley JC, Stewart JW: Cytochemical, ultrastructural, and immunological studies of circulating Reed–Sternberg cells. Br J Haematol 38:485–490, 1978.
75. Kadin ME, Holt L, Najfeld V: Malignant histiocytosis: Establishment and characterization of a permanent cell line. Blood 54 (Supplement 1):173a, 1979.
76. Kamoun M, Martin PJ, Kadin ME, Lum LG, Hansen JA: Human monocyte-histiocyte differentiation antigens defined by monoclonal antibodies: identification of two distinct antigens shared by myeloid and erythroid cells. In press Clin Immunol Immunopath 1983.
77. Poppema S: The diversity of the immunohistological staining pattern of Sternberg–Reed cells. J Histochem Cytochem 28:788–791, 1980.
78. Diehl V, Kirschner HH, Burricter H, Stein H, Fonatsch C, Gerdes J, Schaadt M, Heit W, Uchanska-Ziegler B, Ziegler A, Heintz F, Sueno K: Characteristics of Hodgkin's disease-derived cell lines, Cancer Treat Rep 66:615–632, 1982.
79. Stein H, Uchanska-Ziegler B, Gerdes J, Ziegler A, Weinet P: Hodgkin and Steinberg–Reed cells contain antigens specific to late cells of granulopoiesis. Int J Cancer 29:283–290, ab03 1982.
80. Curran RC, Jones EL: Hodgkin's isease: an immunohistochemical and histological study. J Pathol 125:39–51, 1978.
81. Halie MR, Thiadens J, Eibergin R, an den Brock AA: Hodgkin's disease in the spleen. Investigation of Hodgkin foci and areas for the immune response. Virchows Arch [Cell Pathol] 27:39–48, 1978.
82. Baldwin WM, Cohen N: A giant cell with dendritic cell properties in spleens f the anuran amphibian *Xenopus Laevis*. Dev Comp Immunol 5:461–473, 1981.
83. Hansmann ML, Kaiserling E: Electron microscopic aspects of Hodgkin's disease. J Cancer Res Clin Oncol 101:135–148, 1981.
84. Mulle-Hermelink HR, Schwarting H: Functional studies on the histiocytic and interdigitating reticulum cells from human lymphoid tissue. Virchows Arch [Cell Pathol] 37:217–224, 1981.
85. Lennert K, Kaiserling E, Muller-Hermelink HK: Malignant lymphomas: models of differentiation and cooperation of lymphoreticular cells. *In* Differentiation of normal and neoplastic

88

hematopoietic cells, Clarkson B, Marks PA, Till JE (eds). Cold Spring Harbor Laboratory, Cold Spring Harbor Cold Spring Harbor Conferences on Cell Proliferation, vol 5, book B, sect 8, pp 897–913, 1978.

86. Rausch E, Kaiserling E, Goos M: Langerhans cells and interdigitating reticulum cells in the thymus-dependent region in human dermatopathic lymphadenitis. Virchows Arch [Cell Pathol] 25:327–343, 1977.

87. Watanabe S, Hirohasi S, Takashi N, Shimosato: Cytogenesis of Reed–Sternberg cells in Hodgkin's disease, with special reference to histiocytic cell origin. Jpn J Clin Oncol, in press.

88. Steinman RM, Cohn ZA: Identification of a novel cell type in peripheral lymphoid organs of mice I. Morphology, quantitation, tissue distribution. J Exp Med 137:1142–1162, 1973.

89. Nussenzweig MC, Steinman RM, Unkeless JC, et al.: Studies of the cell surface of mouse dendritic cells and other leukocytes. J Exp Med 154:168–187, 1981.

90. Steinman RM, Lustig DS, Cohn ZA: Identification of a novel cell type in peripheral lymphoid organs of mice. III. Functional properties in vivo. J Exp Med 239:1431–1445, 1974.

91. Steinman RM, Witmer MD: Lymphoid dendritic cells are potent stimulators of the primary mixed leukocyte reaction in mice. Proc Natl Acad Sci USA 75:5132–5136, 1978.

92. Steinman RM, Nussenzweig MC: Dendritic cells: features and function. Immunol Rev 53:127–147, 1980.

93. Muller-Hermelink HK: Characterization of the B-cell and T-cell regions of human lymphatic tissue through enzyme histochemical demonstration of ATPase and 5′-nucleotidase activities. Virchows Arch [Cell Pathol] 16:371–378, 1974.

94. Kadin ME, Gold S, Garratty EM, Stites DP: Immunological membrane markers of Hodgkin's cells. In Modern Trends in Human Leukemia II, Neth R, Gallo RC, Mannweiler K, Maloney WC, (eds). Munich, J.F. Lehmanns, 1976, pp 229–236.

95. Kaplan HS: Patterns of anatomic distribution. In Hodgkin's Disease, 2nd ed, Harvard University Press, Cambridge, MA, 1980, pp 280–339.

96. Schwab V, Stein H, Gerdes J, Lambke H, Kirchner H, Schaadt M, Diehl V: Production of a monoclonal antibody specific for Hodgkin and Sternberg–Reed cells of Hodgkin's disease and a subset in normal lymphoid cells. Nature 299:65–67, 1982.

97. Newcom SR, O'Rourke L: Potentiation of fibroblast growth by nodular sclerosing Hodgkin's disease cultures. Blood 60:228–237, 1982.

98. Ford RJ, Mehta S, Davis F, Maizel AL: Growth factors in Hodgkin's disease. Cancer Treat Rep 66:633–638, 1982.

99. Newcom SR, Hendrickson GR, Barker A: The role of interleukin-1 in nodular sclerosing Hodgkin's disease. Blood 60 (Supplement 1):148a, 1982.

100. Nepom B, Kadin ME, Greenberg P, Diehl V, Antonelli P, Nepom GT: Antigen-presenting function in a Hodgkin's disease cell line, submitted for publication.

101. Miller TP, Byrne GE, Jones SE: Mistaken clinical and pathologic diagnoses of Hodgkin's disease: a Southwest Oncology Group study. Cancer Treat Rep 66:645–651, 1982.

102. Dorfman RF, Colby TV: The pathologist's role in management of patients with Hodgkin's disease. Cancer Treat Rep 66:675–680, 1982.

103. Kadin ME, Donaldson SS, Dorfman RF: Isolated granulomas in Hodgkin's disease. N Engl J Med 283:859–861, 1970.

104. Sacks EL, Donaldson SS, Gordon J, et al.: Epithelioid granulomas associated with Hodgkin's disease. Cancer 41:562–567, 1978.

105. Bergsagel DE, Alison RE, Bean HA, Brown TC, Bush RS, Clark RM, Chua T, Dalley D, DeBoer G, Gospodarowicz M, Hasselback R, Perrault D, Rideout DF: Results of treating Hodgkin's disease without a policy of laparotomy staging. Cancer Treat Rep 66:717–731, 1982.

106. Larson RA, Ultmann JE: The strategic role of laparotomy in staging Hodgkin's disease. Cancer Treat Rep 66:767–774, 1982.

107. Hellman S: Current studies in Hodgkin's disease. What laparotomy has wrought. N Engl J Med 290:894–898, 1974.

108. Rappaport H, Strum SB: Vascular invasion in Hodgkin's disease: its incidence and relationship to the spread of the disease. Cancer 25:1304–1313, 1970.

109. Naeim F, Waisman J, Coulson WF: Hodgkin's disease: the significance of vascular invasion. Cancer 34:655–662, 1974.

110. Lamoureux KB, Jaffe ES, Berard CW, Johnson RE: Lack of vascular invasion in patients with extranodal dissemination of Hodgkin's disease. Cancer 31:824–825, 1973.

111. Bouroncle BA: Sternberg–Reed cells in the peripheral blood of patients with Hodgkin's disease. Blood 27:544–556, 1966.

112. Halie MR, Huiges W, Nieweg HO: Abnormal cells in the peripheral blood of patients with Hodgkin's disease. I. Observations with light microscopy. Br J Haematol 28:317–322, 1974.

113. Schiffer CA, Levi JA, Wiernik PH: The significance of abnormal circulating cells in patients with Hodgkin's disease. Br J Haematol 31:177–183, 1975.

114. Donaldson SS, Kaplan HS: Complications of treatment of Hodgkin's disease in children. Cancer Treat Rep 66:977–989, 1982.

115. Cunningham J, Mauch P, Rosenthal DS, Canellos GP: Long-term complications of MOPP chemotherapy in patients with Hodgkin's disease. Cancer Treat Rep 66:1015–1022, 1982.

116. Coltman CA, Dixon DO: Second malignancies complicating Hodgkin's disease: a southwest oncology group 10-year followup. Cancer Treat Rep 66:1023–1033, 1982.

117. Glicksman AS, Pajak TF, Gottlieb A, Nissen N, Stutzman L, Cooper MR: Second malignant neoplasms in patients successfully treated for Hodgkin's disease: a cancer and leukemia group B study. Cancer Treat Rep 66:1035–1044, 1982.

118. Kaplan HS: Hodgkin's disease: biology, treatment, prognosis. Blood 57:813–822, 1981.

119. Casazza AR, Duvall CP, Carbone PP: Summary of infectious complications occurring in patients with Hodgkin's disease. Cancer Res 26:1290–1296, 1966.

120. Aisenberg AC: Studies on delayed hypersensitivity in Hodgkin's disease. J Clin Invest 41:1964–1970, 1962.

121. Eltringham JR, Kaplan HS: Impaired delayed hypersensitivity responses in 154 patients with untreated Hodgkin's disease. Nat Cancer Inst Monogr 36:107–115, 1973.

122. Young RC, Corder MP, Haynes HA, De Vita VT: Delayed hypersensitivity in Hodgkin's disease. A study of 103 untreated patients. Am J Med 52:63–72, 1972.

123. Winkelstein A, Mikulla JM, Sartiano GP, Ellis LD: Cellular immunity in Hodgkin's disease: comparison of cutaneous reactivity and lymphoproliferative responses to phytohemagglutinin. Cancer 34:549–553, 1974.

124. Levy R, Kaplan HS: Impaired lymphocyte function in untreated Hodgkin's isease. N Engl J Med 290:181–186, 1974.

125. Tan C, de Sousa M, Tan R, Hansen JA, Good RA: In vitro response of peripheral blood and spleen lymphoid cells to mitogens and antigens in childhood Hodgkin's disease. Cancer Res 38:886–893, 1978.

126. Holm G, Mellstedt H, Bjorkholm M, Johansson B, Killander D, Sundblad R, Soderberg G: Lymphocyte abnormalities in untreated patients with Hodgkin's disease. Cancer 37:751–762, 1976.

127. Ziegler JB, Hansen P, Penny R: Lymphocyte defect in Hodgkin's disease: analysis of the intrinsic phytohemagglutinin dose response. Clin Immunol Immunopathol 3:451–469, 1975.

128. Matchett KM, Huang AT, Kremer WB: Impaired lymphocyte transformation in Hodgkin's disease: Evidence for depletion of circulating T-lymphocytes. J Clin Invest 52:1908–1917, 1973.

129. Bobrove AM, Fuks Z, Strober S, Kaplan HS: Quantitation of T and B lymphocytes and cellular immune function in Hodgkin's disease. Cancer 36:169–179, 1975.

130. Posner MR, Reinherz EL, Breard J, Nadler LM, Rosenthal DS, Schlossman SF: Lymphoid subpopulations of peripheral blood and spleen in untreated Hodgkin's disease. Cancer 48:1170–1176, 1981.

131. Romagnani S, Maggi E, Biagiotti R, Giudizi MG, Amadori A, Ricci M: Altered proportion of T and T subpopulations in patient with Hodgkin's disease. Scand J Immunol 7:511–514, 1978.

4. Upon the enigma of Hodgkin's disease and the Reed–Sternberg cell

CLIVE R. TAYLOR

> *All animals are equal, but some are more*
> *equal than others.*
> 'Proclamation of the Pig, Napoleon',
> George Orwell, *Animal Farm*, 1946

1. Introduction

If our hundred year quest for the cell of origin of Hodgkin's disease has taught us anything, it is the importance of maintaining an open mind, preferably with a cheerful capacity for changing it according to the dictates of fashion. Every cell has had its day; as prospective candidates all cells are equal, but (as we shall see) some are more equal than others.

> 'This enlargement of the glands appears to be a primitive affection of those bodies, rather than the result of an irritation propagated to them from some ulcerated surface or other inflamed texture.' (Thomas Hodgkin 1832)

Following this description of 'Some Morbid Appearances of the Absorbent Glands and Spleen' [1], the problems of the nature, nomenclature, diagnosis and clinical definition of tumors of the lymphoid system have promoted fierce controversy among clinicians and pathologists, falling just short of bloodshed. The accumulated literature is now beyond the compass of any one individual, and conflicts abound; the problem is not so much a shortage of data, as a lack of consensus concerning its validity or import.

A matter of philosophy is involved; 'truth' in the biological sciences is less absolute than in the physical sciences. An 'ultimate truth' in molecular physics may be represented by an equation that will be interpreted in a consistent manner by different scientists, in diverse places, subject to disparate educational backgrounds; while in histopathology a single tissue section may be viewed by three different pathologists within a single institution, producing three diagnoses of fundamentally different import. Thus histopathology is a subjective discipline, wherein the search for the truth is an exercise in democracy, a consensus opinion being required. With this in mind we should not forget that Hodgkin's disease continues to be diagnosed, and indeed defined, by histologic opinion, based upon demonstration of typical Reed–Sternberg

Bennett JM (ed), Controversies in the Management of Lymphomas. ISBN 0-89838-586-5.
© *Martinus Nijhoff Publishers, Boston. Printed in the Netherlands.*

cells in an appropriate cellular milieu; and, further, that the recognition of the 'typical Reed–Sternberg cell' is also based solely upon histologic judgment.

In the past decade there have been many attempts to explore Hodgkin's disease using scientific methods that potentially offer more precision and objectivity than conventional histologic techniques. Particularly the methods of the immunochemist and cellular immunologist, that have produced spectacular advances in the understanding of non-Hodgkin lymphomas, have also been applied to Hodgkin's disease. It is, therefore, appropriate to re-examine some established concepts of the nature of Hodgkin's disease and the Reed–Sternberg cell in the light of progress in understanding of the function of the lymphoid system and its component cells.

2. The nature of Hodgkin's disease – Historical aspects

Though previously much debated [2–9], the neoplastic nature of Hodgkin's disease is now generally accepted. Hodgkin, without the advantage of microscopic examination stopped short of claiming the process to be malignant, but clearly thought it to be more than simple inflammation:

'unless the word inflammation be allowed to have a more indefinite and loose meaning, this affection of the glands can scarcely be attributed to that cause.' [1]

Thirty years later Wilks [2], in attaching the eponym of Hodgkin to this disease, was in little doubt:

'It must take its place in the rank of malignant diseases, or amongst those affections that are characterized by new growths in the system.'

Greenfield, in 1978 [10], wrote that, 'Clinically and anatomically there is little distinction from cancer, and it may be regarded as lymphatic cancer,' a viewpoint given all the more credence when Mallory [6] and Warthin [11] added their considerable reputations in support.

Nonetheless, an opposing 'infectious' theory did, at various times, claim some following, including such distinguished disciples of the disease as Sternberg and Reed. Sternberg believed the process to be tuberculosis [4], while Reed [5] felt:

'that the growth differs from malignant tumor in the absence of capsular infiltration and implication of adjacent tissues . . . We believe that closer study will show a greater similarity to inflammatory processes.'

Closer study indeed seemed destined to provide support for this contention, in that many infectious agents were linked with Hodgkin's disease in the succeeding half century [review 12], but having failed to meet Koch's postulates, none have stood the test of time. More recent epidemiologic studies have again raised the spectre of an infectious agent having some role in the causation of

Hodgkin's disease [12], but there has been a subtle shift in emphasis towards an infectious agent as a cause of neoplasia, the neoplasm being Hodgkin's disease.

Thus a democratic consensus now holds that Hodgkin's disease is neoplastic. It is, however, a most peculiar neoplasm; and its very peculiarity provides a major obstacle to scientific study. In a typical case of Hodgkin's disease, a diagnostic microscopic field may contain only a small handful of Reed–Sternberg cells, the putative neoplastic cells; all the remaining cells represent, by current consensus, either residual or reactive normal cellular elements, including lymphocytes, plasma cells, histiocytes, granulocytes and fibrous tissue. That the neoplastic cells should account for 1% or less of the total cell population in typical Hodgkin's disease is, to me, one of the most remarkable and least remarked aspects of Hodgkin's disease, for such an occurrence is exceedingly rare in other malignant neoplasms. The rarity of the malignant cells, and their distribution among so many supposedly normal cells, renders attempts to study pure populations of the malignant cells extremely difficult. This problem is encountered time and time again, and is a significant impediment to controlled studies of the nature and origin of the Reed–Sternberg cells.

In spite of the relative infrequency of the neoplastic Reed–Sternberg cells, the distinction of Hodgkin's disease from other malignant neoplasms of the lymphoidsystem is usually made with some confidence by histologists [review see 13]; indeed, the current consensus supports a clear distinction between Hodgkin's disease and the 'non-Hodgkin lymphomas'. However, the 'truth' was not always so, for beginning with Mallory in 1914 [6], a number of pathologists (see Table 1) have consistently resisted the thesis that Hodgkin's disease is distinct and separate from other lymphomas [14, 15].

Such debate is more than idle semantics, but is fundamental to the problem of Hodgkin's disease – for if the Reed–Sternberg cell, and thus Hodgkin's disease, is lymphocyte derived, then Hodgkin's disease is indeed a 'true lymphoma', more or less closely related to the other lymphomas; whereas if the Reed–Sternberg cell originates from some other progenitor cell, then Hodgkin's disease is not a malignant lymphoma and should not be designated as such.

In the last decade techniques derived from basic immunology (lymphocyte surface marker studies, transformation studies, etc.) have added a new dimension to our understanding of the cellular origin of the neoplastic cells of the non-Hodgkin lymphomas [16] and have profoundly influenced our concepts of the interrelations of these lymphomas one with another [17–19]. It is time to ask the question as to how this radical reappraisal of our knowledge of the form and function of normal and neoplastic lymphocytes might influence current opinion of the relationship of Hodgkin's disease with the true lymphocyte-derived neoplasms. This chapter purports to examine this question.

Table 1. Interrelations of Hodgkin's disease and the non-Hodgkin lymphomas.*

Oliver (1913)	'It is the predominate cell type which allows one to classify the tumour as lymphosarcoma, endothelioma [reticulum cell sarcoma] or Hodgkin's disease ... All constitute a series of neoplastic processes of the lymphatic glands, which differ not so much qualitatively as quantitatively'.
Mallory (1914)	Classified Hodgkin's disease as one of the lymphoblastomas, implying it to be a variant of lymphosarcoma.
Coley (1928)	'These two conditions (lymphosarcoma and Hodgkin's disease) which are usually regarded as quite different and distinct ... bear such a resemblance to one another that in some instances it is impossible to differentiate them either clinically or histologically', so reiterating his views expressed 20 years previously.
MacCarty (1930)	'... a common neoplastic cellular origin'.
Pullinger (1931)	'A group of diseases of the reticulum exists in which proliferation is possible into one or several of the possible cell progeny'.
Warthin (1931)	'Hodgkin's disease is a neoplasm and related genetically to the lymphoblastomas, of which both the aleukaemic and leukaemic forum are identical pathologically. Transition forms exist between all of these groups'.
Levin (1931)	'... phases of the same pathologic entity and the two may co-exist in the same patient'.
Ginsburg (1934)	Extensively reviewed the opinions of Banti (1903), Gibbons (1906), Coley (1908), Mueller (1921), and McCartney (1928), in reaching his own conclusions that 'they [Hodgkin's disease and lymphosarcoma] are merely variations of the same disease'.
Herbut *et al.* (1945)	'These combinations can only be explained by considering the three diseases (Hodgkin's disease, lymphosarcoma, and reticulum cell sarcoma) as not only closely related, but as having a common neoplastic origin'.
Willis (1948)	'I join Warthin, Ginsburg, Herbut *et al.*, and others, who regard all tumors of lymphoid tissue as related variants of one disease.... The names used for the principal variants have descriptive and clinical value but do not denote distinct pathological entities'.
Custer & Bernhard (1948)	'They are all mesenchymal tumors which vary only in degree and type of differentiation ... a striking fluidity in histologic pattern with transitions and combinations'.
Gall (1962)	'To my distress I found that the patterns differed in the same patient in approximately one third of cases. It is true that the variations were often a matter of degree (i.e., Hodgkin's paragranuloma to Hodgkin's sarcoma, differentiated to undifferentiated lymphosarcoma, follicular to diffuse lymphosarcoma); in rare instances, however, the lesions of Hodgkin's disease and of lymphocytic lymphoma were both detectable in the same individual'.

* The originators of these unitarian views were considered by Robb–Smith to follow the 'fluid lymphoma school' [13]. References [14, 15].

3. The Reed–Sternberg cell and the diagnosis of Hodgkin's disease

Today, as ever, the diagnosis of Hodgkin's disease is dependent upon the finding of Reed–Sternberg cells in the appropriate histological setting. Descriptions of the Reed–Sternberg cell abound in the literature. Historically Virchow, in 1863 [20], was perhaps the first to refer to 'large peculiar cells' which he termed lymphadenoma cells. Subsequently Langhans [21] 'grossere Zellen mit 2–4 und mehr Kernen und etwas dunkelkorniger Zellsubstanz,' and Greenfield (10) 'multinucleated cells (containing from four to eight to twelve nuclei) adherent to the trabeculae' provided more detailed descriptions. However, these cells derived their eponymous title from the later more detailed descriptions of Sternberg [4] and of Reed [5]: 'Large giant cells varying from the size of two or three red blood cells to cells twenty times this size. The nucleus is always large in proportion to the size of the cell. It may be single or multiple . . . One or more large nucleoli are always present.'

Subsequently, additional histological features, such as the common presence of a juxtanuclear 'hof', were reported: 'a pale area adjacent to, and often indenting, the nucleus or nuclei' [22], and several variants of the classical Reed–Sternberg cell were described. The mononuclear relative of the Reed–Sternberg cell, having similar nuclear characteristics and one or more large nucleoli, was recognized and was dubbed the 'Hodgkin' cell by Moeschlin and associates [23]. Similar mononuclear variants had previously been observed by others, including both Reed and Sternberg, the latter regarding it as an intermediate type in the development of the classical Reed–Sternberg cell. This concept of the evolution of the Reed–Sternberg cell from a mononuclear progenitor was described minutely, and illustrated beautifully by Favre and Croizat in 1931 [24, for illustration see 25].

There is evidence of RNA synthesis in 'young' forms of the Reed–Sternberg cell (ie, the mononuclear Hodgkin cell), as indicated by cytoplasmic basophilia (or pyroninophilia) [23, 26] and by kinetic studies [27, 28]. Basophilia declines in older forms with lobulate nuclei, and many believe these to be relatively inactive cells with minimal proliferation on the basis of DNA synthesis studies, although some recent reports suggest that these cells may show a greater capacity for nucleic acid synthesis than previously supposed [29, 30]. Thus the relatively quiescent polyploid Reed–Sternberg cell appears to be derived from a proliferating metabolically active mononuclear precursor, the so-called Hodgkin cell. It is the identity and origin of this cell that is in question.

4. Ancillary questions

In answering this fundamental question, one might reasonably expect to shed some light on other, as yet unexplained, aspects of the pathology of Hodgkin's disease: namely the pattern of spread to contiguous lymph node groups, the tendancy to remain confined to the lymphoid system until very late stages, the curious admixture of cells found together in diagnostic tissues, the relative infrequency of occurrence of the malignant cells (ie, Hodgkin and Reed–Sternberg cells) in involved tissues, and the relationship of Hodgkin's disease to the other lymphomas.

5. The cellular origin of the Reed–Sternberg cell – the candidates

> *To give an accurate and exhaustive account*
> *of that period would need a far less brilliant*
> *pen than mine.*
>
> Max Beerbohm, 1872–1956

Over the years the cellular origin of the Reed–Sternberg cell has been a point of much research and more contention, the leading candidates being the reticulum cell (including reticular cell and stem cell), the histiocyte, the lymphoblast, the plasmablast, the megakaryocyte, myeloid cells, and 'special' reticulum cells (Table 2).

5.1. The reticulum cell

The concept of the reticulum cell as the progenitor cell of Hodgkin's disease dates from Maximow [31], who believed that the reticulum cells served as the 'mother lode' or stem cell compartment of all of the lymphoid and hematopietic elements. Simple logic, therefore, related all of the lymphomas one to another through their common relationship to the primordial reticulum cell; this included Hodgkin's disease: 'the reticulum cell is the proliferating cell of Hodgkin's disease ... All the other cellular manifestations (ie, the lymphocytes, plasma cells, histiocytes, granulocytes, etc.) are due to subsequent differentiation of the reticulum cell ... to one or other of the possible cell progeny' [7]. This version of the 'truth' explained almost everything about Hodgkin's disease: the particular involvement of lymphoid tissues, its relationship to other lymphomas, the admixture of cells present; it even avoided the necessity for explaining the scarcity of malignant cells in a malignant neoplasm, since all of the cells were believed to be derived from differentiation of the malignant reticulum cells.

Unfortunately, although esthetically satisfying, the reticulum cell dynasty lasted only a quarter of a century. It saw its last flowering in the beautiful all-embracing flow charts of Custer [32, 33], depicting his vision of the composite

Table 2. Suggested cellular origin for the Reed–Sternberg cell.

Reed	1902	'epithelioid' cells (endothelial)
Mallory	1914	lymphoblast
Lang	1925	adventitial or reticular origin
McJunkin	1928	monocyte–reticular cell
Carballo	1931	plasma cell
Vasiliu, Goia	1927	dual origin–plasma cell and reticuloendothelial cell
Favre, Croizat	1931	haemohistioblast
Medlar	1931	megakaryocyte
Symmers	1927/1948	reticulum cell
Pullinger	1932	reticulum cell
Ross	1933	reticulum cell
Potter	1935	reticulum cell
Robb-Smith	1938	reticulum cell
Lewis	1941	myeloblast
Bessis	1948	histiocyte
Moeschlin *et al.*	1950	reticulum cell
Ackerman *et al.*	1951	reticulum cell
Smetana	1956	reticulum cell
Rebuck	1960	reticulum cell
Rappaport	1966	histiocyte
Dorfman	1964	not histiocyte
Sinkovics, Clein	1966	lymphoid
Leech	1973	lymphoid
Tindle *et al.*	1972	immunoblast (T) cell
Taylor	1974	B cell
Garvin *et al.*	1974	B cell
Kaplan, Gartner	1977	histiocyte
Long *et al.*	1977	histiocyte
Kadin *et al.*	1978	histiocyte
Bernau *et al.*	1978	B cell
Curran, Jones	1978	dendritic histiocyte (reticulum cell)
Reynes *et al.*	1979	B cell
Herva *et al.*	1979	T cell
Poppema	1980	histiocyte some, B cell others
Stein *et al.*	1981/1982	granulocyte
Poppema *et al.*	1982	interdigitating reticulum cell
Schwab *et al.*	1982	hitherto unknown normal cell'

Modified from Taylor [14]; for references prior to 1977 see [14].

lymphomas made clear through the mutual inter-relationship of each of the different lymphomas with the reticulum cell; and it fell, not on a single day, not as a result of a single scientific revelation, and not to the assault of a single dauntless investigator, but rather as a result of mounting frustation with the ill-defined usage of the term 'reticulum cell', coupled with the recognized need for greater precision in cell nomenclature.

If Custer was the last great champion of the reticulum cell, then Gall and Rappaport must be regarded as two of its major detractors, the chief instruments of its demise. Study of the nodular lymphomas resulted in the prototypic Rappaport classification [34], in which it was postulated that the large cell types, perceived previously to take origin from the reticulum cell, might more accurately be thought of as derivatives of the histiocyte. Thus it came to pass that all large cells in lymphoid tissues, whether normal or neoplastic, were histiocytes in one guise or another, including Reed–Sternberg cells.

5.2. The histiocyte

Although McJunkin, Bessis and others (Table 2) had written in support of the monocyte-histiocyte series as precursor to the Reed–Sternberg cell, this viewpoint never really emerged from beneath the umbrella of the reticulum cell concept; understandably since reticulum cells/reticular cells/histiocytes were inextricably interwoven in the folklore of the lymphoreticular system.

Dorfman [35] was among the first to take a hard look at the evidence, and found it wanting; applying then available histochemical techniques for identification of histiocytes in tissues, he concluded that the relationship of the Reed–Sternberg cell to the histiocyte 'is no closer than that of the lymphocyte to the histiocyte'. Partly as a consequence of this work, and partly due to lack of any new initiative, the supporters of the histiocyte, like those of the reticulum cell before them, retired to lick their wounds and to await either the advent of a new candidate for the title or a resurgence of interest in the histiocyte theory.

Thus, there followed an interlude of approximately ten years during which a new classification of Hodgkin's disease was proposed and accepted (Rye classification) [36] for its clinical utility, although it shed no visible light upon the nature of the process. Off stage, however, there were rumors of renewed hostilities, of a return to the trenches, refortified with new evidence in support of the histiocyte or in support of other candidate cells. A wealth of data flowed from the studies of the cellular immunologists and immunochemists, from the development of cell surface marker and immunochemical methods, applied initially to the study of the normal immune system and normal lymphocytes, then to neoplastic lymphocytes, the non-Hodgkin lymphomas, and finally to Hodgkin's disease.

Much of the new evidence cited in support of the histiocytic school was drawn from in vitro studies of Reed–Sternberg cells, either freshly isolated or following short or long term culture.

In 1975 Kay, working with Kadin, penned a letter to the *Lancet* [37], in which the surface characteristics of freshly isolated Reed–Sternberg cells were used as evidence for a macrophage/histiocyte origin. Unfortunately there were some difficulties in morphological definition of the cells in question (normal histiocyte/macrophage versus Reed–Sternberg cell) [38, 39]. In a somewhat longer discourse the next year, Kay [40] reaffirmed support for the macrophage/histiocyte theory, and discussed possible interactions with T lymphocytes (a lymphocyte/macrophage war) in an attempt to develop a unified explanation for the admixture of cell types present in Hodgkin's disease tissue.

The subsequent work of Kaplan and Gartner [41] was based upon tissue culture and cell transplant studies, cultures of Reed–Sternberg cells being identified by morphologic and cytogenetic criteria. Cultured Reed–Sternberg cells were judged to be of histiocytic origin on the basis of phagocytosis of latex particles or red cells, and histochemical stains (particularly nonspecific esterase); this work was open to criticism on the basis of uncertainty in defining the cultured cells as Reed–Sternberg cells rather than an overgrowth of histiocytes. Tissue culture procedures are notoriously open to the induction of artifactual change. Normal cells may radically change their character within a few hours of culture [42]. Even such a standard 'histiocytic marker' as phagocytosis is unreliable; for example, Catanzaro and Graham [43] showed that normal peritoneal lymphocytes were capable of active phagocytosis of latex and red cells following just 24 hours in culture. Nonetheless, Kaplan had sufficient confidence in this data that he later wrote that 'the controversy concerning the origin of the Reed–Sternberg cell was resolved' [44]; the continuing spate of papers, the emergence of brand new candidate cells, and indeed the existence of two chapters in this monograph, serve as notice that not all share Kaplan's opinion.

Kadin and Asbury [29], Long [45], Willson and Pretlow [46] and Roberts [47] and their associates also have succeeded in culturing Reed–Sternberg cells (or Hodgkin cells). Kadin and colleagues appeared to favor a lymphoid origin for their cultured cells [29]. The characteristics of the cells cultured by Long's group were more in keeping with monocytes than lymphocytes; they nevertheless differed dramatically fromm Kaplan's cultured cells in being non-phagocytic; later it transpired that the cells cultured by Long's group represented contaminants [48], reinforcing the concern that conventional criteria for cell identification are extremely unreliable in tissue culture. It should be noted that Pretlow and his collaborators [46], possibly wisest of all, reserved judgment.

Other support for the histiocyte theory was forthcoming in a review bij Desforges and colleagues [49], who surveyed the literature and found 'strong evidence for a macrophage origin of the Reed–Sternberg cell'. This paper evoked a response from Bucsky [50] in which he argued that Reed–Sternberg cells were probably of histiocytic origin, but also cited morphologic evidence that Hodgkin cells might be of B immunoblastic origin (vide infra). Bucsky also discussed the possibility of a 'virus-induced cell fusion' accounting for the 'Janus face of Hodgkin's disease'. Sinkovics and Shullenburger [51] had earlier proposed a similar idea, namely a T lymphocyte-B lymphocyte fusion induced by Epstein–Barr virus. Here again the morphological definition of Reed–Sternberg cells and Hodgkin cells presented a major impediment to study and communication.

The same problem resurfaced in a paper by Peiper and colleagues [52], in which ultrastructural studies were claimed to provide support for the histiocytic nature of Reed–Sternberg cells. Kadin, in a commentary (in the same issue of the journal – 53), expressed some reservations as to whether cells illustrated by Peiper, as having histiocytic features, were indeed Reed–Sternberg cells as opposed to reactive histiocytes.

Kadin has also provided independent evidence for the histiocytic origin of Reed–Sternberg cells, based upon surface and functional characteristics of freshly isolated cell preparations; in some studies there was evidence of surface features and phagocytosis consistent with histiocytes [54], while in other studies there was not [55]; the former study was purported to show internalization of polyclonal immunoglobulin by Reed–Sternberg cells, consistent with a macrophage origin. Since these were freshy isolated cells, the problems of cell identification were considered less severe than in tissue culture studies, and the possibility of functional changes induced by culture conditions was minimized.

5.3. Lymphocytes

> What I tell you three times is true.
> Lewis Carroll, *The Hunting of the Snark*

The idea of a lymphocytic (lymphoblastic) origin for the Reed–Sternberg cell is not new (Table 2). Indeed the idea may be seen again in the teachings of Custer [33], once it is recognized that the term 'reticulum cell', used by Custer, is nothing more than an alias for the transformed lymphocyte, including the large follicular center cells and B and T immunoblasts; if this simple translation is made, then Custer's propasals are seen in a new light, clearly indicating a relationship of Hodgkin's disease and the non-Hodgkin lymphomas to one another and to the immunoblast/reticulum cell. However, such evidence is morphologic and conceptual, lacking independent means of validation. A similar criticism may be leveled at the proposal of Tindle and colleagues [56] relating Reed–Sternberg cells to immunoblasts (probably of T cell type), on the basis of morphologic similarities and the occurrence of Reed–Sternberg-like cells in reactive immunoblastic proliferations.

5.3.1. B Lymphocytes. My own direct involvement in the story began in 1972 with the observation, using immunoperoxidase techniques on paraffin sections, of immunoglobulin in various cells, at that time still considered to be 'malignant reticulum cells', including those cells comprising reticulum cell sarcomas, and the Reed–Sternberg and Hodgkin cells in cases of Hodgkin's disease [57–59]. In the so-called reticulum cell sarcomas, the pattern of light chain staining was usually monotypic (or monoclonal, ie, exclusively kappa or lambda chain), although in some cases a proportion of the neoplastic cells, usually the larger cells, showed bitypic staining (ie, both kappa and lambda in individual cells, as confirmed by serial sections and simultaneous double-staining methods). In Reed–Sternberg and Hodgkin cells the reverse appeared to be true; most cases contained a predominance of bitypic cells, with only a small handful of monotypic (monoclonal) cases. The monoclonal 'malignant reticulum cells' of reticulum cell sarcoma were recognized as malignant B immunoblasts, in keeping with the conceptual reevaluation of non-Hodgkin lymphomas then taking place in the minds and laboratories of Kojima, Lennert, Lukes and others [reviews 17–19]. The possibility was entertained that Reed-Sternberg cells and Hodgkin cells were related to these malignant B immunoblasts on the basis of morphological similarity (Hodgkin cells and B immunoblasts are often indistinguishable on a cell to cell basis) and of their content of immunoglobulin, albeit that in the non-Hodgkin lymphomas B immunoblasts were usually monotypic (and only occasionally bitypic), wereas the converse appeared true of Hodgkin and Reed–Sternberg cells. Other possibilities accounting for the presence of immunoglobulin within these cells were discussed when this work was presented [57, 58 – *vide infra*]. However, with the goal of 'explaining' Hodgkin's disease rather than simply identifying the heritage of the Reed–Sternberg cell, a persuasive factor was the possibility of once again, for the first time since the days of the reticulum cell [Pullinger, Custer and others – *vide supra*], achieving a unified concept for the lymphomas, including Hodgkin's disease, while simultaneously explaining the admixture of cell types in Hodgkin's disease, and the various subtypes of Hodgkin's disease in relationship to prognosis.

The finding of immunoglobulin within Reed–Sternberg cells and its pattern of distribution was confirmed by others working independently [60–63], although interpretation of its significance differed widely.

5.3.2. Immunoglobulin in Reed–Steenberg cells – Significance. Firstly, the presence of immunoglobulin within the cell cytoplasm might be indicative of *in situ* synthesis. Secondly, immunoglobulin might be taken into the cell actively, by pinocytosis or by phagocytosis, possibly in the form of immune complexes following binding to Fc receptors. Thirdly, degenerating cells fail to maintain the integrity of their plasma membranes, thus allowing large molecules freely to enter the cytoplasm. Specific antibody directed against cell surface antigens might, therefore, gain access to cytoplasm, having first induced cell membrane damage; or any nonspecific plasma component might similarly gain entry [57–63].

Other investigators have described the presence of albumin, alpha$_1$-antitrypsin and alpha$_1$-chymotrypsin within Reed–Sternberg cells, in addition to confirming the presence of immunoglobulin. Poppema and collagues [63] attributed the presence of these various proteins within Reed–Sternberg cells to passive absorption by damaged cells. Papadimitriou et al [62] favored *in situ* synthesis on the basis of persuasive evidence of heavy chain subclass restriction within Reed–Sternberg cells.

Thus there was, and indeed still is, conflicting evidence; the monoclonal pattern of staining, observed rarely, favoring *in situ* synthesis of immunoglobulin by Reed–Sternberg cells, but, because of its rarity, raising doubts as to how much weight to give this evidence; the double-staining pattern supporting phagocytosis or passive absorption as the underlying mechanisme.

Examination of the results of immunohistological studies of cases of non-Hodgkin lymphoma and myeloma is of relevance in this respect.

In studies of B lymphocyte-derived neoplasms (eg, large cell follicular center cell lymphomas and immunoblastic sarcomas) particularly those containing bizarre immunoblasts and giant cells resembling Reed–Sternberg cell variants, the expected pattern of monoclonal staining was observed in the majority of cells, but the subpopulation of larger cells showed an anomalous or bitypic pattern with double staining (kappa and lambda) of individual tumor cells [58, 59]. This observation suggested that bizarre polyploid neoplastic B lymphocytes (immunoblasts) in otherwise typical monoclonal B cell lymphomas may contain (parts of) both light chains and thus may not conform to the general thesis of restricted immunoglobulin synthesis; interestingly, such cells are frequently hypodiploid or tetraploid, containing a double, or greater, complement of immunoglobulin-related genes. There is independent evidence for this occurrence from animal studies [64], from *in vitro* cultures of human cell lines [65], and in well-documented human disease, where individual tumors and possibly, though not necessarily, individual tumor cells have been shown to produce both kappa and lambda light chain [66–69].

Finally, ultrastructural immunohistochemical studies favor a B lymphocytic origin. Bernau, Reynes and their respective associates [70, 71] were able to demonstrate, by immunostaining of immunoglobulin at the electron microscopic level, that immunoglobulin in typical Reed–Sternberg cells is localized to free ribosomes and to ribosomes on the endoplasmic reticulum and the perinuclear membranes, a pattern exactly like that seen in B immunoblasts in the early stages of immunoglobulin synthesis.

5.3.3. T lymphocyte. A T lymphocytic origin has also been proposed, based largely upon circumstantial evidence of decreased T cell immune function in Hodgkin's disease, and the apparent predilection of Hodgkin's disease for the T cell zone (paracortex) of lymph nodes [see reviews 12, 53]. There is no direct proof; Reed–Sternberg cells do not form E rosettes, a characteristic of T cells, nor do they react directly with various anti-T cell antisera, including a range of monoclonal antibodies against T and B cell subsets (OKT3, 6, 10, 11; Leul, 2, 3, 4; BA-1, BA-2, B-1 – personal observations).

Independent studies using somewhat different techniques, including histochemistry and autoradiography of lymph node cells from cases of Hodgkin's disease have led to the conclusion that the small lymphocytes intermediate lymphoid cells, immunoblasts, Hodgkin cells and Reed–Sternberg cells all form a 'morphologically continuous DNA synthesizing series' with the histochemical features of T lymphocytes (i.e., punctate staining for acid naphthyl acetate esterase) [72].

Thus again there is no shortage of evidence; the problem is a shortage of agreement as to what it means.

5.4. Interdigitating reticulum cell

The interdigitating reticulum cell, like the immunoblast, has always existed, but only recently has gained recognition, separate from the overall reticulum cell category. This cell type, as defined by Kaiserling and colleagues [73] is found in lymphoid tissues in the T cells areas, including thymus and the T zones of lymph nodes and spleen; similar cells are present in animals in a similar distribution. Their supposed function is in relation to processing of antigen for T cells; as such they are considered analogous to the 'antigen-processing dendritic cells' of the cellular immunologist (it should be noted that Kaiserling has also defined a category of 'dendritic reticulum cells' that are distinct from interdigitating reticulum cells, and are confined to the B cell where they may have a role in antigen processing for B cells [73]).

One characteristic of interdigitating reticulum cells is that they are intimately associated with T cells, forming close surface contacts with T cells in vitro, a phenomenon that some find reminiscent of the 'swarming' of T lymphocytes around isolated Reed–Sternberg cells [74–76]; the ocurrence of this phenomenon has been advocated as a prognostic indicator by some [77].

Poppema and associates [78], in a study of frozen sections from 11 lymph nodes of patients with Hodgkin's disease, utilized a panel of monoclonal antibodies against T cells. They found no evidence of T cell markers on Reed–Sternberg cells, but noted the clustering of T lymphocytes (helper phenotype) around Reed–Sternberg cells and found it 'plausible that

Reed–Sternberg cells are derived from antigen presenting (i.e., interdigitating) reticulum cells in the thymic dependent areas of lymphoid tissue'. Poppema had earlier conducted a variety of immunohistochemical studies of Hodgkin's disease, with a variety of collaborators, producing interesting data and conclusions [review 79]; the Reed–Sternberg cells of lymphocyte–predominant Hodgkin's disease showed patterns of reactivity suggestive of immunoglobulin production and were considered to be derived from B imunoblasts, while the Reed–Sternberg cells of other forms of Hodgkin's disease showed features more consistent with a histiocytic origin.

Prior to leaving the interdigitating reticulum cell, it is worth noting that its sister cell, the dendritic reticulum cell (or histiocyte) of the follicular centers also has been proposed by some investigators as the progenitor cell of Hodgkin's disease. For example, Curran and Jones [80] conducted a histochemical and immunohistochemical study, concluding that the nodules characterizing some forms of Hodgkin's disease represent neoplastic follicles, the neoplastic cells being not lymphocytes, but rather dendritic histiocytes (reticulum cells).

5.5. The ultimate evidence

Thus, in 1980, we had available a wealth of evidence, but appeared no nearer to a consensus that might be considered to approximate to the truth. The last two years have produced still more data, and inevitably new candidate cells, certainly new food for new thoughts; but the process of digestion and assimilation has scarcely begun.

The exhaustive conventional and monoclonal antibody immunohistochemical studies of Stein and colleagues [81–83] fall into two separate, but related, parts. Firstly, conventional, and later monoclonal, antibodies were prepared against a cell line (L428), initially established from the pleural effusion of a patient with Hodgkin's disease (the cell line initially established by Schaadt and colleagues [84] was believed to represent a line of malignant Reed–Sternberg cells). The conventional antiserum was extensively absorbed with a variety of normal cells, following which specificity against Hodgkin and Reed–Sternberg cells was demonstrated, with the exception that reactivity with segmented and mature granulocytes was retained. This observation prompted the authors to study the pattern of reactivity of Reed–Sternberg cells with a panel of monoclonal antibodies known to have activity against granulocytes at various stages of maturation [81]. They observed that Hodgkin cells and Reed–Sternberg cells showed similar patterns of reactivity in the majority of cases of Hodgkin's disease, regardless of subtype; they concluded that the pattern of reactivity more closely resembled granulocytes than any other cell type within the hemato-lymphoid system. The authors stopped just short of claiming a granulocytic origin for the Reed–Sternberg cell, but noted that clarification of the exact relationship between these cells and granulopoietic cells might provide new insights. This, of course, should evoke distinct feelings of dèja vu for all Hodgkin's disease history buffs, in that Lewis, in 1941 [85], had observed 'characteristic writhing movements' of Reed–Sternberg cells *in vitro*, and noted a resemblance to myeloblasts. The production of a monoclonal antibody (dubbed Ki-1) [82, 83] against the L428 Reed–Sternberg cell line served to remove some of the residual doubts concerning the specificity of the conventional antibody. This monoclonal reagent also stained Reed–Sternberg cells, but not the cells of 'more than 50 cases of non-Hodgkin lymphomas', although some staining of large cell lymphomas has now been observed. There are, however, two discrepancies: firstly, the conventional rabbit antibody stains Reed–Sternberg cells and granulocytes, whereas the monoclonal antibody is said 'not to react with cells of normal peripheral blood'; secondly, the monoclonal antibody recognizes a small cell population within normal lymphoid tissues that is not detected by the conventional antibody [81–83]. On the basis of comparative staining with other antibodies (*vide infra*), this population of Ki-1-positive cells was thought not to represent B cells, T cells, macrophages, dendritic or interdigitating reticulum cells, or cells of the granulopoietic, erythropoietic or thrombopoietic series.

As part of their investigation these authors also studied the patterns of reactivity of Reed–Sternberg cells, and normal cells, with an extensive range of monoclonal antibodies, selected for the purpose of identifying all of the major cell types present in lymphoid tissues [81–83]. They included a bewildering array of monoclonal antibodies that, in other hands, have been shown to have reactivity (if not cell specificity) for T lymphocytes, B lymphocytes, monocytes, thymocytes, interdigitating reticulum cells and Langerhans cells, dendritic reticulum cells, granulocytes, platelets and megakaryocytes, cells of the erythroid series, Ia antigens and the $C3_b$ complement receptor; all these in addition to the monoclonal Ki-1 anti-Reed–Sternberg cell antibody. Such a large bolus of evidence proves somewhat indigestible. While some discrepancies exist, the conclusion of the authors that Reed–Sternberg cells are derived from a hitherto unrecognized normal small cell population appears reasonable.

5.6. In conclusion

The pursuit may now shift, at least temporarily, away from the Reed–Sternberg cell itself, towards capture and study of one or more of these unidentified normal cells. As we set out on this new quest for the Grail, we should be cautious. Past experience tells us that for any cell chosen as the progenitor of the Reed–Sternberg cell, the chances that the choice is wrong far outweigh the chances that it is right.

One particular concern is the dawning realization that monoclonal antibodies, though equisitely specific for individual antigenic determinants, are not necesarily specific for individual cell types; it is our experience that the finding in tissue sections of common reactivity of two different cells with a single monoclonal antibody does not prove a developmental relationship (witness the monoclonal antibody OKT6, having reactivity in frozen tissue sections against thymocytes and Langerhans cells of the skin [86]; and the monoclonal antibody BA-1, having reactivity against B lymphocytes and granulocytes in tissue sections [87]. Equally, of course, lack of reactivity with a monoclonal antibody does not disqualify an individual cell from belonging to a particular family (for example, only subsets of B cells react with B-1, BA-1, B-532, or indeed any other B cell antibody, of which I am aware [87]).

6. Current beliefs

*Fere libenter homines id quod volunt credunt.** Julius Caesar, 102–44BC

Thus we are entering an era in which the only certainty is that new information will continue to pour from the 'monoclonal antibody laboratories'. Amid the excitement we should not forget the need for better characterization of these new reagents prior to reaching definitive conclusions as to what they signify. Also, in our zeal for uncovering the identity of the mysterious ancestor of the Reed–Sternberg cell, we should not overlook the larger goals of achieving a better understanding of the disease itself, of explaining the rarity of malignant cells, the characteristic admixture of cell types, the predilection for lymphoid tissues, the relation to other lymphomas and the persisting variations in response to therapy. To my mind, of all the candidates examined, acceptance of the lymphocyte (whether B or T or some subset) would best explain the pecularities of this disease [14, 15, 25], while the interdigitating reticulum cell has intriguing possibilities, somewhat difficult to enunciate since we know so little of the nature of the normal cell. The new UNC candidate (unidentified normal cell) will clearly emerge as the front runner, but only time will tell whether it will stay the course better than its predecessors (Table 2).

Meanwhile histopathologists addicted to the study of Hodgkin's disease will find it difficult to resist playing the scientist, popping down to the laboratory for a quick immunohistochemical fix before dinner.

---

* Men willingly believe whatever they wish.

The world thinks of the man of science as one who pulls out his watch and exclaims 'Ha! half an hour to spare before dinner; I will just step down to my laboratory and make a discovery.'

Sir Ronald Ross, 1857–1932

References

1. Hodgkin T: On some morbid appearance of the absorbent glands and spleen. Trans Med Chir Soc Lond 17:68, 1832.
2. Wilks Sir S: Cases of enlargement of the lymphatic glands and spleen (or, Hodgkin's Disease), with remarks. Guy's Hosp Rep 11:56, 1865.
3. Kundrat: Uber Lympho-Sarkomatosis. Wien klin Wschr 6:211, 1893.
4. Sternberg C: Über eine eigenartige unter dem Bilde der Pseudoleukämie verlaufende Tuberkulose des lymphatischen Apparates. Z Helik 19:21, 1898.
5. Reed DM: On the pathological changes in Hodgkin's disease, with especial reference to its relation to tuberculosis. Johns Hopkins Hosp Rep 10:133, 1902.
6. Mallory FBP: In: The Principles of stPathologic Histology. Philadelphia: WB Saunders Co, 1914, p 333.
7. Pullinger BD: Histology and histogenesis. In: Rose Research in Lymphadenoma. Briol: John Wright, 1932, p 117.
8. Robb-Smith AHT: Reticulosis and reticulosarcoma: a histological classification. J Pathol Bact 47:457, 1938.
9. Kaplan HS, Smithers DW: Auto-immunity in man and homologous disease in mice in relation to the malignant lymphomas. Lancet 2:1, 1959.
10. Greenfield WS: Specimens illustrative of the pathology of lymphadenoma and leucocythaemia. Trans Path Soc Lond 29:272, 1878.
11. Warthin AS: The genetic neoplastic relationships of Hodgkin's disease, aleukaemic and leukamic lymphoblastoma and mycosis fungoides. Ann Surg 93:153, 1931.
12. Howard DR: Hodgkin's disease: Pathology and pathogenesis. CRC Crit Rev Clin Lab Sci 14:109, 1981.
13. Robb-Smith AHT, Taylor CR: An approach to lymph node diagnosis. London: Harvey Miller; New York: Oxford University Press, 1981.
14. Taylor CR: A history of the Reed–Sternberg cell. Biomedicine 28:196, 1978.
15. Taylor CR: The immunopathology of Hodgkin's disease. In: Malignant lymphomas, the pathophysiology of the lymphocyte and its neoplasms, Bosman F, van den Tweel J, Taylor CR (eds.), Leiden: Leiden University Press, 1980, p. 399.
16. Taylor CR, Parker JW: Immuno-methods in diagnostic hematopathology. In: Methods and achievements in experimental pathology, vol 10, Jasmin G, Cantin M (eds.), New York: Karger, 1981, p. 37.
17. Taylor CR: Classification of lymphomas: 'new thinking' on old thoughts Arch Pathol Lab Med 102:549, 1978.
18. Taylor CR: Changing concepts in classification of lymphoma. In: Malignant lymphomas, the pathophysiology of the lymphocyte and its neoplasms, Bosman F, van den Tweel J, Taylor CR (eds.), Leiden: Leiden University Press, 1980, p. 175.
19. Taylor CR: Pathobiology of lymphocyte transformation. In: Pathobiology Annual, Ioachim HL (ed.), New York: Raven Press (in press).
20. Virchow R: Die Krankhaften Geschwultse, vol 1. Berlin, 1863, p. 728.

108

21. Langhans T: Das maligne Lymphosarkom (Pseudoleukämie). Virchows Arch [Pathol Anat] 54:509, 1872.
22. Hoster HA, Dratman MB: Hodgkin's disease (Part I) 1832–1947. Cancer Res 8:1, 1948.
23. Moeschlin S, Schwarz E, Wang H: Die Hodgkinzellen als Tumorzellen. Schweiz med Wschr 80:1103, 1950.
24. Favre M, Croizat P: Caractères généraux du granulome malin, tirés de son étude anatomoclinique. Ann Anat Pathol 8:838, 1931.
25. Taylor CR: Upon the nature of Hodgkin's disease and the Reed–Sternberg cell. In: Recent results in cancer research, vol 64, Mathé G, Seligmann M, Tubiana M (eds.), Berlin: Springer-Verlag, 1978, p. 214.
26. Ackerman GA, Knouff RA, Hoster HA: Cytochemistry and morphology of neoplastic and non-neoplastic human lymph nodes with special reference to Hodgkin's disease. J Natl Cancer Inst 12:465, 1951.
27. Peckham MJ, Cooper EH: Proliferation characteristics of the various classes of cells in Hodgkin's disease. Cancer 24:135, 1969.
28. Peckham MJ, Cooper EH: Cell Biology. In: Hodgkin's disease, Smithers D (ed.), London: Churchill Livingstone, 1973, p. 64.
29. Kadin ME, Asbury AK: Long term cultures of Hodgkin's tissue. A morphologic and radioautographic study. Lab Invest 28:181, 1973.
30. Marinello M, Tkachenko G, Gavilondo J, Baeza B: In vitro incorporation of tritiated thymidine by the Sternberg–Reed cells in Hodgkin's disease. Neoplasma 22:185, 1975.
31. Maximow A: Relation of blood cells to connective tissue and endothelium. In: Special cytology, Cowdry EV (ed.), New York: Hoeber, 1928, 1932; also Physiol Rev 4:533, 1974.
32. Custer RP: Borderlands dim in malignant disease of the blood forming organs. Radiology 61:764, 1953.
33. Custer RP: The changing pattern of lymphocytic malignancies. In: The lymphocyte and lymphocytic tissue. Rebuck JW (ed.), International Academy of Pathology Monograph, New York: Hoeber, 1960, p. 181.
34. Rappaport H, Winter WJ, Hicks EB: Follicular lymphoma: a reevaluation of its position in the scheme of malignant lymphoma, based on a survey of 253 cases. Cancer 9:792, 1956.
35. Dorfman RF: Enzyme histochemistry of normal, hyperplastic, and neoplastic lymphoreticular tissues. In: Symposium on lymphoreticular tumors in Africa. Basel/New York: S Karger, 1964.
36. Lukes RJ, Craver LF, Hall TC, Rappaport H, Ruben P: Report of the nomenclature committee. Cancer Res 26:1311, 1966.
37. Kay MMB, Kadin M: Surface characteristics of Hodgkin's cells. Lancet 1:748, 1975.
38. Kadin ME: Surface characteristics of Hodgkin's cells. Lancet 1:1008, 1975.
39. Kay MMB: Surface characteristics of Hodgkin's cells. Lancet 2:459, 1975.
40. Kay MMB: Hodgkin's disease: a war between T-lymphocytes and transformed macrophages? In: Recent results in cancer research, vol 56, lymphocytes, macrophages and cancer, Mathé G, Florentin I, Simmler MC (eds.), Berlin/New York: Springer-Verlag, 1976, p. 111.
41. Kaplan HS, Gartner S: 'Sternberg–Reed' giant cells of Hodgkin's disease: cultivation in vitro, heterotransplantation, and characterization as neoplastic macrophages. Int J Cancer 19:511, 1977.
42. Krueger GRF, Schaefer JE, Luetzeler J, Fischer R, Kresin V: Spontaneous variations in the cell population of a T-cell lymphoma during tissue culture and transplantation. Z Krebsforsch 84:25, 1975.
43. Catanzaro PJ, Graham RC Jr: Normal peritoneal lymphocytes. A population with increased capacity for endocytosis. Am J Pathol 77:23, 1974.
44. Kaplan HS: Hodgkin's disease: unfolding concepts concerning its nature, management and prognosis. Cancer 45:2439, 1980.

45. Log JC, Zamecnik PC, Aisenberg AC, Atkins L: Tissue culture studies in Hodgkin's disease. Morphologic, cytogenetic, cell surface, and enzymatic properties of cultures derived from splenic tumors. J Exp Med 145:1484, 1977.

46. Willson JKV Jr, Zaremba JL, Pretlow TG II: Functional characterization of cells separated from suspensions of Hodgkin's disease tumor cells in an isokinetic gradient. Blood 50:783, 1977.

47. Roberts AN, Smith KL, Dowell BL, Hubbard AK: Cultural, morphological, cell membrane, enzymatic, and neoplastic properties of cell lines derived from a Hodgkin's disease lymph node. Cancer Res 38:3033, 1978.

48. Harris NL, Gang DL, Quay SC, Poppema S, Zamecnik PC, Nelson-Rees WA, O'Brien SJ: Contamination of Hodgkin's disease cultures. Nature 284:228, 1981.

49. Desforges JF, Rutherford CJ, Piro A: Hodgkin's disease. N Engl J Med 301:1212, 1979.

50. Bucsky P: Origin of Hodgkin's and Reed–Sternberg cells. N Engl J Med 303:284, 1980.

51. Sinkovics JG, Shullenberger CC: Hodgkin's disease. Lancet 2:506, 1975.

52. Peiper SC, Kahn LB, Ross DW, Reddick RL: Ultrastructural organization of the Reed–Sternberg Cell: its resemblance to cells of the monocyte-macrophage system. Blood Cells 6:515, 1980.

53. Kadin ME: A reappraisal of the Reed–Sternberg Cell. A commentary. Blood Cells 6:525, 1980.

54. Kadin ME, Stites DP, Levy R, Warnke R: Exogenous immunoglobulin and the macrophage origin of Reed–Sternberg cells in Hodgkin's disease. N Engl J Med 299:1288, 1978.

55. Kadin ME, Gold S, Garratty EM, Stites DP: Immunological membrane markers of Hodgkin's cells. In: Modern trends in human leukemia II, Neth R, Gallo RC, Manweiler K, Maloney WC (eds.), Munich: JF Lehmanns, 1976, p. 229.

56. Tindle BH, Parker JW, Lukes RJ: 'Reed–Sternberg cells' in infectious mononucleosis? a report of eight cases. Am J Clin Pathol 58:607, 1972.

57. Taylor CR: The nature of Reed–Sternberg cells and other malignant cells. Lancet 2:802, 1974.

58. Taylor CR: An immunohistological study of follicular lymphoma, reticulum cell sarcoma and Hodgkin's disease. Eur J Cancer 12:61, 1976.

59. Taylor CR: Immunocytochemical methods in the study of lymphoma and related conditions. J Histochem Cytochem 26:495, 1978.

60. Garvin AJ, Spicer SS, Parmley RT, Munster AM: Immunohistochemical demonstration of IgG in Reed–Sternberg cells and other cells in Hodgkin's disease. J Exp Med 139:1077, 1974.

61. Landaas TO, Godal T, Halvorsen TB: Characterization of immunoglobulins in Hodgkin cells. Int J Cancer 28:717, 1977.

62. Papadimitriou CS, Stein H, Lennert K: The complexity of immunohistochemical staining pattern of Hodgkin and Sternberg–Reed cells – demonstration of immunoglobulin, albumin. alpha$_1$-antichymotrypsin and lysozyme. Int J Cancer 21:531, 1978.

63. Poppema S, Elema JD, Halie MR: The significance of intracytoplasmic proteins in Reed–Sternberg cells. Cancer 42:1793, 1978.

64. Morse HC II, Pumphrey JG, Potter M, Asofsky R: Murine plasma cells secreting more than one class of immunoglobulin heavy chain. I. Frequency of two or more M-components in ascitic fluids from 788 primary plasmacytomas. J Immunol 117:541, 1976.

65. Litwin SD, Lin PK, Hutteroth TH, Cleve H: Multiple heavy chain classes and light chain types on surfaces of cultured human lymphoid cells. Nature (New Biol) 246:179, 1973.

66. Bouvet JP, Buffe D, Oriol R, Liacopoulus P: Two myeloma globulins IgG1-kappa and IgG1-lambda from a single patient (Im). II. Their common cellular origin as revealed by immunofluorescence studies. Immunology 27:1095, 1974.

67. Oriol R, Huerta J, Bouvet JP, Liacopoulos P: Two myeloma globulins, IgG1-kappa and IgG1-

110

lambda, from a single patient (Im). I. Purification and immunochemical characterization. Immunology 27:1081, 1974.

68. Villiaumey J, Bouvet J-P, Menza C Di, Boccara M: Myélome plasmocytaire 'monoclonal' à deux paraprotéines, IgG kappa et IgG lambda. Nouv Presse Med 3:2707, 1974.

69. Preval C de, Fougereau M: Absence of preferential reassociation between heavy and light chains of two human immunoglobulins from common cellular origin. Biochem Biophys Res Commun 67:236, 1975.

70. Bernuau D, Feldmann G, Vorhauer W: Hodgkin's disease: ultrastructural localization of intra-cytoplasmic immunoglobulins within malignant cells. Br J Haematol 40:51, 1978.

71. Reynes M, Paczynski V, Galtier M. Diebold J: Ultrastructural and immunocytochemical localization of immunoglobulin synthesis in tumor cells in Hodgkin's disease. Int J Cancer 23:474, 1979.

72. Herva E, Ryhänen P, Blanco G, Järvenpää K, Helin H, Alavaikko M: Acid alpha-naphthyl acetate esterase (ANAE) activity and DNA synthesis of lymph node cells in Hodgkin's disease. Scand J Haematol 23:277, 1979.

73. Müller-Hermelink HK, Kaiserling E: Different reticulum cells of the lymph node: micro-ecological concept of lymphoid tissue organization. In: Malignant lymphomas, the pathophysiology of the lymphocyte and its neoplasms, Bosman F, van den Tweel J, Taylor CR (eds.). Leiden: Leiden University Press, 1980, p 57.

74. Stuart AE, Williams ARW, Habeshaw JA: Rosetting and other reactions of the Reed–Sternberg cell. J Pathol 122:81, 1977.

75. Stuart AE: The pathogenesis of Hodgkin's disease. J Pathol 126:239, 1978.

76. Payne SV, Newell DG, Jones DB, Wright DH: Reed-Sternberg cell/lymphocyte interaction. A non-specific adherence phenomenon. Br J Cancer 39:483, 1979.

77. McGuire RA, Pretlow TG, Wareing TH, Bradley EL: Hodgkin's cells and attached lymphocytes. A possible prognostic indicator in splenic tumor. Cancer 44:183, 1979.

78. Poppema S, Bhan AK, Reinherz EL, Posner MR, Schlossman SF: In situ immunological characterization of cellular constituents in lymph nodes and spleens involved by Hodgkin's disease. Blood 59:226, 1982.

79. Poppema S: The diversity of the immunohistological staining pattern of Sternberg–Reed cells. J Histochem Cytochem 28:788, 1980.

80. Curran RC, Jones EL: Hodgkin's disease: an immunohistochemical and histological study. J Pathol 125:39, 1978.

81. Stein H, Uchánska-Ziegler B, Gerdes J, Ziegler A, Wernet P: Hodgkin and Sternberg–Reed cells contain antigens specific to late cells of granulopoiesis. Int J Cancer 29:283, 1982.

82. Stein H, Gerdes J, Schwab U, Lemke H, Mason DY, Ziegler A, Schienle W, Diehl V: Identification of Hodgkin and Sternberg–Reed cells as a unique cell type derived from a newly-detected small-cell population. Int J Cancer 30:445, 1982.

83. Schwab U, Stein H, Gerdes J, Lemke H, Kirchner H, Schaadt M, Diehl V: Production of a monoclonal antibody specific for Hodgkin and Sternberg–Reed cells of Hodgkin's disease and a subset of normal lymphoid cells. Nature 299:65, 1982.

84. Schaadt M, Fonatsch C, Kirchner H, Diehl V: Establishment of a malignant, Epstein-Barr-virus (EBV)-negative cell-line from the pleura effusion of a patient with Hodgkin's disease. Blut 38:185, 1979.

85. Lewis MR: The behavior of Dorothy Reed cells in tissue culture. Am J Med Sci 201:467, 1941.

86. Modlin RL, Hofman FM, Taylor CR, Rea TH: T-lymphocyte subsets in the skin lesions of patients with leprosy. J Am Acad Dermatol 8:182, 1983.

87. Hofman FH, Yanagihara E, Byrne B, Billing R, Baird S, Frisman D, Taylor CR: Analysis of B cell antigens in normal reactive lymphoid tissue using four B cell monoclonal antibodies. (submitted for publication).

5. Selection of an imaging modality for staging abdominal involvement in the malignant lymphomas

Lymphography or computed tomography?

STEPHEN I. MARGLIN and RONALD A. CASTELLINO

1. Introduction

Since the introduction and enthusiastic acceptance of computed tomography (CT), a growing reluctance has emerged towards recommendations for the continued routine utilization of lymphography for the staging of Hodgkin's disease and non-Hodgkin's lymphomas. A number of arguments have been proffered, arguments ranging from adverse time considerations, to technical expertise, to patient preference, and extending ultimately to the all important differences in the sites imaged and the accuracies obtained. In attempting to explain our own approach towards this heterogeneous group of patients, we are constrained to acknowledge that what we propose represents personal opinion rather than irrefutable doctrine, i.e., it is an approach which seems to make sense to us, and which appears to work well in our hands. Because of acknowledged complexities surrounding the selection of an imaging modality, our approach may not be totally applicable to all departments of radiology and to all medical centers.

2. Comparison of imaging modalities

It would be desirable, both from a societal and from an individual patient's perspective, if questions regarding the selection of an imaging modality could be reduced to simple mathematical comparisons of accuracy. Intuitively, however, it is evident that those tests which are considered 'most accurate' are oftentimes not the test which we recommend or choose. Accuracy is, in a sense, a generic term . . . a term which encompasses at least five different facets of the performance of a given imaging system–observer interaction. If one considers a hypothetical test, as illustrated below, i.e., a test which is interpreted as either positive or negative and wherein the presence or absence of

Supported, in part, by Grant CA 05838, NCI.

Bennett JM (ed), Controversies in the Management of Lymphomas. ISBN 0-89838-586-5.
© *Martinus Nijhoff Publishers, Boston. Printed in the Netherlands.*

disease is established pathologically, the following parameters of accuracy can be defined [1].

Presence or absence of disease

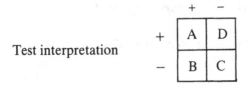

Test interpretation

Overall accuracy = the total number of correct diagnoses divided
  by the total number of patients examined = $(A + C) / (A + B + C + D)$
Sensitivity = number of true positive diagnoses divided by the number
  of patients in whom the disease is actually present =
  A divided by $A + B$
Specificity = number of true negative diagnoses divided by the number
  of patients in whom the disease is absent = C divided by $C + D$
Accuracy of a positive diagnosis = number of true positive diagnoses
  divided by the total number of cases interpreted as 'positive'
  or abnormal = $A / (A + D)$
Accuracy of a negative diagnosis = number of true negative diagnosis
  divided gy the total number of cases interpreted as 'negative'
  or normal = C divided by $B + C$

Reliance upon the single parameter 'overall accuracy' may be misleading, especially in situations where the prevalence of disease is either extremely high or extremely low. Consider, for example, a hypothetical clinical situation where 90% of the patients can be expected *not* to have the disease in question. If every examination in a sample group of 1000 patients were to be interpreted as negative, the entire subset of 100 diseased patients would go totally undetected, this despite the fact that the test would have achieved a 90% (900/1000) overall accuracy!

To deal with the problems associated with disease prevalence, the terms sensitivity and specificity have gained widespread clinical acceptance. Although as a refinement of the concept of 'accuracy' they do represent a more exact assessment of performance, they suffer from the fact that these parameters are not unique reflections of the capability of the methodology, but rather the end product of an interaction between the modality and a group of diagnosticians *using a given set of diagnostic criteria*. If those diagnostic criteria were to be changed, an elastic series of sensitivities and specificities would be produced, ranging fractionally from 0 to 1. When viewed graphically, the sensitivity or true positive fraction can be plotted as a function of the false positive fraction, i.e., D divided by $C + D$ or, its equivalent, 1 minus the specificity, to produce what is known as a receiver operating characteristic (ROC) curve (Fig. 1) [2]. One axiom which this form of depiction tends to emphasize is the fact that when one seeks to increase the sensitivity of the test, i.e., to detect a greater number of diseased patients, an implicit requirement is a likely increase in the number of false positive diagnoses.

ROC curves have been championed for their objectivity and for their ability to assist in the evaluation of competing imaging modalities. If we were to plot ROC curves for two hypothetical forms of abdominal and pelvic lymph node imaging (Fig. 2) it would 'appear' that test A is the test of choice ... i.e., for every level of true positivity, the price paid, i.e., the percentage of false positive diagnoses is less for test A than for test B.

'Appear' is the key word. ROC curves, as elegant as they may seem to some, suffer from a number of serious deficits. They do not, for example, answer the question of whether the test should be done at all. If the incidence of tumor involvement is known to be low, one could easily envision a logical decision not to image. Alternatively, if the incidence of tumor involvement is sizable, and yet it seems unlikely that the results of the test would alter the contemplated therapy, the test should probably be eschewed ... no matter how compelling the anticipated level of accuracy. ROC analysis largely ignores the preferences of the patient. Although autopsies and/or surgical exploration are, generally speaking, both more accurate than almost any form of medical imaging, no sane patient would select the former, and few, if any, the latter, without serious consideration of alternative diagnostic strategies. Lastly, ROC analysis, if it works at all, works best in situations where the tests to be

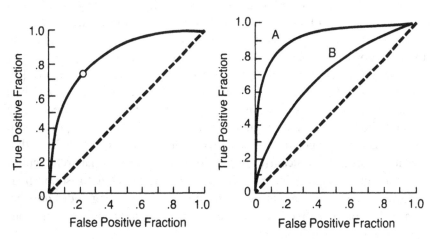

Figure 1 (left). Standard ROC curve, with one point representing the test's 'accuracy' utilizing a single diagnostic decision criterion.
Figure 2 (right). ROC curves for two competing imaging modalities A and B. For every level of diagnostic detection, the incidence of false positive diagnoses is greater for test B than for test A.

compared interrogate precisely the same areas of interest. How to contrast the performance of lymphography, a test which accurately evaluates those lymph nodes which lie adjacent to the aorta, inferior vena cava, as well as the common and external iliac arteries and veins [3], with computed tomography, a modality which surveys the *entire* abdomen and pelvis [4, 5, 6, 7, 8], perhaps with somewhat lesser degrees of accuracy in those nodes opacified by lymphography, is somewhat analogous to the question of which is more desirable, apples or oranges. We make decisions like this all the time ... it's just hard to explain precisely why or how.

3. Lymphography and computed tomography

Although modalities such as excretory urography, gallium scanning and ultrasound, amongst others, have experienced limited periods of enthusiasm in the history of lymph node evaluation, it is probably safe to conclude that the current role of most of these techniques is at best adjunctive. At the time of this writing, the crux of the decision between modalities for assessing abdominal lymph nodes represents a choice between lymphography and computed tomography.

Lymphography, the more established lymph node imaging technique, was first employed as a clinical tool in the mid-1950s, utilizing water soluble contrast media. Within several years Ethiodol®, an oily contrast medium, replaced water soluble agents, thereby permitting both improved visualization of nodal architecture as well as periodic re-imaging over many months and years by virtue of prolonged lumph node retention of the contrast medium. Ethiodol® bathes the sinusoids of lymph nodes with little, if any, incorporation into either normal lymphoid follicles or lymphoid tissue deranged by tumor. The resultant image is a very precise registration of nodal architecture [9]. Evaluation, as is the case with virtually all radiologic examinations, involves an in-depth appreciation of the ranges of normal and an ability to detect subtle deviations from the norm. Although some have emphasized the importance of both the size and the position of opacified nodes, we and others believe that these attributes are significantly less important than the internal architectural appearance of the nodes. Generally speaking, we are reluctant to ascribe great significance to what we cannot see, e.g., to normal appearing nodes *possibly* displaced by non-opacified nodal masses, or to elongated gaps between nodes which appear intrinsically normal.

As indicated earlier, lymphography only opacifies lymph nodes adjacent to the aorta, the inferior vena cava, and the common and external iliac arteries and veins. Although nodes in the femoral/inguinal region are also routinely opacified, we rarely interpret these nodes due to their high incidence of midleading benign reactive changes. Lymphography rarely opacifies lymph nodes cephalad to the level of the renal vascular pedicle, i.e., above L-2.

However high the published accounts of the accuracy of lymphography [3, 10, 11, 12], it is important to recognize that many areas of the abdomen are not interrogated by this technique, areas which include lymph node sites higher than the level of L-2, especially those nodes which lie behind the crux of the diaphragm; nodes adjacent to the spleen, liver, and kidneys; nodes in the mesentery; as well as abdominal organs, e.g., the spleen, liver, pancreas and kidneys.

Some non-statistical parameters of lymphography and computed tomography are presented in Table 1. Without belaboring the obvious, two facets of lymphography are worthy of somewhat greater elaboration. With effort and modest technical aptitude, it is possible for most individuals to master the technical aspects of lymphatic cannulation. This ability notwithstanding, it is also important to acknowledge that lymphatic cannulation may be tedious and time consuming, and can occasionally be quite difficult. For these reasons, many radiologists are distinctly disinclined to perform this examination, especially so since the advent of computed tomography. As the frequency of performance declines, and it would appear to be doing so, the interpretive aspects of lymphography will presumably become more difficult. It is unlikely that a reluctant radiologist who performs this examination infrequently will be able to achieve the high degrees of accuracy which have been reported in the literature, most commonly from medical centers with large cancer populations. The issue of local expertise is significant and must somehow be integrated into management strategies, either to refer patients to centers with high levels of expertise or to perform other, possibly 'less accurate' forms of imaging.

A second important facet of lymphography relates to both follow-up and cost. Because Ethiodol® is retained within the lymphatic sinusoids for upwards of 12–24 months, it is possible to periodically obtain an abdominal radiograph either to evaluate response to treatment or to detect possible nodal relapse [13, 14]. Lymphography *must* be viewed as a dynamic examination,

Table 1. Comparative parameters of lymphography and computed tomography.

	Lymphography	Computed tomography
Skill	Moderate	Minimal
Cost	Moderate for initial exam	Moderate for initial exam
	Minimal for follow-up exam	and for every follow-up exam
Areas imaged	Retroperitoneal nodes below L-2	Entire abdomen and pelvis

i.e., as one whose value is not just related to the initial study, but as one whose value persists for as long as contrast remains detectable within the nodes. Although some centers have expressed pessimism regarding the value of post-lymphography abdominal films [15], we believe this pessimism to be both unfounded and unfortunate. There are distinct physical and financial advantages to following patients with serial abdominal films vis-à-vis serial computed tomographic scans ... the cost is approximately one tenth, the time required is miniscule and neither oral, rectal nor most importantly intravenous contrast is required.

Unlike lymphography, wherein only limited, albeit important, groups of lymph nodes are evaluated, computed tomography has the capability of visualizing virtually all portions of the abdomen and pelvis. The examination is not technically difficult to perform and the images obtained are readily understood and 'accepted' by most clinicians. In contradistinction to lymphography, for which the literature is replete with extensive and carefully designed studies evaluating the accuracy of this technique, equally compulsive studies of the accuracy of computed tomography are notably less numerous.

While lymphography images the fine architectural interstices of opacified nodes, and while interpretation of lymphograms relies upon alterations in internal architecture as a criteria for establishing malignant involvement, computed tomography uses as its only criteria for nodal involvement an increase in lymph node size. Lymph nodes which are normal in size and which contain macroscopic foci of tumor, nodes whose tumor deposition is theoretically detectable by lymphography, would be regarded as normal by computed tomography. The problem is especially relevant to Hodkin's disease, wherein involved nodes may be normal in size or, at times, only modestly enlarged. The converse of this size-related issue is also relevant, i.e., nodes which are increased in size because of benign conditions such as reactive hyperplasia may be correctly recognized as benign by lymphography [10, 16, 17]; these same nodes, however, because they are enlarged, are often judged to contain tumor on the basis of CT criteria.

Lymphography has been utilized successfully in directing surgical oncologists towards the biopsy of *specific* nodes at the time of staging laparotomy [11, 18]. The accuracy of this sampling procedure can be enhanced when intra-operative films are obtained, although such filming is not routinely required. Nodes which are felt to be suspicious on computed tomography are, by definition, abnormally large and are therefore presumably easier to locate. One hopes that this is the case, since there is, at present, no current capability for providing direct intra-operative assistance utilizing CT.

Cost is a factor which is unfortunately rarely integrated into decisions regarding selection of an imaging modality. As mentioned earlier, it is important to recognize that although the cost of an abdominal and pelvic CT is commensurate with the cost of lymphography, the cost of following patients may be many hundreds of dollars less with post-lymphographic abdominal films than with repeated computed tomographic examinations.

4. Hodgkin's disease

The group of diseases which bears the name 'malignant lymphomas' represents a distinctly heterogeneous group of diseases ... diseases with different forms of initial expression and diseases with predictably different forms of biological behavior. Hodgkin's disease, for example, is generally presumed to originate within an isolated nodal focus thereafter, progressing in a predictable 'step-wise' fashion [19]. When patients with presumed supra-diaphragmatic involvement were treated with involved field radiotherapy, alone, relapses were generally noted to occur within the abdomen, usually within either the spleen or within para-aortic lymph nodes. This observation led to the hypothesis of the contiguous spread of Hodgkin's disease and led the Stanford group to suggest the potential importance of surgically staging patients with this disease [18]. Much of the knowledge which we currently possess regarding the behavior of Hodgkin's disease is directly related to the championship of staging laparotomies, as in investigational tool, at Stanford and to the extensive series of carefully controlled clinical trials performed at that institution.

Information obtained from staging laparotomy in a consecutive group of newly diagnosed, previously untreated patients with Hodgkin's disease is presented in Table 2 and is contrasted with comparable data for patients with non-Hodgkin's lymphoma [11, 19-22]. Patients with Hodgkin's disease, unlike their counterparts with non-Hodgkin's lymphoma, rarely exhibit involvement of mesenteric nodes at the time of presentation; if those nodes are involved, it is uncommon for them to be overtly enlarged. Pathologic involvement of retroperitoneal nodes may or may not be associated with nodal enlargement.

Prior to the advent of ultrasound and computed tomography, lymphography

Table 2. Infradiaphragmatic involvement encountered at staging laparotomy in previously untreated patients.

	HD		NHL	
	Adult	Child	Adult	Child
Para-aortic nodes	34%	19%	55%	30%
Mesenteric nodes	<5%		>50%	
Spleen	34%		33%	
Liver	6%		14%	

was accepted as the most accurate form of abdominal lymph node imaging. This persuasion was based upon extensive data, data exemplified by a recently published article which details our experience with 632 consecutive patients with newly presenting Hodgkin's disease and non-Hodgkin's lymphoma [3]. The results of this report are presented in Table 3.

For patients with Hodgkin's disease a negative lymphographic interpretation provides an extraordinarily high likelihood (98%) that the retroperitoneal nodes will be found to be histopathologically free of tumor. Lymphograms which are overtly positive, i.e., with nodes which are enlarged and which exhibit marked derangements in their internal architecture, also provide high likelihood of malignant involvement. Those lymphograms which demonstrate either normal size or slightly enlarged nodes, and which exhibit small filling defects or only slight derangements in internal architecture, are obviously more difficult to interpret. These are the examinations which account, in large part, for the 8% error rate ... the bulk of which represents false positive diagnoses attributed to reactive hyperplasia or partial nodal replacement by fat and/or fibrosis. Few other radiographic examinations, in other clinical settings, have been evaluated so thoroughly as has lymphography in this disease, or have performed so well.

Data similar to that which we have presented for lymphography, i.e., data based upon rigorously controlled clinical trials, has not yet been extensively developed for computed tomography. Although some initial reports have expressed enthusiasm [4-6, 23-31], many have been flawed by a lack of pathological correlation and/or by processes of patient selection which introduced unacceptable bias. Quite clearly the demands placed upon an imaging modality are less severe when patients are at advanced stages of evolution or

Table 3.

		Biopsy results								
		HD			NHL			Total		
		+	−		+	−		+	−	
LAG	+	100	25	+	101	14	+	201	39	
	−	7	284	−	13	88	−	20	372	

	HD	NHL	Total
Sensitivity	93%	89%	91%
Specificity	92%	86%	91%
Accuracy of pos. dx.	80%	88%	84%
Accuracy of neg. dx.	98%	87%	95%
Overall accuracy	92%	88%	91%

when patients are known to be in relapse, than when all patients are newly presenting and untreated. One study which attempts to resolve the issue of the comparative accuracies of CT and lymphography in the evaluation of abdominal and pelvic lymph nodes is an extension of our earlier investigation of the accuracy of lymphography alone. In the current study, consecutive, unselected, newly diagnosed and untreated patients with Hodgkin's disease and non-Hodgkin's lymphoma are evaluated with both lymphography and computed tomography. Within 14 days, unless precluded by medical contraindications or pathologically confirmed stage IV disease, a staging laparotomy is performed. The preliminary results of this head-to-head comparison, for patients with Hodgkin's disease, are presented in Table 4. In this series of 80 patients, lymphography performed slightly better than CT in both overall accuracy, as well as in sensitivity and specificity.

Despite the apparent, albeit slight, superiority of lymphography over CT in assessing retroperitoneal nodal involvement, we would emphasize again that as many as 40% of patients with Hodgkin's disease are know to have splenic involvement at the time of presentation, an organ totally excluded from lymphographic interrogation. This fact, in combination with a quest for occult liver involvement, has served as the impelling rationale for continued emphasis upon routine staging laparotomy. One might have hoped that computed tomography would possess greater ability in evaluating the spleen and the liver than that achieved by other current imaging modalities. Data which attempts to answer this question, again from Stanford, is presented in Table 5. *For interest,* an analysis of the potential value of lymphography in predicting splenic or liver involvement is also presented [32]. In these calculations, lymphograms interpreted as positive were 'extrapolated' to the catagory 'spleen positive' while those interpreted as negative were 'extrapolated' as 'spleen negative.' One readily apparent feature of the data presented in Table 5 is that although computed tomography achieves sensitivities and specificities comparable to previously tested modalities, e.g., nuclear medicine or ultrasound, its accuracy is not yet sufficient to exclude splenic involvement by Hodgkin's disease. In point of fact, computed tomography appears to be less

Table 4. Lymphography/computed tomography/laparotomy correlation for patients with Hodgkin's disease.

| | Retroperitoneal nodes | | Mesenteric nodes |
	LAG	CT	CT
Sensitivity	14/17 = 82%	13/17 = 76%	Only one positive
Specificity	60/60 = 100%	57/63 = 90%	biopsy in 66 patients,
Accuracy	74/77 = 96%	70/80 = 88%	and that was missed by CT

Table 5. Lymphography/computed tomography/laparotomy correlation for patients with Hodgkin's disease.

	Spleen		Liver	
	CT	LAG	CT	LAG
Sensitivity	$23/38 = 61\%$	$58/94 = 62\%$	$1/6 = 17\%$	$14/18 = 78\%$
Specificity	$36/49 = 73\%$	$111/139 = 80\%$	$80/80 = 100\%$	$143/215 = 67\%$
Accuracy	$59/87 = 68\%$	$169/233 = 73\%$	$81/86 = 94\%$	$157/233 = 67\%$

accurate in almost every parameter than the inference drawn from the results of lymphography.

A similar analysis of the data for liver involvement by Hodgkin's disease underscores current problems to be expected from unrealistic reliance upon the results of computed tomography. Although the overall accuracy of this technique is 'high' in evaluating the liver, this statistical aberration is largely a reflection of the relatively low frequency with which hepatic involvement occurs in this disease.

Vermess and associates at the NIH have recently reported on experimental clinical trials with an intravenous contrast agent, EOE-13, an emulsified iodinated ester of poppy seed oil, specifically designed to opacify the spleen and liver [33]. Although reported experience to date is limited, this approach appears promising for increasing the accuracy of computed tomography in the evaluation of the liver and spleen.

Some investigators have recently suggested the importance of further characterizing patients with stage III Hodgkin's disease, in order to identify those patients whose apparently adverse prognosis might argue for primary treatment with chemotherapy [34]. Although an analysis of the data from Stanford does not substantiate the belief that patients with sub-stage III_2A disease do less well than those with sub-stage III_1A [35], should this suggestion ultimately prove to be correct, the importance of precise, anatomically specific, diagnoses would be even greater. Given the data presented, and acknowledging that our experience may not be universally applicable, our current recommendations for radiographic staging of Hodgkin's disease are presented in Table 6. Lymphography continues to represent the most accurate modality for deciding whether Hodgkin's disease is present within the abdomen, in general, and within the retroperitoneal nodes, in particular. It is helpful in planning and performing staging laparotomies and invaluable in the periodic reassessment of the patients under treatment. If patients with stage III_2A disease are to be treated differently than those with more limited disease, we would prefer to place our reliance more upon lymphography, i.e., upon a technique which permits informed judgements of nodes which are

Table 6. Imaging strategy for patients with Hodgkin's disease.

Initial presentation	Lymphography >computed tomography both if possible
Follow-up	Post-lymphographic abdominal film
Diagnostic dilemma	Computed tomography (if post-lymphographic abdominal film not helpful)
Re-staging	1. Post-lymphographic abdominal film 2. Computed tomography 3. Repeat lymphogram, if inadequate contrast remains and CT not diagnostic

normal in size, than upon computed tomography. Because lymphography fails to assess high retroperitoneal and retrocrural nodes, and because it does not provide direct information regarding the status of the liver and spleen, we would also recommend obtaining a CT examination at the time of initial presentation. One might argue for deleting CT in instances where the lymphogram is clearly positive. The risk of so doing relates, in part, to potential mistakes in radiotherapy planning and to the loss of a potentially important baseline for further analysis. Once the retroperitoneal nodes are opacified, we would choose to monitor the patient's subsequent course with periodic abdominal films. Presuming that the patient is asymptomatic or presuming that initially abnormal appearing nodes show improvement while treatment continues, abdominal films will generally suffice. There should, however, be absolutely no reluctance to obtaining CT assessments, if clinical symptoms suggest recurrence and if postlymphographic abdominal films fail to give convincing evidence of same.

For patients treated with chemotherapy, a frequently asked question and a frequently vexing dilemma is whether the prescribed number of courses of chemotherapy is 'adequate'. Imaging to answer this problem is best performed with a combination of computed tomography and plain abdominal films ... lymphography can be repeated with no greater difficulty than that related to the initial examination, if there is insufficient residual contrast to permit diagnostic certainty [36, 37].

5. Non-Hodgkin's lymphoma

The analysis which we employed for selecting an imaging examination for patients with Hodgkin's disease is roughly the same that we propose to utilize for patients with non-Hodgkin's lymphoma. Whereas in Hodgkin's disease involvement of mesenteric nodes is relatively uncommon, i.e., less than 5%, this site can be anticipated to be involved in at least 50% of newly presenting patients with non-Hodgkin's lymphoma [11, 38, 39] (Table 2). For those whose histologies are classified as 'nodular' the rate of involvement may be as high as 70%. Patients with non-Hodgkin's lymphoma are almost twice as likely to experience hepatic involvement at the time of presentation than those with Hodgkin's disease; involvement of the bone marrow is similarly also more common in non-Hodgkin's lymphoma than in Hodgkin's disease. This preponderance of widespread disease at the time of presentation has prompted many oncologists to propose a need for systemic forms of therapy in this disease, except in well documented instances of surgically confirmed localized disease. If this persuasion is correct, radiographic imaging for non-Hodgkin's lymphoma may ultimately be more important as an indicator of response to therapy than as a factor in the selection of a particular form of therapy.

Table 3 presents an analysis of lymphographic accuracy in 216 patients with non-Hodgkin's lymphomas. Table 7, on the other hand, presents the results of a smaller (24 patients), more recent, head-to-head comparison of the ability of lymphography and computed tomography to detect nodal metastases. Although the number of patients is small, and the results roughly comparable, lymphography may still possess a slight edge.

The role of computed tomography *vis-à-vis* lymphography for patients with non-Hodgkin's lymphoma has been championed by some because of CT's presumed ability to assess potential mesenteric lymph node involvement. This ability in an unselected group of newly presenting patients with non-Hodgkin's lymphoma has not been extensively tested. Data from Stanford are compared in Table 8 with a prior analysis in which predictions were made on the basis of the results of the lymphogram [32]. As was the case previously, lymphograms

Table 7. Non-Hodgkin's lymphomas. Evaluation of retroperitonealnodes.

		Biopsy results				
		+	−		+	−
Lymphography	+	14	2		12	6	+ CT
	−	0	6		2	2	−

	Lymphography	CT
Sensitivity	100%	86%
Specificity	75%	75%
Accuracy of pos. dx.	88%	86%
Accuracy of neg. dx.	100%	75%
Overall accuracy	91%	82%

Table 8. Non-Hodgkin's lymphomas. Evaluation for mesenteric adenopathy.

Biopsy results

		+	−		+	−		
CT	+	10	2		32	16	+	Lymphography
	−	5	6		5	24	−	

	CT	Lymphography
Sensitivity	67%	86%
Specificity	75%	60%
Accuracy of pos. dx.	83%	67%
Accuracy of neg. dx.	55%	83%
Overall accuracy	70%	73%

interpreted as positive were 'extrapolated' to the 'mesenteric adenopathy present' category and lymphograms interpreted as negative were 'extrapolated' to the 'mesenteric adenopathy absent' category. Although the numbers are admittedly small, two points appear to warrant some degree of emphasis. First, computed tomography detected only 67% of the surgically proven cases of mesenteric involvement. Second, a negative CT determination carried with it only a 55% likelihood of being correct.

Involvement of the spleen by non-Hodgkin's lymphoma occurs with roughly the same frequency as that which occurs in patients with Hodgkin's disease; the incidence of liver involvement is somewhat higher (Table 2). The ability of CT to detect splenic and hepatic involvement in an unselected, untreated group of patients has also not be extensively evaluated. Our own data is presented in Table 9. Analysis of this data tends to emphasize the relative insensitivity of computed tomography to the presence of splenic involvement in this disease. Although the data for CT detection of liver involvement would appear, at first glance, to suggest acceptable levels of accuracy, this impression, as was the case for CT in patients with Hodgkin's disease, is more a reflection of the infrequency of hepatic involvement than of the accuracy of the test under consideration.

Based upon information concerning the predilection of non-Hodgkin's lymphoma for specific nodal and non-nodal sites, and based upon the results of clinical experiments designed to test the accuracy of lymphography and computed tomography in defining these sites of involvement, we have adopted certain recommendations regarding the radiographic evaluation of newly presenting patients with non-Hodgkin's lymphoma (Table 10). As mentioned in other segments of this chapter, these approaches may not be fully applicable

Table 9. Evaluation of spleen and liver in non-Hodgkin's lymphoma.

Spleen

CT

	+	−
+	5	2
−	6	10

Lymphography

	+	−	
	33	31	+
	6	47	−

Liver

CT

	+	−
+	2	0
−	1	21

Lymphography

	+	−	
	22	42	+
	0	53	−

Non-Hodgkin's lymphoma

	Spleen		Liver	
	CT	LAG	CT	LAG
Sensitivity	45%	85%	67%	100%
Specificity	83%	60%	100%	56%
Accuracy of pos. dd.	71%	52%	100%	34%
Accuracy of neg. dx.	63%	89%	95%	100%
Overall accuracy	65%	68%	96%	64%

Table 10. Imaging strategy for patients with non-Hodgkin's lymphoma.

Initial presentation	Computed tomography >lymphography both if possible
Follow-up	Post-lymphographic abdominal film
Diagnostic dilemma	Computed tomography (if post-lymphographic abdominal film not helpful)
Re-staging	1. Post-lymphographic abdominal film 2. Computed tomography 3. Repeat lymphogram (?) if insufficient contrast remains

to all individuals and to all medical centers. In instances where lymphography is rarely performed and where interpretive confidence in this examination is low, lymphography should probably be eschewed in favor of computed tomography.

If we were restricted to the choice of a single imaging modality for the staging of non-Hodgkin's lymphoma, we would favor computed tomography

... this choice based upon the greater scope of the modality, the larger size of the nodes, when involved, and the greater likelihood of detectable mesenteric involvement. If radiotherapy of bulk disease is contemplated, the rationale for selecting computed tomography would seem to be even stronger. To facilitate follow up and to lessen the financial burden for the patient, we would also recommend that lymphography be performed. As was suggested for patients with Hodgkin's disease, we have absolutely no bias against, nor disinclination to perform, computed tomography, should questions regarding the efficacy of therapy be difficult to resolve with post-lymphographic abdominal films. It should be noted, however, that these situations represent more the exception than the rule. Re-staging, i.e., decisions regarding the need for either more or different forms of therapy, is best performed with a combination of both computed tomography and post-lymphographic abdominal films.

At this juncture one point of caution is perhaps warranted. Residually discernible nodal abnormality, in previously involved nodes, following the completion of a prescribed course of therapy, should not *automatically* be accepted as an indicator of viable tumor [40, 41, 42]. Residual nodal masses may also represent sterilized tumor and/or fibrosis. For this reason, if critical treatment options are being selected on the basis of nodal size, serious consideration should be given to the possibility of histologic verification.

6. Summary

The recommendations which we have formulated for the initial abdominal imaging of patients with Hodgkin's disease and non-Hodgkin's lymphoma are based upon a large body of data ... data which describes the anticipated frequency of disease involvement in differing anatomical sites, as well as data concerning the accuracy of lymphography and computed tomography in interrogating these sites. Data regarding accuracy, especially those which relate to lymphography, are not unique to our experience at Stanford and have been reported from a number of other medical centers [12]. They may not, however, apply to all hospitals and/or all departments of radiology. Ultimately the choice of an imaging modality is an individual decision, one which must take cognizance of such intangibles as local expertise, the quality of equipment, patient preferences, etc. In order to function intelligently in this arena it is incumbent upon clinicians to maintain flexibility and to continually attempt to establish currency with refinements and improvements in imaging modalities, especially newer forms of lymph node imaging. Computed tomography and/or some yet unanticipated form of lymph node imaging may ultimately eliminate the need for lymphography. For the time being, however, we view the predictions of the demise of lymphography as being both unwise and unwarranted.

126

References

1. McNeil BJ, Keeler E, Adelstein SJ: Primer in certain elements of medical decision making. N Engl J Med 293:211–215, 1975.
2. Metz CA: Basic principles of ROC analysis. Sem Nucl Med 8:283, 1978.
3. Marglin S, Castellino R: Lymphographic accuracy in 632 consecutive, previously untreated cases of Hodgkin's disease and non-Hodgkin's lymphoma. Radiology 140:351–353, 1981.
4. Alcorn FS, Mategrano VC, Petnasnick JP, Clark JW: Contributions of computed tomography in the staging and management of malignant lymphoma. Radiology 125:717, 1977.
5. Best JJK, Blackledge G, Forbes WStC, et al.: Computed tomography of abdomen in staging and clinical management of lymphoma. Br Med J 2:1675, 1978.
6. Blackledge G, Best JJK, Crowther D, Isherwood I: Computed tomography in the staging of patients with Hodgkin's disease: a report on 136 patients. Clin Radiol 31:143, 1980.
7. Zornoza J, Ginaldi S: Computed tomography in hepatic lymphoma. Radiology 138:405, 1981.
8. Rubin BE: Computed tomography in the evaluation of renal lymphoma. J Comput Assist Tomogr 3:759, 1979.
9. Tjernberg B: Lymphography: an animal study in the diagnosis of V x 2 carcinoma and inflammation. Acta Radiol (suppl) 214:1–184, 1962.
10. Castellino RA, Billingham M, Dorfman RF: Lymphographic accuracy in Hodgkin's disease and malignant lymphoma with a note on the 'reactive' lymph node as a cause of most false-positive lymphograms. Invest Radiol 9:155, 1974.
11. Goffinet DR, Warnke R, Dunnick NR, et al.: Clinical and surgical evaluation of patients with non-Hodgkin's lymphomas. Cancer Treat Rep 61:981, 1977.
12. Kademian M, Wirtanen G: Accuracy of bipedal lymphography in Hodgkin's disease. AJR 129:1041, 1977.
13. Fabian CE, Nudelman EJ, Abrams HL: Post-lymphangiogram films as an indication of tumor activity in lymphoma. Invest Radiol 1:386, 1966.
14. Castellino RA, Blank N, Cassady JR, Kaplan HS: Roentgenologic aspects of Hodgkin's disease. II. Role of routine radiographs in detecting initial relapse. Cancer 31:316–323, 1973.
15. Lee JKT, Stanley RJ, Sagel SS, Melson GL, Koehler RE: Limitations of the post-lymphangiogram plain abdominal radiograph as an indicator of recurrent lymphoma: comparison to computed tomography. Radiology 134:155, 1980.
16. Castellino RA: Observations on 'reactive (follicular) hyperplasia' as encountered in repeat lymphography in the lymphomas. Cancer 34:2042–2050, 1974.
17. Parker BR, Blank N, Castellino RA: Lymphographic appearance of benign conditions simulating lymphoma. Radiology 111:267–274, 1974.
18. Glatstein E, Trueblood HW, Enright LP, et al.: Surgical staging of abdominal involvement in unselected patients with Hodgkin's disease. Radiology 97:425–432, November 1970.
19. Kaplan HS: Hodgkin's disease. Cambridge: Harvard University Press, 1979.
20. Kadin ME, Glatstein EJ, Dorfman RE: Clinicopathologic studies in 117 untreated patients subjected to laparotomy for the staging of Hodgkin's disease. Cancer 27:1277, 1971.
21. Castellino RA, Bellani FF, Gasparini M, Musumeci R: Radiographic findings in previously untreated children with non-Hodgkin's lymphoma. Radiology 117:657–663, 1975.
22. Castellino RA, Musumeci R, Markovits P: Lymphography. In: Pediatric oncologic radiology, Parker BR, Castellino RA (eds). St. Louis: CV Mosby, 1977.
23. Breiman RS, Castellino RA, Harell GS, Marshall WH, Glatstein E, Kaplan HS: CT – pathologic correlations in Hodgkin's disease and non-Hodgkin's lymphoma. Radiology 126:159, 1978.

24. Jones SE, Tobias DA, Waldman RS: Computed tomographic scanning in patients with lymphoma. Cancer 41:480, 1978.

25. Schaner EG, Head GL, Doppman JL, Young RC: Computed tomography in the diagnosis, staging and management of abdominal lymphoma. J Comput Assist Tomogr 1:176, 1977.

26. Lee JKT, Stanley RJ, Sagel SS, Levitt RG: Accuracy of computed tomography in detecting intraabdominal and pelvic adenopathy in lymphoma. Am J Roentgenol 131:311, 1978.

27. Harell GS, Breiman RS, Glatstein EJ, Marshall WH, Castellino RA: Computed tomography of the abdomen in the malignant lymphoma. Radiol Clin North Am 15:391, 1977.

28. Ellert J, Kreel L: The role of computed tomography in the initial staging and subsequent management of the lymphomas. J Comput Assist Tomogr 4:368, 1980.

29. Castellino RA, Noon M, Carroll BA, et al.: Lymphography, computed tomography and ultrasound in staging Hodgkin's disease and non-Hodgkin's lymphoma. Progress in lymphology. Proceedings of the 7th International Congress of Lymphology, Weissleder H, Bartos V, Clodius L, Malek P (eds), 1981.

30. Earl HM, Sutcliffe SBJ, Kelsey Fry I, Tucker AK, Young J, Husband J, Wrigley PFM, Malpas JS: Computerised tomographic abdominal scanning in Hodgkin's disease. Clin Radiol 31:149, 1980.

31. Crowther D, Blackledge G, Best JK: The role of computed tomography of the abdomen in the diagnosis and staging of patients with lymphoma. Clin Haematol 8:567, 1979.

32. Castellino R, et al., unpublished.

33. Vermess M, Doppman JL, Sugarbaker MD, et al.: Clinical trials with a new intravenous liposoluble contrast material for computed tomography of the liver and spleen. Radiology 137:217, 1980.

34. Golomb HM, Sweet DL, Ultmann JE, Miller JB, Kinzie JJ, Gordon LI: Importance of substaging of stage III Hodgkin's disease. Semin Oncol 7:136, 1980.

35. Hoppe RT: Radiation therapy in the treatment of Hodgkin's disease. Semin Oncol 7:144, 1980.

36. Castellino RA, Fuks Z, Blank N, Kaplan HS: Roentgenologic aspects of Hodgkin's disease: repeat lymphangiography. Radiology 109:53–58, 1973.

37. Dunnick NR, Fuks Z, Castellino RA: Repeat lymphography in non-Hodgkin's lymphoma. Radiology 115:349–354, 1975.

38. Goffinet DR, Castellino RA, Dorfman L, Kim H, Fuks Z, Rosenberg SA, Nelson T, Kaplan HS: Staging laparotomies in unselected patients with non-Hodgkin's lymphomas. Cancer 32:672–681, September 1973.

39. Castellino RA, Goffinet DR, Blank N, Parker BR, Kaplan HS: The role of radiography in the staging of non-Hodgkin's lymphoma with laparotomy correlation. Radiology 110:329–338, 1973.

40. Lewis E, Bernadino ME, Salvador PG, Cabanillas FF, Barnes PA, Thomas JL: Post-therapy CT-detected mass in lymphoma patients: is it viable tissue? J Comput Assist Tomogr 6:792–795, 1982.

41. Markovits P, Blanche R, Charbit A: Radiologic aspects of lymphangiography after chemotherapy for malignant lymphomas. Anatomic-radiologic correlations. Ann Radiol 13:539–558, 1970.

42. Markovits P, Blanche LR, Gasquet C, Charbit A: Radiologic appearance of lymphograms performed after radiotherapy. Ann Radiol 12:835–847, 1969.

6. The definitive management of limited and intermediate stages of Hodgkin's disease with radiation therapy alone

RICHARD T. HOPPE

1. Introduction

Advances in pathology, staging, and treatment of Hodgkin's disease have provided for a dramatic improvement in patient prognosis during the past three decades [1]. With current treatment programs, the majority of patients with all stages of Hodgkin's disease may now be cured. For patients with limited or intermediate stages of Hodgkin's disease (I–IIA/B, and favorable IIIA) initial treatment may be with irradiation alone and the majority of these patients will be cured. The realization of a high degree of success in the management of these patients, however, is dependent upon precise staging and careful attention to every detail of patient management. This chapter will review the essentials for the development of an effective program of curative irradiation treatment for patients wth limited or intermediate stages of Hodgkin's disease. It will daw primarily upon the Stanford experience in discussions of staging, treatment techniques, complications, and outcome.

2. Staging considerations

The Ann Abor staging system has been applied successfully to patients with Hodgkin's disease [2]. It provides prognostic information and helps define appropriate treatment programs. Both the stage (I–IV) and the presence of constitutional (B) symptoms influence treatment choice. The concept of 'bulk of disease', not included in the Ann Arbor system, is nevertheless important, since patients with bulky masses require very individualized therapy.

The Ann Arbor system defines both a clinical stage (CS) and pathologic stage (PS). The CS is based on the sites of disease identified by the initial diagnostic biopsy(-ies), physical examination, and radiographic studies. The PS includes results of all subsequent biopsies such as bone marrow biopsy or staging laparotomy and splenectomy.

Routine staging studies should include a thorough history and physical.

Bennett JM (ed), Controversies in the Management of Lymphomas. ISBN 0-89838-586-5.
© *Martinus Nijhoff Publishers, Boston. Printed in the Netherlands.*

complete hemogram, platelet count, and serum chemistries. The erythrocyte sedimentation rate and serum copper are measured since they may be useful indications of disease activity in individual patients. Radiographic studies include a PA and lateral chest X-ray. If any abnormality is noted on the chest X-ray further radiographic examinations should be obtained to define the extent of disease. Hilar oblique tomograms are useful to detect hilar lymph node enlargement [3] and thoracic CT scanning is helpful both to identify pulmonary parenchymal disease and to define the extent of intrathoracic disease as an aid to radiation treatment planning [4].

Subdiaphragmatic sites are evaluated by bipedal lymphography and abdominal–pelvic CT scan. These examinations are complimentary. The lymphogram is the most reliable means for assessing involvement of retroperitoneal or pelvic lymph nodes [5]. In addition, the lymphogram is essential for assessing the degree of response to therapy and the maintenance of that response during the follow-up period. The CT scan is a better study for assessing the upper paraaortic and celiac nodes. Mesenteric nodes may also be visualized by CT scan, but they are rarely involved in Hodgkin's disease [5].

In patients with B-symptoms or any clinical evidence of subdiaphragmatic disease, a percutaneous needle bone marrow biopsy is performed. In patients with disease clinically limited to supradiaphragmatic sites and who have no B-symptoms a marrow biopsy can be deferred until the time of staging laparotomy.

In the absence of medical contraindications, a laparotomy with splenectomy is a routine part of our staging evaluation for patients with CS I–IIA/B or IIIA disease. The information obtained by laparotomy is essential to define the optimal treatment program and irradiation fields. There are some clinical situations in which the yield from laparotomy is too low to warrant its use. For example, patients with lymphocyte predominant Hodgkin's disease restricted to the high neck [6] or patients with Hodgkin's disease limited clinically to intrathoracic sites (no palpable lymph nodes in the neck or axilla and a negative lymphogram) may be staged reliably by clinical studies alone [7].

The technique of laparotomy includes a thorough exploration [8]. A splenectomy is performed with the splenic hilum dissected and clipped as medially as possible. The nodes along the celiac axis are sampled and, based upon the lymphogram, selected retroperitoneal lymph node biopsies are obtained, with intraoperative radiographic confirmation if appropriate. Wedge and needle biopsies are obtained from both lobes of the liver and an open bone marrow biopsy is performed. A bilateral midline oophoropexy is completed in all women [9].

Laparotomy findings which *often* influence the treatment program include the detection of Hodgkin's disease in the spleen, the extent of splenic involvement, and presence of disease in the celiac or retroperitoneal nodes [1]. The laparotomy procedures which facilitate later irradiation treatment include the splenectomy and oophoropexy (9–10).

3. Irradiation techniques

Important concepts in the curative management of patients with Hodgkin's disease include: the use of a tumoricidal dose of irradiation; the prophylactic treatment of clinically uninvolved sites adjacent to sites of known involvement; the design of large fields which encompass multiple lymph node regions; the use of megavoltage equipment to provide skin sparing and permit the treatment of large fields at extended distance; and the use of field simulation and verification during treatment.

When using irradiation alone, tumoricidal doses (4000–4400 rad) should be delivered to all initially involved sites [11]. While data support this dose for clinically apparent disease, less information is available concerning the dose needed to control microscopic disease. In the prophylactic treatment of uninvolved lymphoid regions, we utilize a dose of at least 3600 rad. Extralymphoid sites such as the lungs and liver may be considered at high risk for involvement in the presence of disease in the ipsilateral pulmonary hilum or spleen respectively. Since a dose of 3600 rad cannot be delivered safely to these organs, we utilize 'partial transmission lead blocks'. A 37% transmission block permits lung irradiation to 1650 rad during the time that the mantle field receives 4400 rad [12]. A 50% transmission liver block permits treatment to 2200 rad during the time required to treat the paraaortic nodes to 4400 rad [13].

Another important consideration in effective irradiation management is the utilization of large fields shaped to conform to the patient's anatomy and designed to treat multiple contiguous lymph node regions. This minimizes the risk of either 'overlap' or 'under-dosage' which could result in serious normal tissue toxicity or inadequate therapy. Field blocking is provided by individually contoured cerrobend or lead blocks.

The ability to treat these large fields requires treatment at 'extended distance'. This capability is available primarily with contemporary linear accelerators. A 6 MeV beam seems optimal. It provides substantial 'skin sparing', since the maximum ionization occurs at an approximate depth of 1.5 cm.

Essential to treatment accuracy and reproducibility is the use of field simulation and verification. Design of fields using a simulator permits careful tumor and normal tissue localization with diagnostic-quality imaging. Routine beam verification or 'port' films confirm that the desired areas are being treated and facilitate any adjustments.

The mantle field is designed to treat the cervical, supraclavicular, axillary, infraclavicular, mediastinal, *and* pulmonary hilar lymph nodes. The lymphoid regions encompassed by this field are usually involved or at high risk for involvement in most patients with Hodgkin's disease. This field is treated by evenly weighted anterior-posterior opposed technique to 4400 rad in 4–5 weeks. Unless otherwise indicated clinically, the larynx is protected throughout the course of treatment. In the posterior field, a block is placed over the cervical spinal cord throughout treatment and over the thoracic spinal cord after 2000 rad. The infraclavicular lymph nodes are treated only by the anterior field and therefore, when involved, must be 'boosted' anteriorly with orthovoltage X-rays or electrons. In the absence of mediastinal disease, the apex of the heart is protected throughout treatment. When the mediastinum is involved, the entire cardiac silhouette is treated initially. A block is then inserted over the apex of the heart at 1500 rad and over the subcarinal portion of the heart (two vertebral bodies below the carina) at 3000–3500 rad. When the mediastinal mass extends onto the pericardium (usually evidenced by a pericardial effusion), the entire cardiac silhouette should be treated to 3000 rad [1, 14]. When the pulmonary hilum is involved, the ipsilateral lung is treated by a partial transmission (37%) lung block. Areas of extralymphatic extension into the pulmonary parenchyma must be treated to the same high doses utilized for involved lymphoid tissue.

The design of the mantle field is often modified during therapy. As enlarged mediastinal lymph nodes regress, wider lung blocks are cut in order to protect more of the pulmonary parenchyma (shrinking field technique) [1, 14]. If the initial mediastinal mass is large, treatment is given slowly, i.e. 150 rad per day to a total dose of 1500 rad. Therapy is then interrupted for 7–10 days to permit regression of the mediastinal adenopathy and design of larger lung blocks. In appropriate patients, low dose mantle irradiation is completed prior to staging laparotomy in order to avoid problems with intubation and anesthesia.

The Waldeyer field utilized in Hodgkin's disease is actually intended to treat the preauricular lymph nodes. It is treated with opposed lateral megavoltage photon or unilateral electron fields with the inferior border matched to the top of the mantle. Because of the xerostomia induced by treating this area, prophylactic treatment (3600 rad/4 weeks) is restricted to patients being treated with irradiation alone who have involvement of high cervical nodes (above the level of the thyroid notch). Occasional patients present with a major component of Hodgkin's disease in jugulodigastric, submandibular, or high cervical lymph nodes. In these patients, these nodes are treated through larger opposed lateral fields matching to a mantle field in the low neck, inferior to the sites of bulky disease [15]. Since the oropharynx and larynx cannot be shielded using this technique, after 2000 rad the treatment is changed to a standard mantle (upper border near the edge of the mandible) and small Waldeyer (preauricular) field.

The spade field and the inverted-Y field are the major subdiaphragmatic fields. These fields are matched to the mantle in the midplane and a skin gap calculated based upon field size, beam divergence, and patient thickness. A posterior block is inserted over the spinal cord (to the bottom of L1) at 2000 rad. In the design of these fields, the location of the kidneys is important. Normal kidney position is confirmed by pretreatment staging studies such as the CT scan. In some instances, an IVP is obtained to rule out the possibility of a horseshoe or pelvic kidney which would lie within the radiation field. The subdiaphragmatic field is treated by anterior-posterior opposed technique, four days a week, at a dose of 150–200 rad per day depending upon the field size and patient tolerance.

When the spleen is intact, the subdiaphragmatic field must encompass the entire spleen. Careful localization of the left kidney is required in those cases and no more than the upper 1/3 of the left kidney should be included in the treatment field. In patients with a risk of liver involvement (documented splenic involvement at laparotomy) being treated with irradiation alone, the subdiaphragmatic field is extended over the right lobe of the liver and the liver is treated by means of a partial transmission (50%) block [13].

The spade field includes the paraaortic, common iliac nodes, and the splenic hilum. The inverted-Y field extends down into the pelvis to encompass the external iliac and inguinal–femoral nodes. A generous size midline block is utilized in the pelvis to protect the bladder and rectum. In females, a double thickness midline pelvis block provides protection to the ovaries which were transposed to the midline during laparotomy [16].

Total lymphoid irradiation (TLI) for Hodgkin's disease implies sequential treatment to the mantle and inverted-Y fields. *Subtotal lymphoid irradiation* (STLI) indicates treatment to the mantle and spade fields. After completion of irradiation to one field (i.e. mantle) and before treating the next, a 'split' (break) is provided to permit hematologic recovery. These splits average 10 days–2 weeks. When the subdiaphragmatic field is an inverted-Y, especially if the intact spleen or liver is being irradiated, the field can be divided into two portions at the level of the iliac crests and treated sequentially.

4. Outcome

Between 1968 and 1980 at Stanford University, our standard initial management for patients with PS I–IIA/B, IIIS/A included the staging studies outlined above followed by treatment with radiation alone [6]. Patients with PS IA, IIA and IIEA were usually treated with subtotal lymphoid irradiation. Patients with PS IB, IIB, or IIEB were treated with total lymphoid irradiation. Patients with PS IIIA were treated with total lymphoid irradiation including prphylactic liver treatment if the spleen was involved (PS IIISA). Although these treatments were considered 'standard', during the same period of time a large number of patients who presented with stage I–III disease were entered onto prospective clinical trials and were randomized to treatment with either irradiation alone or irradiation followed be adjuvant chemotherapy [17]. Most of these patients received adjuvant chemotherapy consisting of nitrogen mustard, vincristine, procarbazine and prednisone (MOPP) [18] but between 1974 and 1980 there was a randomization of adjuvant chemotherapy between MOPP and a combination which included procarbazine, alkeran, and vinblastine (PAVe) [19]. Experience in treating these two populations of patients – one with irradiation alone and the other with combined modality therapy – has permitted an analysis of outcome for similarly staged patients treated in either fashion. These analyses have also permitted the identification of important prognostic factors within each stage of disease. As a result of these analyses, we have been able to modify our standard treatment programs and develop new clinical trials.

All of the patients included in these analyses were staged as outlined in section 2. Regular follow-up visits after completion of therapy included a physical examination, routine blood studies, PA and lateral chest film, and abdominal X-ray. Most patients underwent repeat bipedal lymphography if there was inadequate contrast remaining for follow-up examination of retroperitoneal or pelvic lymph nodes for 2–3 years following initial therapy. In most instances, first recurrences were documented pathologically.

Survival, freedom-from-relapse, and freedom-from-second-relapse were calculated from the date of first visit to Stanford according to the actuarial technique of Kaplan and Meier [20]. The generalized Wilcoxon test of Gehan [21] was used to assess significance of differences between the actuarial curves. The prognostic significance of selected covariates was also evaluated using the multivariate regression technique of Cox [22].

4.1. Stage I–II

Included in this analysis are all stage I–II patients treated on the Stanford prospective randomized clinical trials between 1968 and 1979 [23]. Twenty-three patients on early clinical protocols who were treated with limited irradiation alone were excluded from analysis. The ramaining 230 patients were treated with either subtotal or total lymphoid irradiation alone (109 patients) or involved field, subtotal, or total lymphoid irradiation followed by six cycles of adjuvant chemotherapy with MOPP or PAVe (121 patients). Irradiation techniques utilized in the two different groups were the same with the exception that prophylactic treatment of the preauricular lymph nodes or lung, was not included if adjuvant chemotherapy treatment was planned.

For the purpose of this analysis, in addition to the review of the routine staging studies, the extent of involvement of the mediastinum by Hodgkin's disease was assessed by calculating a 'mediastinal mass ratio'. This ratio was determined by dividing the maximum width of the mediastinal mass, excluding the hila, by the maximum intrathoracic width as visualized on the pretreatment standing PA chest radiograph [24]. A mediastinal mass ratio $>1/3$ was considered large while one $\leq 1/3$ was considered small.

The pre-treatment characteristics of the two different patient groups are summarized in Table 1. The extent of disease as measured by pathologic stage or the presence of constitutional symptoms was similar in each. The distribution of histologic subtypes, age and sex distribution, sites of lymphoid involvement were also similar. A larger proportion of patients treated with combined modality therapy had 'E' lesions – a reflection of treatment protocols in use between 1974 and 1980, in which all such patients were treated with combined modality therapy.

All patients are included in the outcome analysis including two who refused to complete their initial course of irradiation, four who refused treatment with adjuvant chemotherapy, and two who had extension of their Hodgkin's disease to unirradiated sites prior to the initiation of adjuvant chemotherapy. Among the patients treated with adjuvant chemotherapy, the mean number of drug cycles completed was 5.4 and 88% of these patients received at least 5 cycles. The average dose of alkylating agent was 66% of the calculated dose and the average dose of procarbazine received was 57% of the calculated dose.

Table 1. Pretreatment characteristics of patients with PS I–II Hodgkin's disease treated with either irradiation alone (XRT) or irradiation followed by adjuvant combination chemotherapy (XRT + CHX).

	XRT (n = 109)	XRT + CHX (n = 121)
Male	59 (54%)	60 (50%)
Age ≥ 40	15 (14%)	18 (15%)
MCHD	15 (14%)	18 (15%)
PS II	89 (82%)	99 (82%)
B-symptoms	26 (24%)	38 (31%)
E-lesions	9 (8%)	31 (26%)
Mediastinum involved	72 (66%)	84 (70%)
Mediastinal mass ratio $>1/3$*	14 (13%)	27 (22%)
Subdiaphragmatic	4 (4%)	8 (7%)
Lymphoid sites ≥ 4	29 (27%)	46 (38%)

* See text for definition.

Table 2. Clinical characteristics, prognostic factors, and their influence on survival and freedom from relapse among patients with PS I–II Hodgkin's disease.

Subgroup	No. of patients	5-y survival (%)			5-y freedom from relapse		
		XRT	XRT + CHX	p(Gehan)	XRT	XRT + CHX	p(Gehan)
All PS I–II	230	96	92	0.39	79	87	0.09
PS I	42	100	100	0.47	100	90	0.91
PS II	188	95	90	0.25	75	86	0.07
A	166	97	95	0.75	77	89	0.07
B	64	92	85	0.59	83	84	0.97
Female	111	97	90	0.05	79	84	0.46
Male	119	94	94	0.47	78	90	0.15
Age <40 y	197	96	94	0.47	77	88	0.07
Age ≥40 y	33	93	81	0.66	93	80	0.58
LP, NS*	197	95	92	0.54	78	86	0.17
MC, UN	33	100	93	0.52	83	94	0.52
Supradiaphragmatic	218	96	92	0.47	78	88	0.08
Subdiaphragmatic	12	100	88	0.24	100	66	0.43
Non-E	190	95	93	0.75	79	86	0.18
E	40	100	88	0.24	78	90	0.33
Mediastinum involved	156	93	91	0.37	73	86	0.05
Mediastinum uninvolved	74	100	93	0.91	89	87	0.87
No. sites <4	155	97	95	0.99	84	87	0.53
No. sites >4	75	92	87	0.38	61	86	0.04
Mediastinal mass ratio ≤1/3	99	97	93	0.27	83	90	0.58
Mediastinal mass ratio >1/3	41	84	84	0.92	45	81	0.03

Table 2 shows the survival and freedom-from-relapse according to treatment modality for the entire treatment group as well as specific prognostic subgroups. The ten year survival is 84% for treatment with either irradiation alone or combined modality therapy (p = 0.39). Freedom-from-relapse at ten years is 77% and 84%, respectively (p = 0.09). A high 'salvage rate' has been reported using combination chemotherapy after patients have failed irradiation treatment for early stage Hodgkin's disease [25]. The effect of salvage treatment may be measured by determination of freedom-from-second-relapse. Patients are not scored as treatment failures in this analysis unless they have failed to enter a complete remission, have failed to enter second complete remission after relapse, or have relapsed after a second complete remission [26]. The freedom from second relapse at 10 years is 89% among patients treated initially with irradiation alone and 94% among patients treated initially with combined modality therapy (p = 0.56).

Specific prognostic factors were analyzed in more detail. Although systemic symptoms have been considered and adverse factor, in this analysis restricted to stage I–II patients, the presence of systemic symptoms had no influence on outcome for patients treated with irradiation alone. In fact, the ten year freedom-from-relapse in this group was superior to that of patients who presented without systemic symptoms (83% *vs.* 77%). In addition, the use of adjuvant chemotherapy failed to improve either the freedom-from-relapse or the survival of patients with systemic symptoms (p = 0.59, p = 0.97).

Traditionally, histologic subtype has also been considered an important prognostic factor in Hodgkin's disease. This impression results from the longer natural history associated with nodular sclerosing or lymphocyte predominant compared to mixed cellularity or lymphocyte depleted Hodgkin's disease and also to the fact that the latter two histologic subtypes more commonly present with advanced stage disease. Within this analysis restricted to stage I–II patients, however, histologic subtype was not an important prognostic factor. In fact, freedom-from-relapse and survival were slightly superior for the unfavorable histologic subtypes.

Approximately 5% of patients presented with Hodgkin's disease limited to subdiaphragmatic sites (excluding the spleen). The staging and treatment policies for this group were similar to those for patients presenting with supradiaphragmatic disease, except that the pelvic lymph nodes were always irradiated. Location of disease above or below the diaphragm had no significant influence on outcome and failed to identify a subgroup of patients requiring systemic treatment.

Occasional reports have indicated that patients with limited extranodal involvement (E-lesions) have a poorer prognosis than patients whose disease is restricted to lymphoid sites. In this analysis, 40 patients presented with E-lesions, some with multiple sites of extension. The most common sites of involvement included the lung (28 patients) and pericardium (13 patients). When irradiation alone was utilized in these patients, high doses were employed to the extralymphatic sites. Table 2 shows that limited extranodal involvement was not an important prognostic factor within either treatment group and failed to identify a subgroup of patients in whom even the freedom-from-relapse could be significantly improved by the use of adjuvant chemotherapy. The five-year survivals were 100% and 88%, respectively, after treatment with either irradiation alone or combined modality therapy (p = 0.24).

Retrospective determination of bulk of disease is difficult for most sites but can be done quite readily for the mediastinum by the measurement of the mass size on pretreatment radiographic studies. We were able to confirm in this series that patients with large mediastinal masses (>13 of the maximum intrathoracic width) have a much higher risk for relapse after treatment with irradiation alone than those patients who present with smaller masses (five-year freedom-from-relapse 45% *vs.* 83%). Furthermore, the relapse risk of patients with large mediastinal masses could be reduced significantly by the addition of chemotherapy to the treatment program (five-year freedom-from-relapse 45% *vs.* 81%, p = 0.03). However, despite the substantial difference in relapse rate for patients with large mediastinal masses treated by the two different techniques, the five-year survivals are equivalent (83%). This is again related to the efficacy of salvage chemotherapy.

The initial sites of relapse in the two different treatment groups are listed in Table 3. The most common site of relapse among patients treated with irradiation alone was in previosuly treated lymphoid regions, usually initially involved mediastinal or axillary lymph nodes. In addition, 4/53 patients (8%) treated with subtotal lymphoid irradiation had their initial site of relapse limited to untreated pelvic lymph nodes. The addition of adjuvant chemotherapy appeared to decrease the likelihood of relapse in each region about equally.

Significant complications observed in these patients are noted in Table 4. Symptomatic radiation pericarditis was most frequent among patients with large mediastinal masses in whom inadequate protection of the heart are pericardium could be provided during the course of irradiation [27]. There were two cases of fatal post treatment sepsis and one fatal case of herpes encephalitis. Subsequent malignancies were identified in five patients. The leukemia, melanoma, and sarcoma were all fatal.

Table 3. Initial sites of relapse in patients with PS I–II Hodgkin's disease treated with either irradiation alone (XRT) or irradiation followed by adjuvant chemotherapy (XRT + CHX).

	XRT (33/109 patients)	XRT + CHX (19/121 patients)
Lymph nodes		
Initially involved	10	4
Initially uninvolved		
Irradiated	8	3
Unirradiated	5	6
Extranodal		
Lung/pleura	6	4
Bone	1	–
Marrow	1	–
Other	2	2

Table 4. Serious complications among patients with PS I–II Hodgkin's disease treated with either irradiation alone (XRT) or irradiation followed by adjuvant chemotherapy (XRT + CHX).

	XRT (n = 109)	XRT + CHX (n = 121)
Radiation pneumonitis (requiring therapy)	0	2
Radiation pericarditis (requiring therapy)	1	5
Fatal sepsis	0	2
Duodenal ulcer	1	2
Hemolytic anemia	1	0
Idiopathic thrombocytopenic purpura	0	1
Aseptic necrosis of femoral head	0	2
Herpes encephalitis	0	1
Subsequent malignancy		
Leukemia	0	1
Melanoma	0	1
Sarcoma	0	1
Uterine carcinoma	1	0
Lymphoma cutis (non-Hodgkin's)	1	0

Table 5. Current status of patients with PS I–II Hodgkin's disease treated with either irradiation alone (XRT) or irradiation followed by adjuvant chemotherapy (XRT + CHX).

	XRT (n = 109)	XRT + CHX (n = 121)
Alive		
No relapse	84 (77%)	98 (81%)
Prior relapse		
Currently NED*	10 (9%)	7 (6%)
With disease	5	3
Dead		
No relapse	2	7
Prior relapse, NED at death	1	1
With disease	7	5

* No evidence of disease.

Current patient status is summarized in Table 5. Overall, 87% of the patients are alive without evidence of disease. Most of the patients (7/10) who died after initial treatment with irradiation alone died with active Hodgkin's disease. The three intercurrent deaths in the group were due to myocardial infarction, cerebral vascular accident, and probable sepsis. There were five deaths due to Hodgkin's disease among patients treated initially with combined modality therapy. The eight intercurrent deaths included three instances of second malignancies, two cases of sepsis and one case each of idiopathic pneumonitis and probable pancarditis.

A detailed analysis of patients with extensive mediastinal involvement reveals that relapse occurred in 50% of patients treated initially with irradiation alone and 19% of those treated initially with combined modality therapy. Recurrent intrathoracic disease was a component of the initial relapse in 7 of the 12 patients (5/7 treated with irradiation alone, 2/5 treated with combined modality therapy). Both patients with large mediastinal masses who were treated with irradiation alone and subsequently died had active Hodgkin's disease at the time of death. In contrast, the three deaths in the combined modality group were due to intercurrent causes (herpes encephalitis, pneumonitis, and acute myelogous leukemia).

These data suggest that radiation therapy alone is appropriate initial treatment for nearly all patients with PS I–II Hodgkin's disease. Treatment with subtotal or total lymphoid irradiation is necessary, however, since earlier studies have shown a high relapse rate in asymptomatic patients treated with involved field irradiation and both a high relapse rate and poor survival after such limited therapy in patients with B-symptoms [28].

In this study, the presence of systemic symptoms did not have an effect on prognosis. The excellent survival (92% at 5 years) and freedom-from-relapse (83% at 5 years) observed in these 26 symptomatic patients treated with total lymphoid irradiation is better than has been reported in other series [29–32]. This difference may be accounted for by either the use of staging laparotomy and splenectomy or by the treatment of total lymphoid fields, rather than more limited therapy. Staging laparotomy in clinical stage IIB is essential to rule out subdiaphragmatic involvement, since patients who have disease on both sides of the diaphragm (PS IIIB) will require chemotherapy in their management [33]. However, even in those series which incorporate staging laparotomy, the results utilizing only extended field treatment are inferior to those reported here [29, 34–35].

These data confirm the observation that histologic subtyping of Hodgkin's disease has little influence on prognosis when careful staging and optimal therapy are employed. Furthermore, the occasional difficulties that pathologists encounter in subclassifying cases of Hodgkin's disease makes any subclassification of limited value [36]. Nevertheless, histologic subtype remains important in predicting natural history.

The influence of extralymphatic extension on prognosis in Hodgkin's disease is controversial. The initial data of Musshoff [37] suggested that extralymphatic extension did not confer a worse prognosis and the concept of 'E-lesion' was therefore incorporated into the Ann Arbor staging classification system [2]. The validity of this decision has been challenged by some investigators who report a poor survival for patients with extralymphatic extension who were treated with irradiation alone [38]. Reports which have drawn this conclusion have failed to account for the independent effects of E-lesions and large mediastinal masses. This is unfortunate, since pulmonary extension may often accompany a large mediastinal mass. It is important to assess the relative impact of these two factors. In our experience, not only did the presence of an E-lesion fail to influence curability and survival in patients treated with irradiation alone, but when a multivariate analysis was performed, the only significant prognostic factor predictive of relapse in patients with stage I–II disease treated with irradiation alone was the presence of a large mediastinal mass [23]. Extralymphatic extension *alone* is not a significant factor.

Extensive mediastinal disease has been reported by several authors to adversely affect the prognosis the patients with Hodgkin's disease treated with irradiation alone [24, 38–39], however, the data reported in those series were inadequate to conclude that the prognosis of these patients could be significantly improved by the addition of adjuvant chemotherapy. Nevertheless, the recommendation for routine chemotherapy was made for those patients. This analysis shows that the freedom-from-relapse of patients with large mediastinal masses can indeed be improved by the addition of chemotherapy (10 year freedom-from-relapse 45% *vs.* 81%). However, despite the marked improvement in freedom-from-relapse, a survival benefit was not achieved. The lack of a survival benefit is a result of two factors. First of all, even with large mediastinal disease, the majority of patients who fail initial radiation treatment were successfully salvaged with subsequent MOPP therapy and are currently without evidence of disease. Secondly, intercurrent deaths were more frequent in the group of patients with large mediastinal disease treated with combined modality therapy and, in fact, accounted for all deaths in that group. The improved freedom-from-relapse but identical survival achieved by the routine use of chemotherapy in these patients has now been confirmed by others [40].

At Stanford University, the general philosophy in the management of patients with PS I–II Hodgkin's disease is to maximize staging in order to minimize therapy and thereby minimize significant long term complications. In the absence of medical contraindications, nearly all patients undergo thorough staging including lymphography and staging laparotomy with splenectomy. The final treatment program is then based upon the staging information derived from these studies. Two-thirds of the clinical stage I–II patients will have pathologic stage I–II disease and can be treated with subtotal or total lymphoid irradiation utilizing the techniques summarized in section 3. One-third of the asymptomatic patients who present with clinical involvement restricted to supradiaphragmatic sites will have subdiaphragmatic involvement documented by laparotomy. Most of these patients will have either subdiaphragmatic lymph node disease or minimal splenic involvement identified and will still be managed by irradiation alone, although the extent of the subdiaphragmatic irradiation portals must be extended (see section 4.2). All patients with extensive splenic disease or pathological stage IIIB will be treated with combined modality therapy.

In patients who present with large mediastinal masses the therapy is more individualized. We often deliver a dose of 1500–2000 rad to the mantle field and assess response to that treatment before deciding to proceed with a staging laparotomy and possible treatment with irradiation alone or, if the response is poor, to utilize combined modality therapy.

Careful followup of these patients is mandatory. Even with optimal irradiation approximately 10–15% of patients can be expected to develop new manifestations of Hodgkin's disease. These should be identified as soon as possible in order to optimize the efficacy of salvage therapy.

4.2. Stage IIIA

Included in this analysis are all stage IIIA patients treated at Stanford University between 1968 and 1980 [41]. All patients underwent the standard staging evaluation as specified in Section 2. In addition, the extent of splenic involvement was defined according to the laparotomy pathology report. Extensive splenic involvement included all cases in which five or more nodules (irrespective of size) were identified grossly in the sectioned splenectomy specimen. Patients were treated with either total lymphoid irradiation alone (102 patients) or total lymphoid irradiation followed by six cycles of adjuvant chemotherapy with MOPP or PAVe (99 patients). Irradiation techniques utilized in the two different groups were the same with the exception that prophylactic treatment of the preauricular lymph nodes, lung, or liver was not included if adjuvant chemotherapy was planned.

Table 6. Pretreatment characteristics of patients with PS IIIA Hodgkin's disease treated with either irradiation alone (XRT) or irradiation followed by adjuvant combination chemotherapy (XRT + CHX).

	XRT (n = 102)	XRT + CHX (n = 99)
≥5 total sites	54 (53%)	64 (65%)
CS III	45 (44%)	42 (42%)
III$_2$	43 (42%)	44 (44%)
S+	86 (84%)	87 (88%)
S+ extensive	40 (39%)	41 (41%)

The pretreatment characteristics of the two different groups are summarized in Table 6. The extent of disease as measured by clinical stage, number of sites of involvement, extent of splenic involvement, and number of sites involved were similar in each group. The distribution of histologic subtypes, age and sex were also similar. Among patients who received adjuvant chemotherapy, five or more cycles of chemotherapy were administered to 81% of the patients and the average drug doses were about 70% of the calculated optimum dose [19].

Table 7 shows the survival and freedom-from-relapse according to treatment modality for the entire group as well as specific prognostic subgroups. The ten year survival was 83% after treatment with combined modality therapy and 70% after treatment with irradiation alone (p = 0.3). A marked difference in freedom-from-relapse is noted at 10 years (80% *vs.* 50%,

Table 7. Clinical characteristics, prognostic factors, and their influences on survival and freedom from relapse among patients with PS IIIA Hodgkin's disease.

Subgroup	No. of patients	5-y survival (%)			5-y freedom from relapse (%)		
		TLI	TLI + CHX	P (Gehan)*	TLI	TLI + CHX	P (Gehan)*
All IIIA	201	.82	.91	0.30	.61	.83	<0.00008
LP,NS	146	.90	.90	0.38	.62	.85	<0.0005
MC,LD, unclassified	55	.82	.87	0.88	.61	.86	<0.09
<5 total sites	83	.91	.91	0.92	.65	.94	<0.01
⩾5 total sites	118	.84	.89	0.20	.59	.81	<0.0009
CS I, II	114	.91	.88	0.91	.57	.88	<0.0003
CS III	87	.83	.92	0.19	.67	.81	<0.11
'Anatomic substage III$_1$'	114	.91	.89	0.66	.59	.92	0.00003
'Anatomic substage III$_2$'	87	.83	.90	0.29	.63	.77	0.13
S−	28	.81	.92	0.62	.69	.74	0.49
S+	173	.88	.89	0.47	.60	.87	0.00006
S+ minimal	92	.95	.89	0.70	.80	.87	0.40
S+ extensive	81	.81	.90	0.23	.37	.87	<0.00001
S− or S+ minimal	120	.91	.89	0.86	.77	.84	0.25

LP, lymphocyte predominance; NS, nodular sclerosis; MC, mixed cellular; LD lymphocyte depleted; UN, unclassified Hodgkin's disease.

* The P (Gehan) value compares survival or freedom from relapse for treatment with total lymphoid irradiation (TLI) alone versus treatment with total lymphoid irradiation followed by adjuvant chemotherapy (TLI + CHX).

p <0.01), however, because of the efficacy of salvage chemotherapy the freedom-from-second-relapse at 10 years is quite similar in the two treatment groups (87% vs. 83%, p = 0.3) [41].

Specific prognostic factors were again analyzed in more detail. As summarized in Table 7, many potential prognostic factors were found to be clinically unimportant. These included histology, clinical stage, and 'anatomic substage'. Previous analyses also indicated that age and sex were also unimportant prognostic variables [42].

The 'anatomic substage' of PS IIIA patients has been reported by some investigators to influence prognosis [43–44]. Our experience utilizing the substaging criteria is shown in Table 7. Freedom-from-relapse is better after combined modality therapy compared to TLI alone; however, the difference is significant only for patients with substage III_1, a conclusion exactly opposite that which has been described in another study [44]. Moreover, the survival of neither substage III_1 or III_2 patients is improved significantly by the use of combined modality therapy. This suggests that substaging is not an adequate means for defining treatment policy. As demonstrated in previous analyses, the extent of splenic involvement was the single factor with the greatest influence or prognosis in our patients with PS IIIA disease [42]. As the table shows, patients with minimal splenic disease had a similar prognosis irrespective of initial treatment type. On the other hand, patients with extensive splenic involvement had a five year freedom-from-relapse of only 37% after TLI alone, compared with 87% after treatment with combined modality therapy (p =0.01). However, despite this disparity in freedom-from-relapse, the survival difference is still not statistically significant (p = 0.23).

The distribution and extent of subdiaphragmatic disease exclusive of splenic involvement failed to show any impact on prognosis [41]. The prognosis was similar for patients with subdiaphragmatic involvement limited to the spleen, the spleen and splenic hilar lymph nodes, or the spleen and subdiaphragmatic nodes other than the splenic hilar nodes.

Table 8. Correlation of clinical stage and extent of splenic involvement in patients with PS IIIA Hodgkin's disease.

Splenic involvement	No. of patients in clinical stage	
	I–II	III
Uninvolved	6	22
Minimal	69	23
Extensive	39	42
Total	114	87

Unfortunately, despite the importance of splenic involvement as a prognostic factor, the extent of splenic disease could not be predicted by clinical studies alone. The correlation between extent of splenic involvement and clinical stage is shown in Table 8. Patients with extensive splenic involvement had an equal likelihood of having clinical stage I–II or III disease. The application of newer staging techniques such as ultrasound and computerized tomographic scanning is not expected to significantly improve our ability to identify the extent of splenic involvement [5]. Many extensively involved spleens contain nodules less than 1 cm in diameter, beyond the resolution of those imaging modalities. Furthermore, even an assessment of splenic size, possible with computerized tomographic scanning, is an unreliable predictor of splenic involvement. The median, mean and range of weight of the spleen as a function of the extent of splenic involvement are shown in Table 9. The overlapping ranges of splenic weight prohibit the determination of splenic involvement based exclusively on size.

Table 10 summarizes the sites of initial relapse in the two different treatment

Table 9. Correlation of splenic weight with extent of splenic involvement in patients with PS IIIA Hodgkin's disease.

Splenic involvement	Spleen weight (g)		
	Range	Median	Mean
Uninvolved	50–400	142	161
Minimal	65–450	153	172
Extensive	60–450*	180	197

* 750 g in one additional patient.

Table 10. Initial sites of relapse in patients with pathological stage IIIA Hodgkin's disease treated with either total lymphoid irradiation alone (TLI) or TLI followed by adjuvant chemotherapy (TLI + CHX).

Relapse sites	TLI (34/102 patients)	TLI + CHX (14/99 patients)
Nodal only	17	6
Extranodal only	8	4
Nodal plus extranodal	9	4
Supradiaphragmatic only	10	8
Subdiaphragmatic only	6	3
Generalized	18	3

One patient in each group who failed to achieve an initial complete remission has been excluded.

groups. Extranodal relapse was more common in these stage IIIA patients than in the stage I–II patients (c.f. Table 3). The distribution of relapse sites is more generalized in the TLI group, 53% of the patients having a component of relapse on both sides of the diaphragm, while only 21% of the patients in the combined modality group have similar extent of relapsing disease. Relapse limited to supradiaphragmatic sites was much more common than at sub-diaphragmatic sites.

The causes of death are summarized in Table 11. The number of deaths due to Hodgkin's disease was quite small, accounting for only 7.5% of the patients in this analysis. The two patients who died from thrombocytopenia and hemorrhage had been treated with colloidal ^{198}Au as a component of their liver irradiation. They developed hematologic complications shortly after ^{198}Au administration. This technique of liver irradiation was discontinued in 1972.

There is substantial controversy regarding the importance of different prognostic factors in pathological stage IIIA Hodgkin's disease. The results of different studies are difficult to compare because of differences in treatment modalities and techniques. Even minor variations in therapy may influence results. For example, at Stanford we employ low dose irradiation to the liver in the presence of splenic involvement, and there have been no initial relapses in the liver in these patients. In contrast, at centers where liver irradiation is not used routinely, initial relapses in the liver may account for as many as 30% of relapses in PS IIIA patients [45]. Our retrospective experience indicates that the extent of splenic involvement is the most important prognostic factor in PS IIIA disease. This interpretation is supported by multivariate analysis which considers all potential prognostic factors [42]. We hypothesize that there is an

Table 11. Causes of death in patients with pathological stage IIIA Hodgkin's disease treated with either total lymphoid irradiation alone (TLI) or TLI followed by adjuvant combination chemotherapy (TLI + CHX).

Cause of death	No. of patients	
	TLI	TLI + CHX
Active Hodgkin's disease	9	6
Infection or sepsis	2[a]	2
Acute myelogenous leukemia	1[a]	1
Thrombocytopenia and hemorrhage	2[b]	–
Solid tumors	3[c]	–
Other	2[d]	–

[a] These three patients received MOP(P) as salvage therapy.
[b] Both patients developed severe thrombocytopenia after treatment with colloidal ^{198}Au (see text).
[c] Lung cancer (two cases) and colon cancer.
[d] Hypertension, automobile accident.

increased likelihood of occult extranodal disease in the presence of extensive splenic involvement, and management of irradiation alone is therefore often unsuccessful.

We were unable to confirm any prognostic influence whatsoever for the concept of 'anatomic substage'. This is in disagreement with other reports in the literature [43–44] and may be a reflection of different treatment techniques. Policies involving routine treatment of the pulmonary hilar and pelvic lymph nodes and prophylactic treatment of the preauricular nodes, lungs, and liver under appropriate circumstances generally are not followed at those centers where 'anatomic substage' has been found to be an important prognostic factor. It may be that our more aggressive and effective initial treatment program obscures the prognostic significance of the 'anatomic substage'. Furthermore, although at Stanford we have not observed a correlation between 'anatomic substage' and the extent of splenic involvement (36% III_1 and 43% III_2 have extensive involvement of the spleen), at the University of Chicago there appears to be a strong correlation [46]. In their experience with 76 patients, 76% of III_2 patients had extensive splenic involvement while only 44% of III_1 patients have extensive splenic disease. It is possible that it is the extensive splenic involvement that confirms an unfavorable prognosis on their substage III_2 patients. A multivariate analysis of these data might confirm that suspicion.

Unfortunately, although the extent of splenic involvement was clearly the most important prognostic factor in our PS IIIA patients, clinical staging studies were inadequate for its determination; staging laparotomy was always required. Although standard ultrasonography and CT scanning are not expected to improve upon this ability, potential new modalities such as CT scanning done with contrast media taken up selectively by the reticulo–endothelial system [47], nuclear magnetic resonance, or ultrasound tissue characterization studies [48] may, in the future, provide us with the ability to detect excessive involvement of the spleen without splenectomy.

Based on these retrospective observations, we have modified our approach to PS IIIA Hodgkin's disease. After laparotomy to define the distribution of subdiaphragmatic disease and the extent of splenic involvement, we feel confident in managing patients with negative or minimally involved spleens with total lymphoid irradiation alone. Low dose irradiation to the liver is included whenever the spleen is involved. For patients with extensively involved spleens, however, we utilize systemic therapy in every instance. Our standard treatment protocol involves alternating combination chemotherapy and total lymphoid irradiation in a fashion identical to that which we have described for the management of patient with stage IIIB disease [49].

In conclusion, radiation therapy remains the most effective single agent in

148

the treatment of Hodgkin's disease. A management program which includes intensive staging followed by aggressive irradiation treatment that is individually tailored to each patient and his disease will achieve cure in the majority of patients with PS I–IIA/B and IIIA favorable Hodgkin's disease. When performed properly these staging and treatment programs will be associated with minimal but acceptable morbidity. Less intensive management programs may compromise patient outcome and thereby necessitate utilization of combination chemotherapy as salvage treatment.

Acknowledgements

This study was supported in part by Grant CA05838 from The National Cancer Institute, National Institutes of Health.

The author is grateful to Marge Keskin for secretarial assistance.

References

1. Kaplan H: Hodgkin's Disease. 2nd edition. Cambridge, Mass., Harvard University Press, 1980.
2. Carbone PP, Kaplan HS, Mushoff K, Smithers DW, Tubiana M: Report of the committee on Hodgkin's disease staging classification. Cancer Res 31:1860–1861, 1971.
3. Favez G, Willa C, Heinzer F: Posterior oblique tomography at an angle of 55° in chest roentgenology. Am J Roentgenol 120:907–915, 1974.
4. Rostock RA, Giangreco A, Wharam MD, Lenhard R, Siegelman SS, Order SE: CT scan modifications in the treatment of mediastinal Hodgkin's disease. Cancer 49:2267–2275, 1982.
5. Castellino RA: Imaging techniques for staging abdominal Hodgkin's disease. Cancer Treat Rep 66:697–700, 1982.
6. Kaplan HS, Rosenberg SA: The management of Hodgkin's disease. Cancer 36:796–803, 1975.
7. Johnson DW, Hoppe RT, Cox RS, Rosenberg SA, Kaplan HS: Hodgkin's disease limited to intrathoracic sites. Cancer 52:8–13, 1983.
8. Enright LP, Trueblood HW, Nelsen TS: The surgical diagnosis of abdominal Hodgkin's disease. Surg Gynec Obstet 130:853–858, 1970.
9. Ray GR, Trueblood HW, Enright LP, Kaplan HS, Nelsen TS: Oophoropexy: A means of preserving ovarian function following pelvic megavoltage radiotherapy for Hodgkin's disease. Radiology 96:175–180, 1970.
10. Salzman JR, Kaplam HS: Effect of prior splenectomy on hematologic tolerance during total lymphoid radiotherapy of patients with Hodgkin's disease. Cancer 27:471–478, 1971.
11. Kaplan HS: Evidence for a tumoricidal dose level in the radiotherapy of Hodgkin's disease. Cancer Res 26:1221–1224, 1966.
12. Palos B, Kaplan HS, Karzmark CJ: The use of thin lung shields to deliver limited whole-lung irradiation during mantle-field treatment of Hodgkin's disease. Radiology 101:441–442, 1971.
13. Schultz HP, Glatstein E, Kaplan HS: Management of presumptive or proven Hodgkin's disease of the liver: A new radiotherapy technique. Int J Radiat Oncol 1:1–8, 1975.

14. Hoppe RT: Radiation therapy in the treatment of Hodgkin's disease. Semin Oncol 7:144–154, 1980.
15. Hoppe RT, Burke JS, Glatstein E, Kaplan HS: Non-Hodgkin's lymphoma-involvement of Waldeyer's ring. Cancer 42:1096–1104, 1978.
16. LeFloch O, Donaldson SS, Kaplan HS: Pregnancy following oophoropexy and total nodal irradiation in women with Hodgkin's disease. Cancer 38:2263–2268, 1976.
17. Rosenberg SA, Kaplan HS, Hoppe RT, Kushlan P, Horning S: The Stanford randomized trials of the treatment of Hodgkin's disease: 1967–1980. In: Malignant lymphomas. Etiology, immunology, pathology, treatment, Rosenberg SA, Kaplan HS (eds). New York: Academic Press. 1982, pp. 513–522.
18. DeVita VT, Serpick AA, Carbone PP: Combination chemotherapy in the treatment of advanced Hodgkin's disease. Ann Intern Med 73:881–895, 1970.
19. Wolin EM, Rosenberg SA, Kaplan HS: A randomized comparison of PAVe and MOP(P) as adjuvant chemotherapy for Hodgkin's disease. In: Adjuvant Therapy of Cancer II, Jones SE, Salmon SE (eds). New York: Grune and Stratton. 1979, pp. 119–127.
20. Kaplan ES, Meier P: Non-parametric estimation from incomplete observation. Am Stat Assoc J 53:457–480, 1958.
21. Gehan EA: A generalized Wilcoxon test for comparing arbitrarily singly-censored samples. Biometrika 52:203–233, 1965.
22. Cox DR: Regression models and life tables. J R Stat Soc B 34:187–220, 1972.
23. Hoppe RT, Coleman CN, Cox RS, Rosenberg SA, Kaplan HS: The management of stage I–II Hodgkin's disease with irradiation alone or combined modality therapy: the Stanford experience. Blood 59:455–465, 1982.
24. Mauch P, Goodman R, Hellman S: The significance of mediastinal involvement in early stage Hodgkin's disease. Cancer 42:1039–1045, 1978.
25. Portlock CS, Rosenberg SA, Glatstein E, Kaplan HS: Impact of salvage treatment on initial relapses in patients with Hodgkin's disease, stages I–III. Blood 51:825–833, 1978.
26. Rosenberg SA, Kaplan HS, Glatstein EJ, Portlock CS: Combined modality therapy of Hodgkin's disease, A report on the Stanford trials. Cancer 42:991–1000, 1978.
27. Stewart JR, Fajardo LF: Dose response in human and experimental radiation-induced heart disease. Radiology 99:403–408, 1971.
28. Kaplan HS, Rosenberg SA: Current status of clinical trials: the Stanford experience, 1962–1972. International Symposium on Hodgkin's Disease, NCI Monograph 36, Bethesda, 1973, p. 363–371.
29. Mintz U, Miller JB, Golomb HM, Kinzie J, Sweet DL Jr, Lester EP, Variakojis D, Roth NO, Blough RR, Ferguson DJ, Ultmann JE: Pathologic stage I and II Hodgkin's disease, 1968–1975. Relapses and results of retreatment. Cancer 44:72–79, 1979.
30. Thar TL, Million RR, Hausner RJ, McKetty MHB: Hodgkin's disease, stages I and II. Relationship of recurrence to size of disease, radiation dose, and number of sites involved. Cancer 43:1101–1105, 1979.
31. Stoffel TJ, Cox JD: Hodgkin's disease stage I and II. A comparison between two different treatment policies. Cancer 40:90–97, 1977.
32. Aisenberg AC, Linggood RM, Lew RA: The changing face of Hodgkin's disease. Am J Med 67:921–928, 1979.
33. Rosenberg SA, Kaplan HS, Brown BW: The role of adjuvant MOPP in the therapy of Hodgkin's disease: an analysis after ten years. In: Adjuvant therapy of cancer II, Jones SE, Salmon SE (eds). New York: Grune and Stratton, 1979, pp. 109–117.
34. Fuller LM, Madoc-Jones H, Gamble JF, Butler JJ, Sullivan MP, Fernandez CH, Gehan EA: New assessment of the prognostic significance of histopathology in Hodgkin's disease for laparotomy-negative stage I and stage II patients. Cancer 39:2174–2182, 1977.

35. Coltman CA, Fuller LA, Fisher R, Frei E: Extended field radiotherapy versus involved field radiotherapy plus MOPP in stage I and II Hodgkin's disease. In: Adjuvant therapy of cancer II, Jones SE, Salmon SE (eds): New York, Grune and Stratton, 1979, pp. 129–136.
36. Coppleson LW, Factor RM, Strum SB, Graff PW, Rappaport H: Observor disagreement in the classification and histology of Hodgkin's disease. J Natl Cancer Inst. 45:731–740, 1970.
37. Musshoff K: Prognostic and therapeutic implications of staging in extranodal Hodgkin's disease. Cancer Res 31:1814–1828, 1971.
38. Levi JA, Wiernik PH: Limited extranodal Hodgkin's disease – unfavorable prognosis and therapeutc implications. Am J Med 63:36–372, 1977.
39. Timothy AR, Sutcliffe SBJ, Stansfeld AG, Wriley PFM, Jones AE: Radiotherapy in the treatment of Hodgkin's isease. Br Med J 1:1246–1249, 1978.
40. Mauch P, Gorshein D, Cunningham J, Hellman S: Influence of mediastinal adenopathy on site and frequency of relapse in patients with Hodgkin's disese. Cancer Treat Rep 66:809–817, 1982.
41. Hoppe RT, Cox RS, Rosenberg SA, Kaplan HS: Prognostic factors in pathologic stage III Hodgkin's disease. Cancer Treat Rep 66:743–749, 1982.
42. Hoppe RT, Rosenberg SA, Kaplan HS, Cox RS: Prognostic factors in pathologic stage IIIA Hodgkin's disease. Cancer 46:1240–1246, 1980.
43. Desser RK, Golomb HM, Ultmann JE, Ferguson DJ, Moran EM, Griem ML, Vardiman J, Miller B, Oetzel N, Sweet D, Lester EP, Kinzie JJ, Blough R: Prognostic classification of Hodgkin's disease in pathologic stage III, based on anatomic considerations. Blood 49:883–893, 1977.
44. Stein RS, Golomb HM, Diggs CH, Mauch P, Hellman S, Wiernik PH, Ultmann JE, Rosenthal DS: Anatomic substage of stage III-A Hodgkin's disease. A collaborative study. Ann Intern Med 92:159–165, 1980.
45. Mauch P, Goodman R, Rosenthal DS, Botnick L, Piro AJ, Hellman S: An evaluation of total nodal irradiation as treatment for stage III A Hodgkin's disease. Cancer 43:1255–1261, 1979.
46. Larson RA, Ultmann JE: The strategic role of laparotomy in staging Hodgkin's disease. Cancer Treat Rep 66:767–774, 1982.
47. Vermess M, Doppman JL, Sugarbaker PH, Fisher RI, O'Leary TJ, Chatterji DC, Grimes G, Adamson RH, Willis M, Edwards BK: Computed tomography of the liver and spleen with intravenous lipoid contrast material: review of 60 examinations. AJR 138:1063–1071, 1982.
48. Sommer FG, Joynt LF, Carroll BA, Macovski A: Ultrasonic characterization of abdominal tissues via digital analysis of backscattered waveforms. Radiology 141:811–817, 1981.
49. Hoppe RT, Portlock CS, Glatstein E, Rosenberg SA, Kaplan HS: Alternating chemotherapy and irradiation in the treatment of advanced Hodgkin's disease. Cancer 43:472–481, 1979.

7. The role of combination chemotherapy alone or as an adjuvant to radiation therapy in limited stages of Hodgkin's disease

LEONARD R. PROSNITZ

1. Introduction

The treatment of Hodgkin's disease has become a very successful and satisfying endeavor for both the radiation oncologist and medical oncologist. Cure rates of 90–95% may be achieved for the patient with pathologic stages I and II disease [1, 2, 3]. For patients with more advanced stages, chemotherapy alone or, as our data suggest, preferably in combination with radiation, will succeed in curing 65–75% of patients [4, 5]. This chapter, however, will not discuss in any detail the therapy of advanced disease. Our purpose is to evaluate the role of combination chemotherapy either alone or with radiation in the management of more limited stage disease.

Limited stage disease is a rather vague term but, for the purposes of this report, we will define it as those stages of Hodgkin's disease amenable to an attempt at curable treatment with radiation therapy alone. Clearly, stages IIIB and IV do not fit this category but virtually every other stage does, i.e. stages I and II, A and B, E subtype, and stage IIIA. Although one may attempt a cure for limited stage disease with radiation therapy alone, it may not always be appropriate to do so. That issue is the subject of this report.

The impetus for applying chemotherapy to the earlier stages of Hodgkin's disease stems, of course, from the success of chemotherapy in the treatment of advanced disease. Logic suggests that if chemotherapy is effective in advanced disease, it should be even more so in limited disease. However, students of Hodgkin's disease are becoming increasingly sensitive to the long term complications that may result from either drugs, radiation, or the combination of the two. Before recommending any treatment for any patient with Hodgkin's disease, it is necessary to examine the risk:benefit ratio with some care. The following questions appear to be the important ones to ask:

1. What is the cure rate with limited disease with radiation therapy alone, with chemotherapy reserved for those patients who relapse after a curative attempt with radiation?
2. What cure rate might be expected with chemotherapy alone, or in combina-

Bennett JM (ed), Controversies in the Management of Lymphomas. ISBN 0-89838-586-5.
© *Martinus Nijhoff Publishers, Boston. Printed in the Netherlands.*

tion with radiation for limited stage disease?

3. Are there subsets of patients within the larger group of patients with limited disease who have a worse prognosis and who might benefit from chemotherapy or from combined modality therapy at the onset?

4. What are the long term toxicities of chemotherapy, radiation therapy and the combined modality program?

2. Results of radiation therapy alone in limited stage disease

This subject is covered in detail by Dr. Hoppe elsewhere in the symposium. Nevertheless, it is critical to the issue of the role of combination chemotherapy and will be discussed briefly here. At Yale University since 1969, 168 patients with pathologic stage IA and IIA disease have had subtotal nodal irradiation as their initial therapy. Included are patients with large mediastinal masses and E disease. Results are shown in Fig. 1 [1]. The 10 year actuarial survival is 94% with only 7 patients having died of Hodgkin's disease. 77% of patients are continually free of disease from the onset of therapy. Of a total of 33 patients who relapsed after initial radiation, 26 appear to have been cured with subsequent combined modality therapy. These results in PS IA and IIA patients

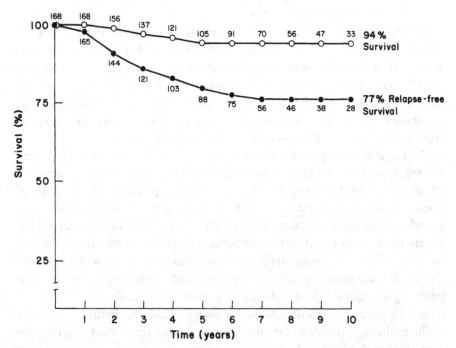

Figure 1. Actuarial survival and relapse-free survival of PS IA and IIA patients treated initially with radiation alone.

are in close agreement with survival rates of 90–95% obtained by a number of other centers [2, 3].

For patients with PS IIIA disease, results with initial management with radiation therapy alone have not been as good. [See Dr. Stein's article elsewhere in this symposium as well]. 52 patients were treated in this fashion at Yale since 1969 and the outcome shown in Fig. 2 [1]. The actuarial 10 year survival is 72% with only 32% of patients being continuously free of disease. Because of this experience, we began a program in 1977 of combined modality therapy for most patients with IIIA disease. Of 15 patients treated in this fashion, 14 are alive and continuously free of disease (93% actuarial survival and relapse-free survival). Our results with radiation therapy alone for the treatment of IIIA disease are similar to those reported from the Joint Center at Harvard and the University of Chicago [6, 7] but contrast with those from Stanford, where the 5-year survival for patients treated with radiation therapy alone was 86% and the relapse-free survival 66% [8]. Reasons for these differences are not clear but seem unlikely to be due just to technique differences – the major one being the use of prophylactic liver radiation by the Stanford group for patients with splenic involvement.

Our data suggest two categories of patients with stage IIIA disease. Those

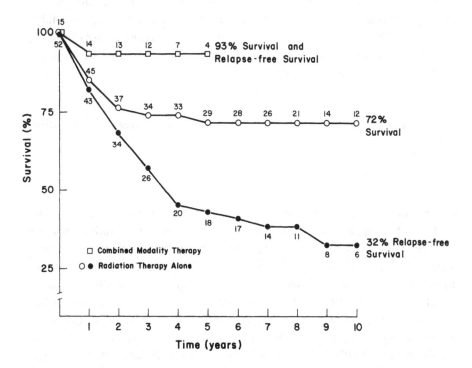

Figure 2. Actuarial survival and relapse-free survival of stage IIIA patients treated with radiation alone and with combined modality therapy.

individuals with clinically evident stage III disease prior to staging laparotomy (CS IIIA), i.e. a positive lymphangiogram, seem clearly to be a worse category than those who become IIIA only subsequent to a staging laparotomy (CS I, IIA/PS IIIA) [9]. In the former group, actuarial relapse-free survival was 18% at 5 years compared with approximately 50% for patients who were CS IA, IIIA/PS IIIA. This subdivision into CS IA, IIIA/PS IIIA and CS IIIA/PS IIIA corresponds roughly to the University of Chicago division into III_1 and III_2 and again our experience is similar to that of the Chicago and Harvard groups, where the III_2 category had a considerably worse outlook than the III_1 category in terms of relapse-free survival following radiation therapy alone.

Patients with PS IB and IIB disease comprise another uncommon subgroup, only 33 such patients having been treated at Yale between 1969 and 1980. 28 of the 33 received subtotal nodal irradiation (STNI) or total nodal irradiation (TNI) as therapy, and 5 were treated with combined modality therapy. The 5- and 10-year actuarial survival rates were 90% with 51% of patients being continuously free of disease. The 5 patients treated with combined modality therapy are all alive and free of disease.

In summary, PS IA and IIA patients comprise the majority of patients with limited stage disease, and these patients have done quite well (94% 10-year survival) with a treatment policy of initial radiation alone with chemotherapy reserved for relapsing patients. IIIA and I and IIB patients have acceptable survivals, (72% and 90%, respectively), but fairly high relapse rates (50–80%) when treated initially with radiation therapy alone, and should be considered for alternative therapeutic strategies.

3. Results of chemotherapy alone or combined modality treatment in limited stage disease

3.1. PS IA and IIA disease

Experience with chemotherapy alone in these patients or with combined modality therapy, is quite limited, largely because results of radiation alone have been so satisfactory that there is little motivation to change therapies. Some data are available from Stanford where, between 1968 and 1979, eight different protocols were in use for PS I and II patients, mostly comparing radiation alone versus radiation and a chemotherapeutic combination [2]. Results from these protocols were pooled to make some general comparisons. Actuarial 10-year survival was 84% in both patients receiving radiation alone and those treated with combined modality therapy. Freedom from relapse was 84% in the combined modality group and 77% in the radiation alone group (not significantly different).

In an attempt to identify specific patients at a high risk for relapse following radiation alone, several prognostic variables were examined, including systemic symptoms, age, histologic subtype, E lesions and large mediastinal masses. Only the group of patients with large mediastinal masses had a significantly worse relapse-free survival (45%) when treated with radiation alone compared with those receiving combined modality therapy (81% at 10 years). Overall survival was the same in both groups, however. The authors concluded that no firm rules could be established for the management of patients with large mediastinal masses and that treatment ought to be individualized.

A number of trials of combined modality therapy for stage IA and IIA disease have been conducted in European centers [10, 11, 12]. These studies are somewhat difficult to compare to the U.S. experience, since many of the patients did not undergo staging lapratotomy and/or the chemotherapy program was not as vigorous as the usual six months of MOPP (nitrogen mustard, vincristine, prednisone, procarbazine) that would be considered standard in the United States. Nevertheless, several conclusions emerge: (a) patients treated with combined modality therapy have a lesser relapse rate compared with radiation therapy alone; (b) the use of combined modality therapy probably obviates the need for staging laparotomy; (c) survival is not improved due to the ability to treat successfully with chemotherapy those patients relapsing after treatment with radiation alone. These studies for the most part do not discuss in any detail the long term effects of the different therapy programs, nor do they attempt to assess the risk-benefit ratio of the alternate therapies.

Chemotherapy alone without radiation for IA or IIA disease was utilized in a small series of children treated in Uganda [13]. Nine patients were treated with 6 months of MOPP, all achieved complete remission but actuarial survival at 5 years was 75%. The small numbers involved obviously prevent drawing any firm conclusions.

Hodgkin's disease in children, in general, represents a special situation because of the growth and development problems. An approach to treatment employing combination chemotherapy and low dose radiation (approximately 2000 rad) is being increasingly explored in an attempt to decrease the complications of full dose radiation in growing children. 15 patients have been treated with such a program at the Princess Margaret Institute in Toronto, with 14 of 15 remaining in remission for periods of 1–5 years [14]. 17 IA and IIA patients treated at Stanford University with 6 months of MOPP and low dose radiation are all alive and free of disease for periods of 1–10 years [15].

3.2. PS IIIA disease

We have already mentioned that the results in our experience and at most centers with the treatment of most PS IIIA patients with radiation therapy alone are not satisfactory, with relapse rates from 50–80%. In contrast, combined modality therapy in our institution has been very satisfactory, with 14 of 15 entering complete remission and remaining in complete remission from periods of 1–5 years. The British National Lymphoma Study compared patients with IIIA disease treated with chemotherapy alone versus radiation alone [16]. The patients treated with chemotherapy had a 72% complete response rate and a 53% relapse-free survival at two years, compared with a 90% complete response rate for patients treated with total nodal irradiation and a 71% two year relapse-free survival (the complete response rate differences were significant statistically, the relapse-free survivals were not).

At the National Cancer Institute, 7 patients with IIIA disease are included among the 198 patients treated with MOPP chemotherapy that comprise the well known NCI series [5]. We do not know precisely what happened to these 7, but amongst the somewhat larger group of 23 asymptomatic patients in the NCI series (stages IIA, IIIA and IVA), 22 of 23 remain without evidence of disease. This has led DeVita to suggest a study of chemotherapy alone as a treatment modality for stage IIIA disease.

A combined modality trial at the M.D. Anderson Hospital for IIIA disease included 55 patients who were treated with two cycles of MOPP and full dose total nodal irradiation [17]. The actuarial 5-year survival was 85% and the relapse-free survival was 76%.

3.3. PS I and IIB disease

As mentioned, this is an infrequent subset of patients, less than 10% of the overall Hodgkin's disease experience at Yale, with a similar frequency in other institutions. Therefore, there are not much data available as a guide to managing these patients. Our series comprises 33 patients. Five received combined modality therapy, all of whom are continuously free of disease. Twenty-eight patients were treated with radiation alone, 11 with subtotal nodal irradiation (7 have relapsed) and 17 with total nodal irradiation (9 have relapsed).

The experience at Stanford University was somewhat different. 38 patients treated with total nodal irradiation and chemotherapy had a virtually identical 10-year survival and relapse-free survival when compared to 26 patients treated with total nodal irradiation alone, both groups having an 80% 10-year relapse-free survival [2].

The Harvard group reported 11 patients with IIB disease treated with chemotherapy and total nodal irradiation, all of whom have subsequently been disease-free, compared with 11 patients treated with subtotal nodal irradiation or total nodal irradiation alone, 9 of whom have remained disease-free, one has relapsed and died and one has relapsed and subsequently become disease-fee with chemotherapy [18].

In summary then, the experience with chemotherapy alone in limited stage disease is in itself quite limited. Somewhat more data are available for the evaluation of combined modality therapy in limited stage disease. These data indicate no real survival advantage for the addition of chemotherapy to radiation for most patients, a probable exception being many stage IIIA patients. Relapse-free survival is improved by the addition of chemotherapy in most instances but this seldom conveys an improvement in overall survival, due to the ability to salvage most patients who relapse after radiation alone with subsequent chemotherapy.

4. Are there subsets of patients with limited stage disease who do not do well with radiation therapy alone and who should be considered for combined modality therapy as initial treatment?

We have already touched upon this question in some of the above sections, but will explore the issue in some detail here. The following groups of patients with limited stage disease are the ones most often alleged to have a worse outlook and/or perhaps in need of combined modality therapy at the onset: (1) patients with IA and IIA disease but with large mediastinal masses; (2) IB and IIB disease; (3) IIIA disease, most notable CS IIIA disease or III_2 disease; (4) limited E stage disease.

4.1. Mediastinal masses

About one half of the patients with IA and IIA disease will have mediastinal involvement and approximately one third of those with mediastinal involvement will have a mass lesion greater than one third the transverse diameter of the chest. Mauch *et al.* were the first to point out that patients with a large mediastinal mass appeared to have a higher relapse rate than those with either no mediastinal mass or a small one [19]. In their series, 50% of such patients relapsed. There was, however, no adverse effect on survival as the great majority of the relapsed patients were subsequently salvaged with combination chemotherapy. This observation has subsequently been confirmed in a number of other series. Patients with IA and IIA disease and large mediastinal masses had a 45% relapse-free survival at 10 years in the Stanford series [2], a relapse rate of 39% in the M.D. Anderson experience [20], 74% relapse rate in the Minnesota experience [21] and a 45% relapse rate in our experience at Yale [22]. In all of the above series survival was not adversely affected, however. Nevertheless, this relapse rate is cause for concern, since not all patients who relapse can be expected to be cured with subsequent chemotherapy.

Our own observations suggest that the larger the mass the worse the problem, that patients with a mediastinal mass greater than one half the transverse diameter of the chest should almost certainly have combined modality therapy at onset. Those with masses between one third and one half may perhaps be given a therapeutic trial of radiation and if rapid shrinkage occurs, radiation alone may be appropriate, but if not, one is almost forced to employ combined modality therapy because of the inability to properly shield from radiation the vital structures such as the heart and lungs. The patterns of failure in patients with mediastinal masses are of interest. In our series, of the 19 patients with mediastinal masses who relapsed, 12 of the 19 did so in the lungs or pleura. Prophylatic lung irradiation may decrease the relapse rate. This approach is being explored by several groups but additional data are needed.

These patients with large mediastinal masses constitute difficult management problems in a number of ways. The size of the mass may preclude a staging laparotomy at onset. It is our practice to evaluate the abdomen with lymphangiography and computed tomography. If these studies are negative and the mediastinal mass is between one third and one half the transverse diameter of the chest, then a trial of radiation therapy up to approximately 2000 rad is given. If there is good shrinkage, the patient then goes on to staging laparotomy, but if there is no appreciable reduction in the size of the mass, chemotherapy will be added. With chemotherapy and a negative clinical evaluation of the abdomen, staging laparotomy does not appear to be necessary.

Chemotherapy alone does not seem to be adequate for patients with large mediastinal masses. It is precisely this group of patients that had the highest relapse rate following induction of complete remission in the NCI series and it is a tendency of most centers to employ both radiation and chemotherapy for this group.

In our view, patients with large mediastinal masses and other stages of Hodgkin's disease besides I and IIA, i.e. IB or IIB or IIIA, should definitely receive combined modality treatment.

4.2. IB and IIB disease

The randomized Stanford trial showing no benefits for combined modality therapy compared with radiation alone, has already been mentioned. The relapse rate in our somewhat smaller series was 60%, however, for patients treated with radiation alone. Our bias is that IB and IIB patients with other factors that might also imply a worse prognosis, i.e. large mediastinal masses, should be treated with combined modality therapy from the onset. Total nodal irradiation is reserved for patients with either no mediastinal mass or a small one.

4.3. IIIA disease

In our experience this has been the worst category for Hodgkin's disease patients, both in terms of relapse rate and absolute survival, even worse than stage IIIB and IV because of the high relapse rate that has been observed when these patients were treated with radiation therapy alone (see section on results of radiation alone for details). Patients identified as IIIA prior to staging laparotomy did especially poorly, with an 82% relapse rate. Combined modality therapy without staging laparotomy is the recommended treatment for these patients. Patients with IIIA disease detected only subsequent to laparotomy with minimal involvement below the diaphragm would appear to be suitable for radiation alone, i.e. patients with upper paraaortic node involvement only or splenic hilar node involvement of minimal splenic involvement. The Stanford data [8] and a recent small series from the University of Minnesota suggest that prophylactic liver irradiation may be of benefit [23]. Therefore, those patients with splenic involvement who are treated with radiation therapy alone are now also receiving 1750 rad to the liver using a 50% transmission block during the course of 3500 rad to the inverted Y field.

4.4. E disease

There exists considerable confusion in the literature about this category of disease, its prognosis and suitability for treatment with radiation therapy alone. As we pointed out in a recent editorial [24], some of the confusion stems from labeling patients as stage IIE when they might be more appropriately termed stage IV, e.g. a patient with a mediastinal mass and a non-contiguous solitary pulmonary nodule. This type of patient is not suitable for curative radiation alone and one should not even make the attempt. The E category should be restricted to Musshof's original precepts, i.e. patients with a localized extranodal extension of disease but of a relative limited nature and technically suitable for curative radiation therapy alone.

The Baltimore Cancer Research Group has been the main proponent of the concept that E stage disease should not be treated with radiation alone but more appropriately with combined modality therapy [25]. However, most of the 11 patients in their series who received radiation alone received only 2000 rad to part of the tumor, usually because of very large mediastinal masses and concern for lung tolerance. These patients are probably more appropriately assessed in the large mediastinal mass category. The Stanford data as well as our own do not indicate any worse outlook for E disease, provided the definition is restricted in the way described.

5. What are the long term consequence of radiation alone, chemotherapy alone, and combined modality therapy?

This question has become central since we are now fortunate enough to have several curative modalities available for the treatment of Hodgkin's disease. It is no longer enough, however, to cure a patient with Hodgkin's disease. One must also attempt to do so with a minimum of complications. Sufficient experience has now accumulated with the various forms of treatment so that we have a fairly good idea of the long term toxicities of each modality. These will be enumerated below.

5.1. Radiation complications

The experience with supervoltage radiation for Hodgkin's disease now extends back more than 20 years and accordingly the long-term complications are reasonably well defined. They have been reviewed recently in a symposium on Contemporary Issues in Hodgkin's Disease [26]. Second malignancies following radiation alone are rare. In our protocol patients treated since 1969, among 253 patients that received radiation alone, there were a total of four second malignancies, only one of which appeared to be related to the radiation. This was a woman who developed thyroid cancer at age 28, 41/2 years after subtotal nodal irradiation for stage IIA Hodgkin's disease. Two patients, both in their 50's and both of whom were heavy smokers, developed carcinoma of the lung, three and 10 years after radiation for Hodgkin's disease, with the carcinoma appearing outside the high dose radiation field. One woman developed breast cancer at age 38, 18 months after treatment for IIA Hodgkin's disease. Two additional patients treated prior to 1969 and therefore not a part of the protocol group, developed basal cell skin carcinomas with the treatment fields. There have been no cases of leukemia or other second hematologic malignancies. This experience pretty much parallels that of other major centers. Second hematological malignancies are very rare and only a scattering of miscellaneous solid tumors have been recorded, many of which do not seem to be clearly related to the radiotherapy [2].

Other complications of radiation observed in our series have included a 4% frequency of radiation pneumonitis, pericarditis in 3%, hypothyroidism in 16%. One patient with radiation pneumonitis died from this complication, but otherwise all patients have recovered without permanent sequelae. None of the patients with radiation pericarditis has required surgical intervention.

Three patients have sustained fatal myocardial infarctions. One of these was a 23-year old man with no prior history of heart disease who had been treated with subtotal nodal irradiation for IIA Hodgkin's disease; three years later at age 26 he had a fatal myocardial infarct (autopsy confirmed). Another patient was treated at age 46 for IIB Hodgkin's disease with total nodal irradiation and sustained a fatal myocardial infarct six years later. The third patient had a preceding history of arteriosclerotic heart disease. He was treated with subtotal nodal irradiation for IIA Hodgkin's disease at age 52, and died of a myocardial infarct four years later. It seems reasonable to attribute the first patient's death to a radiation complication but probably not patients 2 and 3.

A major consequence of radiation in growing children is retardation of growth in whatever bones are included in the radiation field. With full therapeutic doses for Hodgkin's disease in a prepubertal child, this will result in marked stunting of growth in the irradiated bones in virtually all patients.

The other principal problem that may occur as a consequence of radiation therapy is impaired fertility. Patients with limited stages of Hodgkin's disease treated with subtotal nodal irradiation generally have no impairment of fertility except in the rare instances of women whose ovaries are unusually high in the pelvis and therefore may be inadvertently included in the lower end of the paraaortic field. This problem may be avoided by appropriately clipping and moving the ovaries at the time of staging laparotomy.

Male patients who receive total nodal irradiation may receive significant doses of radiation to the gonads (150–250 rad) if no special precautions are taken. If appropriate testicular shielding is used, however, doses are usually reduced well below 100 rad with transient effects on sperm production.

Women who receive total nodal irradiation will all have ablation of ovarian function if the ovaries are not surgically repositioned away from the pelvic nodes so that they can be shielded from radiation. Even with ideal positioning and subsequent shielding from the direct radiation beam, the ovaries receive approximately 10% of the treatment dose due principally to scatter. Most patients, however, will retain normal menstrual function or regain it after variable periods of amenorrhea, if the ovaries are properly positioned and shielded [27].

5.2. Chemotherapeutic complications

Short term problems such as gastrointestinal symptomatology or bone marrow depression will not be discussed, except to say that there is an approximately 1% frequency of fatal septicemia in most large series of patients treated with chemotherapy (including our own). Other serious long term problems include second malignancies, effects on gonadal function, and avascular necrosis of joints.

The most frequently observed second malignancy is acute non lymphocytic leukemia (ANLL). Following MOPP chemotherapy or similar combinations containing both an alkylating agent and procarbazine, the actuarial frequency of ANLL is about 5% at 5 years and may increase somewhat between the 5th and 10th year of follow-up [28, 29]. A similar risk of developing a non-Hodgkin's lymphoma (NHL) is present [30]. A variety of miscellaneous solid tumors have also been observed, but it is less clear that there is a causative relationship between these cancers and the antecedent chemotherapy. Some earlier reports suggested that the greatest frequency of second malignancies was in patients treated with combined modality therapy or those who had been initially treated with radiation for localized disease, subsequently relapsed and then received combination chemotherapy [31]. More recent studies, however, do not show significant differences in frequency of second hematologic malignancies for patients receiving chemotherapy alone compared with those receiving both radiation and chemotherapy [28, 29, 32]. Patients treated with the ABVD (adriamycin, bleomycin, vinblastine, DTIC) combination may not be at as great a risk for the development of a second malignancy. Thus far, the Milan group has not observed any second malignancies in patients receiving either ABVD alone or ABVD in combination with radiation [33].

The effects of chemotherapy on gonadal function are profound. With MOPP and related combinations, i.e. those that contain an alkylating agent and procarbazine, at least 80–90% of men will be rendered permanently sterile [34]. Again, ABVD may be less harmful in this regard [35]. Similarly, MOPP is apt to cause permanent amenorrhea in premenopausal women [36]. About one half of women treated will have this complication with the frequency increasing with the age of the patient. A promising investigational approach to the prevention of this problem is the use of oral contraceptives while the patient is receiving chemotherapy [37].

Avascular necrosis of bone has been reported with chemotherapy alone, probably more frequently with the combination of chemotherapy and radiation [38]. It is a non-fatal but potentially disabling complication whose exact frequency is unknown.

5.3. Complications of combined modality therapy

The complications of combined modality treatment are qualitatively very similar, if not identical to, those that are observed following chemotherapy or radiation therapy alone. They would thus include second malignancies, sterility, fatal septicemia, avascular necrosis, hypothyroidism, pneumonitis, pericarditis, and growth disturbances. The usual procedure in administration of combined modality therapy is to employ full doses of chemotherapy and thus the usual complications of chemotherapy will be expected. The dose of radiation therapy may be the full tumoricidal dose used for Hodgkin's disease when radiation therapy alone is being employed (i.e. 4000 rad) or may be reduced ('low dose' radiation therapy, approximately 2000 rad). The radiation complications will obviously be less in the latter situation.

In most organ systems, the frequency of a given complication will be increased by combining the two treatment modalities. For example, it is well established that the radiation tolerance of the lungs and heart is reduced by the concomitant administration of certain chemotherapeutic agents, such as alkylating agents, adriamycin and bleomycin [39]. A clear increase in a complication known to result from one modality caused by a combination of the two, e.g. increased frequency of radiation pneumonitis in patients receiving both drugs and radiation, has not been reported as yet in Hodgkin's disease patients treated with combined modality therapy. The lack of such reports, however, may be due to precautionary measures on the part of the radiation therapist or medical oncologist such as careful tailoring of treatment volumes, reduction in the radiation therapy dose, etc. It is our clinical impression that bone abnormalities are enhanced by the use of combined modality therapy both as far as the production of avascular necrosis is concerned, and growth impairment.

A critical question is the effect of combined modality therapy on the induction of second malignancies compared with the effects of either radiation or chemotherapy alone. It has been pointed out that second malignancies following radiation alone are very uncommon. Earlier studies in the literature suggested a frequency of ANLL and NHL of approximately 2–3% following chemotherapy alone, 5–7% after combined modality therapy [31]. More recent and larger studies, however, indicate a 5% five-year actuarial frequency for both ANLL and NHL after chemotherapy alone (again provided the combination contains both an alkylating agent and procarbazine) and a similar frequency after combined modality therapy [28, 29]. Additional follow-up will be necessary to resolve the question of whether there is a difference in this respect between chemotherapy alone and combined modality therapy.

6. Summary

Limited stage Hodgkin's disease is usually best treated with extended field radiation therapy alone. This results in a high cure rate and a relatively low long term complication rate. Combination chemotherapy is reserved for those patients who relapse and thus the majority of patients will be spared long term complications associated with the use of combination chemotherapy. With this approach, the frequency of relapse will be higher than if combined modality therapy were given to all patients from the onset, but the morbidity and mortality from treatment will be considerably less.

In certain subcategories of patients with limited stage disease, there is a high relapse rate following radiation therapy alone (greater than 50%) and, in these categories, the use of combined modality treatment may be appropriate from the onset since it would appear that such a high relapse rate will eventually translate into an increased morbidity as well.

Children constitute a special situation because of the profound effects of high dose radiation on growth. In most instances the risks of combined modality therapy seem preferable to the certainty that growth impairment will occur if full dose radiation is used.

There would appear to be little role for chemotherapy alone in limited stage disease. The few studies that are available in this regard suggest that combined modality treatment is superior to chemotherapy alone and that furthermore the complication rate is not significantly increased for combined therapy compared with chemotherapy alone.

References

1. Kapp DS, Prosnitz LR, Farber LR, et al.: Patterns of failure in Hodgkin's disease: the Yale Universty experience. Am J Clin Oncol, in press.
2. Hoppe RT, Coleman CN, Cox RS, et al.: The management of stage I/II Hodgkin's disease with irradiation alone or combined modality therapy: the Stanford experience. Blood 59:455–465, 1982.
3. Hellman S, Mauch P: Role of radiation therapy in the treatment of Hodgkin's disease. Cancer Treat Rep 66:915–923, 1982.
4. Prosnitz LR, Farber LR, Kapp DS, et al.: Combined modality therapy for advanced Hodgkin's disease: long term followup data. Cancer Treat Rep 66:871–879, 1982.
5. DeVita VT, Simon RM, Hubbard SM, et al.: Curability of advanced Hodgkin's disease with chemotherapy. Ann Intern Med 92:587–595, 1980.
6. Mauch P, Goodman R, Rosenthal DS, et al.: An evaluation of total nodal irradiation as treatment for stage IIIA Hodgkin's disease. Cancer 43:1255–1261, 1979.
7. Stein RS, Golomb HM, Diggs CH, et al.: Anatomic substages of stage IIIA Hodgkin's disease. Ann Intern Med 92:159–165, 1980.
8. Hoppe RT, Rosenberg SA, Kaplan HS, Cox RS: Prognostic factors in pathological stage IIIA Hodgkin's disease. Cancer 46:1240–1246, 1980.

9. Prosnitz LR, Montalvo RL, Fischer DB, *et al.*: Treatment of stage IIIA Hodgkin's disease: is radiotherapy alone adequate? Int J Oncol 4:781–787, 1978.

10. Tubiana M, Henry-Amar M, Hayat M, *et al.*: Long term results of the E.O.R.T.C. randomized study of irradiation and vinblastine in clinical stages I and II of Hodgkin's disease. Eur J Canc 15:645–657, 1979.

11. Andrieu JM, Montagnon B, Asselain B, *et al.*: Chemotherapy–radiotherapy association in Hodgkin's disease, clinical stages IA, II₂A. Cancer 46:2126–2130, 1980.

12. Nissen NI, Nordentoft AM: Radiotherapy versus combined modality treatment of stage I and II Hodgkin's disease. Cancer Treat Rep 66:799–803, 1982.

13. Olweny CLM, Katongole-Mbidde E, Kiire C, *et al.*: Childhood Hodgkin's disease in Uganda. Cancer 42:787–792, 1978.

14. Jenkin D, Chan H, Freedman M, *et al.*: Hodgkin's disease in children: treatment results with MOPP and low dose extended field irradiation. Cancer Treat Rep 66:949–960, 1982.

15. Donaldson SS: Pediatric Hodgkin's disease: focus on the future. In: Status of the curability of childhood cancers, Van Eys J, Sullivan MP (eds), New York: Raven Press, 1980.

16. British National Lymphoma Investigation: Initial treatment of stage IIIA Hodgkin's disease: comparison of radiotherapy with combined chemotherapy. Lancet 2:991–995, 1976.

17. Rodgers RW, Fuller LM, Hagemeister FB, *et al.*: Reassessment of prognostic factors in stage IIIA and IIIB Hodgkin's disease treated with MOPP and radiotherapy. Cancer 47:2196–2203, 1981.

18. Goodman R, Mauch P, Piro A, *et al.*: Stages IIB and IIIB Hodgkin's disease: results of combined modality treatment. Cancer 40:84–89, 1977.

19. Mauch P, Goodman R, Hellman S: The significance of mediastinal involvement in early stage Hodgkin's disease. Cancer 42:1039–1045, 1978.

20. Fuller LM, Madoc-Jones H, Hagemeister FB, *et al.*: Further follow-up of results of treatment in 90 laparotomy-negative stage I and II Hodgkin's disease patients: significance of mediastinal and non-mediastinal presentations. Int J Rad Oncol 6:799–808, 1980.

21. Lee CKK, Bloomfield CD, Levitt SH: Results of lung irradiation for Hodgkin's disease patients with large mediastinal masses and/or hilar disease. Cancer Treat Rep 66:819–826, 1982.

22. Prosnitz LR, Curtis AM, Knowlton AH, *et al.*: Supradiaphragmatic Hodgkin's disease: significance of large mediastinal masses. Int J Rad Oncol 6:809–813, 1980.

23. Lee CK, Bloomfield CD, Levitt SH: Liver irradiation in stage IIIA Hodgkin's disease patients with splenic involvement. Int J Rad Oncol 8:67, 1982.

24. Prosnitz LR: The Ann Arbor staging system for Hodgkin's disease: does 'E' stand for error? Int J Rad Oncol 2:1039, 1977.

25. Levi JA, Wiernik PH, O'Connell MJ: Patterns of relapse in stages I, II and IIIA Hodgkin's disease: influence of initial therapy and implications for the future. Int J Rad Oncol 2:853–862, 1977.

26. Kinsella TJ, Fraass BA, Glatstein E: Late effects of radiation therapy in the treatment of Hodgkin's disease. Cancer Treat Rep 66:991–1002, 1982.

27. Horning SJ, Hoppe RT, Kaplan HS, Rosenberg SA: Female reproductive potential after treatment for Hodgkin's disease. N Eng J Med 304:1377–1382, 1981.

28. Coltman CA, Dixon DO: Second malignancies complicating Hodgkin's disease: a Southwest Oncology Group 10-year followup. Cancer Treat Rep 66:1023–1034, 1982.

29. Glicksman AS, Pajak TF, Gottlieb A, *et al.*: Second malignant neoplasms in patients successfully treated for Hodgkin's disease: a cancer and leukemia group B study. Cancer Treat Rep 66:1035–1044, 1982.

30. Krikorian JG, Burke JS, Rosenberg SA, Kaplan HS: Appearance of non-Hodgkin's lymphoma after therapy for Hodgkin's disease. N Eng J Med 300:452–458, 1979.

166

31. Arseneau JC, Canellos GP, Johnson R, DeVita VT: Risk of new cancers in patients with Hodgkin's disease. Cancer 40:1912–1916, 1977.
32. Pedersen-Bjergaard J, Larsen SO: Incidence of acute non-lymphocytic leukemia, pre-leukemia and acute myeloproliferative syndrome up to 10 years after treatment of Hodgkin's disease. N Eng J Med 307:965–971, 1982.
33. Valagussa P, Santoro A, Bellani FF, et al.: Absence of treatment-induced second neoplasms after ABVD in Hodgkin's disease. Proc Am Assoc Cancer Res 22:197, 1981.
34. Whitehead E, Shalet SM, Blackledge G, et al.: The effects of Hodgkin's disease and combination chemotherapy on gonadal function in the adult male. Cancer 49:418–422, 1982.
35. Santoro A, Bonadonna G, Zucali R, et al.: Therapeutic and toxicologic effects of MOPP versus ABVD when combined with RT in Hodgkin's disease. Proc Am Soc Clin Oncol 22:522, 1981.
36. Chapman RM, Sutcliffe SB, Malpas JS: Cytotoxic-induced ovarian failure in women with Hodgkin's disease: 1. Hormone function. JAMA 242:1877–1881, 1979.
37. Chapman RM, Sutcliffe SB: Protection in of ovarian function by oral contraceptives in women receiving chemotherapy for Hodgkin's disease. Blood 58:849–851, 1981.
38. Prosnitz LR, Lawson JP, Friedlaender GE, et al.: Avascular necrosis of bone in Hodgkin's disease patients treated with combined modality therapy. Cancer 47:2793–2797, 1981.
39. Phillips TL, Fu KK: Quantification of combined radiation therapy and chemotherapy effects on critical normal tissues. Cancer 37:1186–1200, 1976.

8. Chemotherapy for stage III-A Hodgkin's disease: The proper role

RICHARD S. STEIN

1. Introduction

Despite the availability of results from a large number of clinical trials, therapy of stage III-A Hodgkin's disease remains a subject of controversy as chemotherapy alone, radiotherapy alone, and combined modality therapy have all been advocated as optimal treatment for patients with stage III-A Hodgkin's disease. In this paper I will review the data which supports each of these therapeutic recommendations. However, the majority of this paper will review the evidence that there is no one optimal therapy for stage III-A Hodgkin's disease, and that, instead, anatomic substage – the extent of nodal disease within the abdomen – should be the critical factor in allocating stage III-A Hodgkin's disease patients to different therapies.

2. Chemotherapy alone as initial therapy

The argument that chemotherapy alone is the optimal treatment for all patients with stage III-A Hodgkin's disease is based on limited data. In the large MOPP series reported from the National Cancer Institute [1], 175 of 198 patients were symptomatic. Of the 23 asymptomatic patients (III-A and IV-A), 94% were alive and free of disease at both five and ten years. This is the best clinical result reported in stage III-A Hodgkin's disease, and if this data had been replicated, the only argument against chemotherapy alone as optimal treatment would be that it is unnecessarily toxic, i.e. chemotherapy is associated with nausea, vomiting, and a high incidence of undesirable late side effects such as sterility. This toxicity would be especially hard to justify in view of the fact that for stage III patients with limited disease, mantle and upper abdominal radiotherapy ports, without the inclusion of pelvic radiotherapy, may be adequate therapy.

However, the major argument against chemotherapy alone as the optimal treatment for all stage III-A patients is that the excellent results achieved in the

Bennett JM (ed), Controversies in the Management of Lymphomas. ISBN 0-89838-586-5.
© *Martinus Nijhoff Publishers, Boston. Printed in the Netherlands.*

NCI series have not been replicated. In a British study [2] of patients with stage III-A Hodgkin's disease randomized to either total nodal irradiation or MOPP, complete remissions were achieved in only 75% of patients receiving MOPP. At 2 years, relapse-free survival in patients receiving MOPP was less than 50%, although with salvage therapy the overall survival at 4 years was 90%, equivalent to the results achieved with radiotherapy alone.

These studies suggest that MOPP is a reasonable option for patients with stage III-A Hodgkin's disease but do not establish it as the optimal therapy for all patients. Results obtained with chemotherapy alone are not clearly superior to results obtained with other approaches (Table 1). As will be discussed in detail, for patients in substage III_1, chemotherapy alone as initial therapy probably represents overtreatment. However, in view of the poor results obtained in substage III_2 with radiotherapy alone (Table 2), therapy with chemotherapy alone or with chemotherapy plus radiotherapy is a very reasonable therapeutic option for these patients.

3. Radiotherapy alone as initial treatment

Considering all stage III-A patients as a single group, results using radiotherapy alone, with chemotherapy reserved for salvage, have been comparable to the results achieved with chemotherapy alone. Some of the best results using radiotherapy alone (Table 1) have been achieved at Stanford University where the standard total nodal radiotherapy ports are generally modified to include the liver (when splenic involvement is present) and the ipsilateral lung (when mediastinal disease is present). Researchers at Stanford have reported 5-year relapse-free survival of 66% in stage III-A patients, and a 5-year overall survival rate of 86% [3, 4]. Using standard radiotherapy, the results we have

Table 1. Therapeutic results in stage III-A Hodgkin's disease.

Treatment	Author	5-y relapse-free survival	5-y survival
MOPP	DeVita *et al.* [1]	94%	94%
MOPP	Strickland [2]	50%	85%
Radiotherapy	Hoppe *et al.* [3, 4]	66%	86%
Radiotherapy	Stein *et al.* [5, 6]	49%	76%
Radiotherapy & chemotherapy	Hoppe *et al.* [3, 4]	86%	89%
Radiotherapy & chemotherapy	Stein *et al.* [5, 6]	89%	89%

previously reported in a collaborative study are a 5-year relapse-free survival of 49% and a 5-year survival of 76% [5, 6].

While these results may at first glance suggest that the radiotherapy approach employed at Stanford is optimal for all stage III-A patients, this is probably not the case. As shown in Table 2, for patients in substage III_1, equivalent results – and presumably less toxicity – have been obtained with smaller ports than those used at Stanford. Only for substage III_2 does the modified radiotherapy approach used at Stanford seem to be superior to standard total nodal radiotherapy. However, it remains to be established that radiotherapy alone is the optimal approach to stage III_2 disease. Clearly, *standard* total nodal radiotherapy is inadequate therapy for stage III_2–A Hodgkin's disease. As Table 2 deals only with results at 5 years, this latter point may be underscored by noting that using total nodal radiotherapy as initial treatment we have reported an 8-year relapse-free survival of only 19% and an 8-year overall survival of only 41% in patients with stage III_2–A disease [6].

While the majority of this discussion is concerned with therapy of stage III-A disease it is relevant at this point to note that there is precedent for defining subsets of stage III disease for which radiotherapy alone is inadequate therapy – specifically stage III-B disease. Relapse-free survival at 5 years following radiotherapy alone in stage III-B has been reported to be as low as 7% [7]. In essence this means that nearly all patients assigned to radiotherapy for stage III-B disease will eventually require chemotherapy. Since it is optimal to administer chemotherapy when the tumor burden is minimal, combined modality therapy as initial therapy seems preferable to radiotherapy alone as the initial treatment of these patients, and, generally, chemotherapy alone or chemotherapy plus radiotherapy are used in these patients (Table 3). The data to which I have alluded above, and which will be presented in detail, suggests that similar considerations may be made for stage III_2-A as for stage III-B disease.

Table 2. Results with radiotherapy alone in stage III-A Hodgkin's disease as related to substage.

Stage	Author	5-y relapse-free survival	5-y survival
III_1	Hoppe *et al.* [3, 4]	62%	90%
III_1	Stein *et al.* [5, 6]	64%	90%
III_2	Hoppe *et al.* [3, 4]	69%	88%
III_2	Stein *et al.* [5, 6]	32%	53%

Table 3. Therapeutic results in stage III-B Hodgkin's disease.

Treatment	Author	5-y relapse-free survival	5-y survival
Radiotherapy & chemotherapy	Rosenberg et al. [7]	50%	62%
Radiotherapy	Rosenberg et al. [7]	7%	44%
MOPP	DeVita et al. [1]*	63%	61%

* Includes stage IV-B as well as III-B.

4. Combined modality therapy (chemotherapy plus radiotherapy) as initial treatment

One solution to the controversy regarding therapy for stage III-A Hodgkin's disease has been to advocate the use of combined modality therapy. Simply speaking, the rationale of this approach is that the patient with stage III-A disease is at risk of relapse following total nodal radiotherapy, and that this risk may be reduced by systemic therapy which might effectively deal with occult disease outside the radiotherapy ports.

There are several drawbacks to this approach. First, combined modality therapy is unnecessarily toxic to those patients who could be cured by radiotherapy alone. This toxicity includes not only the morbidity of nausea, vomiting, myelotoxicity and potential sterility, but the mortality of a very refractory form of acute myelogenous leukemia. This risk, which is clearly higher in patients receiving combined modality therapy than in patients receiving chemotherapy alone or radiotherapy alone, has been estimated at four percent at seven years [8]. While it has been suggested that the use of ABVD rather than MOPP in combined modality therapy may be associated with a lesser risk of leukemia [9], the limited duration of follow-up in the radiotherapy plus ABVD study limits the acceptance of that approach.

The risk of leukemogenesis associated with combined modality therapy would be acceptable, however, if such therapy was clearly associated with superior results. In fact, despite the handicap of being associated with a risk of fatal acute leukemia, long term survival with combined modality therapy has been *superior* to the results obtained with radiotherapy alone in stage III-A Hodgkin's disease. For stage III-A patients we have reported an 8-year relapse-free survival of 88% and an 8-year survivial of 86% using combined modality therapy [6]. For similar combined modality therapy plus radiotherapy, Stanford has reported a 5-year relapse-free survival of 86% and a 5-year survival of 89% [4]. When compared to radiotherapy alone, these improvements with combined modality therapy have been statistically significant in some studies [5, 6] and not significant in others [3, 4]. This suggests, however, that if a single approach were to be taken for all stage III-A patients, combined modality therapy would probably be the most logical approach. Nevertheless, while combined modality therapy might produce the best results for the population of patients, choosing therapy based on anatomic substage can limit the morbidity and mortality associated with treatment while not compromising clinical results.

5. Anatomic substage as a basis for determining therapy in stage III-A Hodgkin's disease

In a number of recent studies [5, 6, 10, 11] investigators have attempted to resolve the controversy regarding therapy of stage III-A Hodgkin's disease by considering anatomic substage. In summary, these studies have suggested that:

a) Patients with stage III-A Hodgkin's disease can be divided into anatomic substages based on the extent of abdominal nodal disease. Stage III_1 is defined as including stage III patients with abdominal involvement limited to the lymphatic structures in the upper abdomen, i.e. spleen, or splenic, celiac, or hepatic portal node, or any combination of these. Stage III_2 is defined as including stage III patients with involvement of lower abdominal nodes, i.e. para-aortic, iliac, or mesenteric nodes, with or without involvement of upper abdominal sites.

b) Patients in the two substages have markedly different prognoses. In fact, the survival curves for the two substages are so different when patients are treated with radiotherapy alone that they may be considered as different stages.

c) Anatomic substage is a rational basis for determining therapy for patients with stage III-A Hodgkin's disease. For patients in substage III_1-A, radiotherapy alone – with chemotherapy reserved for salvage – is adequate therapy as this approach has produced results equivalent to the best results achieved with combined modality therapy. For patients in stage III_2-A, the results of radiotherapy alone are not adequate; these patients require either combined modality therapy or chemotherapy alone.

The data for the above statements comes from a number of independent clinical trials [10–13]. However, since some of those studies used slightly different definitions of substage, and also included some patients with stage III-B disease, raw data from those studies was pooled in a collaborative effort [5]. This data has recently been updated [6]. While the data from any of the individual institutions would support the same conclusions, I will use the data from the collaborative study [6] as the basis for the following discussion.

All 130 stage III-A patients in the study [6] had undergone pathologic staging including laparotomy. Follow-up was greater than 5 years for 128 patients and greater than 8 years for 100 patients. Details of therapy have been previously reported [5, 6]. Eighty-five patients received radiotherapy alone. These patients received chemotherapy only at the time of relapse; combination chemotherapy was identical to that used in the combined modality group. Forty-five patients received combined modality therapy, i.e. chemotherapy plus radiotherapy. Combination chemotherapy was either the standard MOPP regimen [1, 14] or a minimal variant, i.e. cyclophosphamide substituted for mechlorethamine or vinblastine for vincristine. Although most patients received chemotherapy after radiotherapy, seven patients received three to four cycles of chemotherapy before radiotherapy.

The composition of the entire series, and of the various treatment and substage groups is shown in Table 4. Clearly, differences attributed to substage in this study cannot be attributed to differences in gender, age, or histologic type of Hodgkin's disease.

For the entire series, 8-year relapse-free survival was 59% and 8-year survival was 69%. If patients are pooled with respect to therapy and stratified only on the basis of substage, the clinical results are superior in stage III_1-A as compared to III_2-A. Relapse-free survival was 70% for stage III_1-A as com-

Table 4. Characteristics of patient groups.*

	Stage III_1	Stage III_2	Stage III_1		Stage III_2	
			RT	RT/CT	RT	RT/CT
Patients studied	74	56	48	26	37	19
Sex						
Male	41	34	27	14	24	10
Female	33	22	21	12	13	9
Median age (years)	28	27	28	29	28	26
Histology						
Lymphocyte predominant	5	5	1	4	1	4
Nodular sclerosis	46	32	30	16	22	10
Mixed cellularity	23	19	17	6	14	5
Therapy						
RT	48	37				
RT/CT	26	19				
Spleen						
Involved	68	37				
Not involved	6	19				

* RT = radiotherapy alone; RT/CT = radiotherapy and chemotherapy. Unless specified otherwise, values = no. of patients.

pared to 40% for stage III$_2$-A, p<.001. Overall survival was 80% for stage III$_1$-A as compared to 54% for stage III$_2$-A, p<.001.

Stratifying on the basis of therapy, and considering only those patients who received radiotherapy as initial treatment, the differences again strongly favor stage III$_1$-A (Fig. 1). Both relapse-free survival (60% *vs*. 19%, p<.001) and overall survival (76% *vs*. 41%, p<.001) are significantly better in III$_1$-A as compared to III$_2$-A (Table 5). These differences are of the same order of magnitude as the differences in relapse-free survival and survival which are observed when stage II and stage III are compared. It should also be noted that the overall survival in stage III$_2$-A is similar to that reported for stage IV patients treated with MOPP [1].

The differences in survival between substage III$_1$ and substage III$_2$ support the idea that these substages could meaningfully be regarded as separate stages. In fact, throughout this discussion we use the terms stage and substage as equivalent terms in describing substage (stage) III$_1$ and III$_2$. However, my primary concern is not merely to show that these substages are different, but to illustrate that different therapies are appropriate for each substage.

While this was not a randomized trial, as shown in Table 4, within each substage, patients receiving radiotherapy and patients receiving combined modality therapy are comparable with respect to age, sex, and histology. Thus, it is reasonable to stratify on the basis of substage and analyze for the effects of therapy.

For the entire series, both relapse-free survival (88% *vs*. 43%, p<.001) and survival (86% *vs*. 61%, p<.001) are better in patients receiving combined modality therapy. As previously noted, if one therapy had to be chosen for all

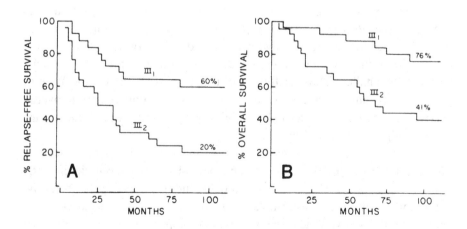

Figure 1. Actuarial relapse free survival (A) and overall survival (B) for all stage III$_1$ and III$_2$ patients treated with radiotherapy alone. P < .001.

Table 5. Relapse-free survival and overall survival as related to substage and treament groups

Stage	Therapy*	No. of patients	8-y relapse-free survival	8-y overall survival
III_1	RT, RT/CT	74	71%	80%
			$p < 0.001$	$p < 0.001$
III_2	RT, RT/CT	56	40%	54%
III_1	RT	48	60%	76%
			$p < 0.002$	$p = 0.20$
III_1	RT/CT	26	92%	88%
III_2	RT	37	19%	41%
			$p < 0.001$	$p < 0.01$
III_2	RT/CT	19	84%	84%
III_1 and III_2	RT	85	43%	61%
			$p < 0.001$	$p < 0.01$
III_1 and III_2	RT/CT	45	88%	86%

*RT = radiotherapy alone; RT/CT = radiotherapy and chemotherapy.

stage III-A patients, combined modality therapy would be the logical choice. However, a careful examination of the data suggests that this is not the optimal approach as the differences in favor of combined modality therapy are primarily limited to stage III_2.

For patients in substage III_1, relapse-free survival was superior in patients receiving combined modality therapy as compared to patients receiving radiotherapy alone, 92% *vs.* 60%, p<.002. However, because of the efficacy of salvage chemotherapy in stage III_1 patients who relapsed following radiotherapy alone, overall survival was not significantly different for the two treatment groups. Specifically, in stage III_1 patients, actuarial overall survival at 8 years was 76% with radiotherapy alone (with chemotherapy salvage as needed) as compared to 88% with combined modality as initial therapy, p = .20. With further follow-up beyond 8 years, this difference has become numerically smaller. Thus, at this time, it appears that the combination of chemotherapy and radiotherapy offers no significant improvement in overall survival to the results which can be achieved with radiotherapy alone in stage III_1-A Hodgkin's disease (Fig. 2).

For stage III_2-A disease, however, radiotherapy alone is not adequate therapy. Both relapse-free survival and overall survival were significantly better in patients receiving combined modality therapy than in patients receiving radiotherapy alone. In substage III_2-A patients, relapse-free survival at 8 years was only 19% with radiotherapy alone as compared to 84% for combined modality therapy, p<.001. Overall survival in stage III_2 was 84% in patients receiving combined modality therapy as compared to 41% in patients receiving

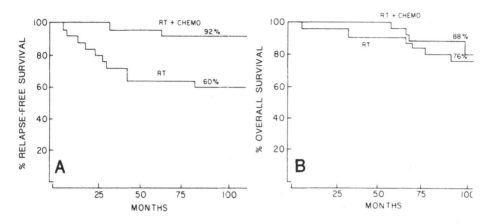

Figure 2. Actuarial relapse free survival (A) and overall survival (B) for stage III₁ patients given either radiotherapy alone or radiotherapy plus chemotherapy. For A, p < .002; for B, p = .20.

radiotherapy alone, p<.01 (Fig. 3). This 41% survival figure is inferior to the results which should be achievable with chemotherapy alone in *stage IV*. Thus, standard total nodal radiotherapy is inadequate for stage III₂, and these patients require either combined modality therapy or chemotherapy alone.

This study also provides some insights into why stage III₂-A disease is associated with a poor prognosis when radiotherapy alone is given. There is probably no negative prognosis associated with involvement of lower abdominal nodes *per se*; stage I and II Hodgkin's disease presenting below the diaphragm has been shown to carry a prognosis equivalent to stage I or II disease presenting above the diaphragm [15]. However, it seems reasonable that – compared to III₁ disease – stage III₂ disease involves a greater tumor burden and reflects either poorer control of disease by the patient or greater time elapsed since the onset of the illness. Either of these factors might be associated with a greater tendency to dissemination and while the incidence of nodal relapses were similar for patients in III₁ and in III₂, visceral relapses were significantly more frequent in the III₂ patients receiving radiotherapy (51%) than in the stage III₁ patients receiving radiotherapy (23%), p = .007. Since survival following visceral relapses is poorer than survival following nodal relapses, it is not surprising that overall survival was worse in stage III₂.

Since stage III₂ has a relatively poor prognosis because of the higher risk of visceral dissemination, it would be expected that therapeutic measures designed to limit visceral dissemination may eliminate the negative prognosis associated with stage III₂ disease. In our series, stage III₂ disease was associated with an overall survival equivalent to that observed in stage III₁ when one considers *only* the patients who received combined modality therapy. Also, using radiation ports which included the lung and liver, physicians at Stanford

176

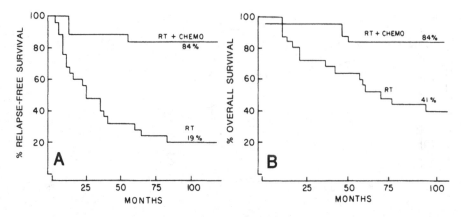

Figure 3. Actuarial relapse free survival (A) and overall survival (B) for stage III$_2$ patients given either radiotherapy alone or radiotherapy plus chemotherapy. For A, p < .001; for B, p < .01.

have produced results in stage III$_2$, equivalent to those achieved in stage III$_1$ [3, 4]. Since the lungs and liver accounted for many of the visceral relapses in our series, this result with radiotherapy is not unexpected. However, in addition to the fact that the long term sequellae of that radiation approach are not known, it is also true that the lungs and liver are not the sole sites of visceral failure. In patients with a high risk of visceral dissemination, i.e. stage III$_2$, systemic chemotherapy would seem a more rational addition to radiotherapy than the use of modified radiotherapy ports.

6. Anatomic substage: implications for staging

All the studies regarding the utility of substage come from series which have employed staging laparotomy. These studies have shown an inaccuracy of clinical substaging in as many as 30% of cases [5]. While this suggests that staging laparotomy should be performed routinely, this is probably *not* the case.

For patients with clinical stage I or II Hodgkin's disease – nodular sclerosis type – excellent results can be obtained using radiotherapy alone following clinical staging [16, 17]. While up to a third of these patients might be found to be in stage III at laparotomy, analysis of laparotomy findings suggests that most of these patients would have disease limited to the upper abdomen, i.e. stage III$_1$ [18]. Without a laparotomy, these patients would receive extended field radiotherapy which would include the upper abdomen. Unless pelvic radiotherapy is somehow critical in stage III$_1$, this would be adequate treatment.

As for patients with a positive lymphangiogram, if chemotherapy is to be employed, staging laparotomy to detect stage IV disease seems pointless, and the only value of laparotomy would be to detect the false positive lymphangiogram, i.e. the patient who is truly less than stage III$_2$.

While no firm data on this point exist, it is my opinion that lymphangiograms can generally be divided into those which are unequivically positive and those which are 'probably positive.' In the former group it seems reasonable to proceed on the basis of clinical staging; in the latter group staging laparotomy may be valuable. It should be noted in this regard that Hodgkin's disease tends to spread in a contiguous fashion within the abdomen [10]. When a lymphangiogram is read as positive based on a single node which would suggest a 'skip' pattern of disease, it is probably best to regard the lymphangiogram as equivocal no matter how 'positive' the solitary node appears.

7. Splenic involvement in Hodgkin's disease: a re-evaluation

One of the major facts to emerge from early studies of staging laparotomy in Hodgkin's disease was that splenic involvement was a necessary condition for hepatic involvement [18]. Also demonstrated, but not particularly emphasized in these early reports on the relationship between splenic involvement and hepatic involvement was the fact that the greater the weight of the involved spleen, the higher the risk of hepatic involvement (Table 6) [19–25]. A decade marked by only sporadic cases of hepatic involvement in the absence of splenic involvement [26] has served to establish the reliability of these observations. Nevertheless, two of the assumptions drawn from this association of splenic involvement and hepatic involvement have not borne fruit and probably should be laid to rest.

First, the demonstration that splenic involvement was necessary for liver

Table 6. Liver involvement in Hodgkin's disease as related to splenic involvement and splenic weight.*

	Liver involved/No. of cases
Spleen involved	
Weight > 400 grams	10/27
Weight < 400 grams	6/61
Spleen not involved	
Weight > 400 grams	0/4
Weight < 400 grams	0/112

* Source: references 19–25.

involvement supported the idea that splenic involvement was a sign of hema-togenous spread and as such an indicator for systemic therapy. Such a hypoth-esis is attractive, especially as there are no obvious lymphatic channels into the spleen. However, while splenic involvement in Hodgkin's disease may indi-cate hematogenous spread, a decade of clinical trials [3–6] has clearly established that splenic involvement is compatible with clinical cure by radi-otherapy alone. In fact, as has been discussed, for patients with stage III$_1$ disease this appears to be the optimal approach. In these patients, visceral disease is either not present, or not beyond the ability of the host to produce a cure once radiotherapy has dealt with the bulk of the disease.

The second idea to emerge from the association of splenic involvement and hepatic involvement was the idea that within stage III, splenic involvement should be used as a basis for stratifying patients and for making clinical decisions. The high water mark for this idea was the Ann Arbor Conference on Hodgkin's disease, when stage III disease was separated into III and III-S based on whether or not splenic involvement was present.

However, despite the Ann Arbor modification of the staging system for Hodgkin's disease, there is little evidence that splenic involvement is a critical prognostic factor within stage III. Among radiotherapy series, relapse free survival has only occasionally been significantly better in stage III patients *without* splenic involvement [2, 27]. Furthermore, overall survival has gener-ally been equivalent in stage III patients with and without splenic involvement, or else has been slightly *better* in patients with splenic involvement [3, 6] (Table 7).

It may seem paradoxical that splenic involvement, an indicator of possible hepatic involvement, would not be a prognostic factor in stage III disease. However, a bit of analysis quickly suggests why this might be the case. Patients with splenic involvement include both patients with hepatic disease as well as patients without evidence of hepatic disease. When staging laparotomy is

Table 7. Therapeutic results in stage III Hodgkin's disease as related to splenic involvement in patients receiving radiotherapy only.

Stage	Author	5-y relapse-free survival	5-y survival
IIIS +	Stein *et al.* [6]	49%	80%
IIIS −	Stein *et al.* [6]	57%	53%
IIIS +	Hoppe *et al.* [3]	61%	85%
IIIS −	Hoppe *et al.* [3]	71%	68%
IIIS +	Strickland [2]	40%	80%
IIIS −	Strickland [2]	75%	80%

performed, many - if not most - of the patients with both splenic and hepatic disease are detected and correctly categorized astæ as stage IV. Once these patients have been identified, and separated from the stage III patients, splenic involvement loses its prognostic value in stage III.

While splenic involvement *per se* has not proven to have prognostic significance in stage III Hodgkin's disease, splenic involvement is not totally irrelevant. A number of studies [3, 4, 6] have suggested that the number of splenic nodules may provide useful prognostic information. In two series [3, 6], the number of splenic nodules has predicted an increased risk of relapse following radiotherapy alone. However, because of effective salvage therapy, the number of splenic nodules has not been shown to predict a significantly inferior survival if radiotherapy alone is used.

In our series [6], patients were stratified with respect to both substage and the extent of splenic involvement. Limited splenic involvement was defined as four or fewer nodules; extensive involvement was defined as five or more nodules. Within substage III_2, the prognosis conferred by substage was such that radiotherapy alone appeared inadequate regardless of the number of splenic nodules. For substage III_1, however, results were different. Substage III_1 patients with limited splenic involvement who received radiotherapy alone had a response much like that seen in *stage II*; 8-year relapse-free survival was 86% and 8-year survival was 91%. For stage III_1 patients with extensive splenic disease 8-year relapse-free surivæ survival was 41% and 8-year survival was only 72%. These differences with respect to survival as related to the number of splenic nodules are not statistically significant. However, the chance of finding a significant difference is limited by the fact that the number of patients in any subset is small when one stratifies by treatment, substage, and number of splenic nodules. Thus, it is not clear whether or not therapy in stage III_1 should be modified based on the number of splenic nodules. Further studies will be needed to resolve this point. One factor does emerge from these recent studies [3–6]; once one has separated stage III patients from stage IV patients by performing staging laparotomy, the number of splenic nodules is a far more important prognostic factor than splenic involvement *per se*.

8. Summary

Anatomic substage is a major prognostic indicator in stage III Hodgkin's disease and can serve as a rational basis for allocating patients to receive radiotherapy alone as opposed to chemotherapy with or without irradiation. While excellent results have been achieved in some series using radiotherapy alone, or chemotherapy alone for all stage III patients, such approaches likely represent undertreatment for some patients and overtreatment for others.

Basing therapy on anatomic substage is a rational means of minimizing toxicity while maximizing clinical benefits.

References

1. DeVita VT, Simon RM, Hubbard SM, *et al.*: Curability of advanced Hodgkin's disease with chemotherapy. Ann Intern Med 92:587–595, 1980.
2. Strickland P: Radiotherapy or chemotherapy as the initial treatment for stage IIIA Hodgkin's disease (Report No. 13). Clin Radiol 32:527–530, 1981.
3. Hoppe RT, Rosenberg SA, Kaplan HS, *et al.*: Prognostic factors in pathologic stage IIIA Hodgkin's disease. Cancer 46:1240–1246, 1980.
4. Hoppe RT, Cox RS, roseæ Rosenberg SA, Kaplan HS: Prognostic factors in pathologic stage III Hodgkin's disease. Cancer Treat Rep 66:743–749, 1982.
5. Stein RS, Golomb HM, Diggs CH, *et al.*: Anatomic substages of stage III-A Hodgkin's disease. A collaborative study. Ann Intern Med 92:159–165, 1980.
6. Stein RS, Golomb HM, Wiernik PH, *et al.*: Anatomic substages of stage IIIA Hodgkin's disease: followup of a collaborative study. Cancer Treat Rep 66:733–741, 1982.
7. Rosenberg SA, Kaplan HS, Glatstein EJ, *et al.*: Combined modality therapy of Hodgkin's disease: a report on the Stanford trials. Cancer 42:991–1000, 1978.
8. Coleman CN, Williams CJ, Flint A, *et al.*: Hematologic neoplasia in patients treated for Hodgkin's disease. N Engl J Med 297:1249–1252, 1977.
9. Valagussa P, Santoro A, Fossati F, *et al.*: Absence of treatmentinduced second neoplasms after ABVD in Hodgkin's disease. Blood 59:488–494, 1982.
10. Desser RK, Golomb HM, Ultmann JE, *et al.*: Prognostic classification of Hodgkin's disease in pathologic stage III, based on anatomic considerations. Blood 49:883–893, 1977.
11. Levi JA, Wiernik PH: The therapeutic implications of splenic involvement in stage IIIA Hodgkin's disease. Cancer 39:2158–2165, 1977.
12. Hellman S, Mauch P, Goodman RL, *et al.*: The place of radiation therapy in the treatment of Hodgkin's disease. Cancer 42:971–978, 1978.
13. Stein RS, Hilborn RM, Flexner JM, *et al.*: Anatomical substages of stage III Hodgkin's disease. Cancer 42:429–436, 1978.
14. DeVita VT, Simon RM, Hubbard SM, *et al.*: Curability of Advanced Hodgkin's disease with chemotherapy. Ann of Intern Med 92:587–595, 1980.
15. Krikorian JG, Portlock CS, Rosenbert SA, *et al.*: Hodgkin's disease, stages I and II coæ occurring below the diaphragm. Cancer 43:1866–1871, 1979.
16. Griffin T, Gerdes A, Parker R, *et al.*: Are pelvic irradiation and routine staging laparotomy necessary in clinically staged IA and IIA Hodgkin's disease? Cancer 40:2914–2916, 1977.
17. Johnson RE, Zimbler H, Berard CW, *et al.*: Radiotherapy results for nodular sclerosing Hodgkin's disease after clinical staging. Cancer 39:1439–1444, 1977.
18. Desser RK, Moran EM, Ultmann JE: Staging of Hodgkin's disease and lymphoma: diagnostic procedures including staging laparotomy and splenectomy. Med Clin N Am 57:479–498, 1973.
19. Aisenberg AC, Goldman JM, Baker JW, *et al.*: Spleen involvement at the onset of Hodgkin's disease. Ann Intern Med 74:544, 1971.
20. Farrer-Brown G, Bennett MH, Harrison CV, *et al.*: Pathological findings following laparotomy in Hodgkin's disease. Br J Cancer 25:499, 1971.
21. Glatstein E, Guernsey JM, Rosenberg SA, *et al.*: The value of laparotomy and splenectomy in the staging of Hodgkin's disease. Cancer 24:709, 1969.

22. Glatstein E, Trueblood HW, Enright LP, *et al.*: Surgical staging of abdominal involvement in unselected patients with Hodgkin's disease. Radiology 97:425, 1970.
23. Hanks GE, Newsome JF, Lewis NT: The value of laparotomy in staging lymphomas. South Med J 64:585, 1971.
24. Lowenbraum S, Ramsey H, Sutherland J, *et al.*: Diagnostic laparotomy and splenectomy for staging Hodgkin's disease. Ann Intern Med 72:655, 1970.
25. Prosnitz LR, Nuland SB, Kiligerman MM: Role of laparotomy and splenectomy in the management of Hodgkin's disease. Cancer 29:44, 1972.
26. Fialk MA, Jarowski CI, Coleman M, Mouradian J: Hepatic Hodgkin's disease without involvement of the spleen. Cancer 43:1146–1147, 1979.
27. Prosnitz LR, Montalvo RL, Fischer DB, *et al.*: Treatment of stage IIA Hodgkin's disease: Is radiotherapy alone adequate? Int J Radiat Oncol Biol Phys 4:481–787, 1978.

9. The Rappaport classification of the non-Hodgkin's lymphomas: Is it pertinent for the 1980's?

BHARAT N. NATHWANI

1. Rappaport classification (1956)

Prior to the proposal of the so-called 'Rappaport classification' [1] malignant lymphomas were divided into four types – Hodgkin's disease [2], lymphosarcoma [3], reticulum cell sarcoma [4, 5], and follicular lymphoblastoma [6]. The morphologic criteria for recognition of the latter three types of malignant lymphoma were vague, and different investigators often designated the same tumor by different names. Because of a lack of uniformity in diagnoses, no meaningful correlations could be established between the histologic types of lymphomas and their clinical behavior.

In 1956, Rappaport, Winter, and Hicks proposed a classification of malignant lymphomas [1]. This classification divided lymphomas into five types and was subsequently used as a basis for extensive elaboration in the fasicle [7] published by the Armed Forces Institute of Pathology (Table 1). The terminology of the classification took into account the presumed cellular origin, the degree of differentiation of the tumor cells, the cellular composition, and growth pattern of the tumor [7]. The terms 'lymphocytic' and 'histiocytic' indicated the cellular origin of these lymphomas. 'Histiocytic' was employed for lymphomas in which the tumor cells resembled the nonneoplastic benign histiocytes of reactive follicles [7]. The modifying terms 'well-differentiated', 'poorly differentiated', and 'undifferentiated' indicated the degree of differentiation of these tumors in comparison with mature lymphocytes and based on the predominating type of cellular proliferation, lymphomas were classified as lymphocytic, histiocytic, or mixed lymphocytic–histiocytic. Finally, according to the growth pattern of the tumor, each type of lymphoma was considered to have a nodular and/or a diffuse pattern [7]. It was also shown that the natural history of nodular lymphomas consisted of progression to a diffuse phase [7]. 'Nodular' was preferred over the term 'follicular' because of a lack of conclusive evidence at that time that the neoplastic cells of nodular lymphomas originated from reactive follicles [7].

Soon after publication of this classification, however, it became evident that

Bennett JM (ed), Controversies in the Management of Lymphomas. ISBN 0-89838-586-5.
© *Martinus Nijhoff Publishers, Boston. Printed in the Netherlands.*

Table 1. Rappaport classification of non-Hodgkin's lymphomas (1956).

Nodular and/or diffuse	
Well differentiated lymphocytic	Histiocytic
Poorly differentiated lymphocytic	Undifferentiated
Mixed (lymphocytic–histiocytic)	

Table 2. Rappaport classification of NHL as modified by Berard in 1975 [9].

Nodular (follicular) lymphomas	Diffuse lymphomas
Lymphocytic, poorly differentiated	Lymphocytic, well differentiated
Mixed lymphocytic–histiocytic	Lymphocytic, intermediate differentiation
Histiocytic	Lymphocytic, poorly differentiated
	Mixed lymphocytic–histiocytic
	Undifferentiated, Burkitt's type
	Undifferentiated, pleomorphic (non-Burkitt's) type
	Histiocytic

undifferentiated lymphoma of the Burkitt type was a distinct clinicopathologic entity and required a separate position in the classification scheme of NHL [8]. Moreover, it was learned that undifferentiated lymphomas and the well-differentiated lymphocytic lymphomas rarely had a nodular pattern. In view of these findings, minor modifications of the Rappaport classification were suggested [9] (Table 2) and this modified classification has generally been referred to as the 'Rappaport classification'.

In their initial study, Rappaport *et al.* showed that the morphologic subdivision of the follicular lymphomas into five subtypes was related to the clinical course [1]. Subsequent studies at several major centers repeatedly demonstrated the clinical usefulness of the classification leading to its wide popularity and utilization as a basis for clinical trials [10–16]. For example, each of the different Rappaport conceived subtypes of NHL was found to be associated with a distinctive natural history, response to therapy, and median survival. The classification therefore aided clinicians in the formulation of meaningful treatment protocols. In addition, because the Rappaport classification was relatively uncomplicated, pathologists found it applicable in their clinical practice.

2. The current Rappaport classification (1976)

In the 1970's, newer methods were developed for the study of human lymphomas [17–48]. These techniques included the use of immunofluorescence

[22–28] in cell suspensions and frozen sections, immunoperoxidase [29–35] staining of paraffin sections as well as frozen sections, cell surface receptors [36, 37] and the application of monoclonal antibodies [38–41], cytochemistry [21], immunocytochemistry [42–43], electron microscopy [17–20], and flow microfluorometry [44–46]. Based on the results obtained with these techniques, lymphomas were related to the immune sysem and the majority could be designated either as a B or T lymphocyte immunophenotype. It became evident that nodular lymphomas were neoplasms of follicular center cells, and that most cells within follicles were lymphoid [17–20, 27, 28, 36, 47, 48]. Follicular center cells were found to have a distinctive morphology, on the basis of which their cellular origin could be predicted even with a diffuse growth pattern [47]. Burkitt's tumor also was shown to be of B-cell follicular center origin [49, 50], and most lymphomas previously designated as diffuse 'histiocytic' were proven to be of lymphoid and not histiocyte origin [26, 28, 47, 48]. Moreover, it was discovered that many of the diffuse lymphomas were clinically [15, 51–58], morphologically [47, 59–68], and immunologically [69–76] heterogeneous and that the concept of differentiation previously applied to lymphocytes was no longer applicable to lymphomas [27, 77–80].

The new evidence suggested that the terminology of the Rappaport classification was scientifically inaccurate. In addition to the new immunologic data, several morphologic types of lymphoma were described that had not been designated by the original or modified Rappaport classification. For example, it was recognized in 1975 that lymphoblastic lymphoma was a distinct clinicopathologic entity requiring a separate position in the schema of non-Hodgkin's lymphomas [81]. Intermediate lymphocytic lymphoma [9, 82, 83] with morphologic features intermediate between well-differentiated and poorly differentiated lymphomas was proposed; this lymphoma was thought to originate in the mature lymphocytes of mantle zones. As a result, the Pathology Panel for Lymphoma Clinical Studies [84, 85] modified the Rappaport classification of NHL to make provision for the intermediate lymphocytic and lymphoblastic histologic subtypes.

Based on the studies of others [8, 9, 27, 47–49, 80, 86–90] and our own studies [34, 42, 43, 59, 91–96], several further modifications of the Rappaport classification were suggested. In 1976, during a symposium on NHL held in San Francisco, Rappaport proposed his own modification of his classification which included the addition of categories of lymphoblastic, Burkitt's lymphomas, mycosis fungoides and non-Hodgkin's lymphomas with epithelioid histiocytes [97]. He also employed 'immunoblastic' to describe lymphomas that had plasmacytoid features and for those arising from pre-existing lympho- and immunoproliferative diseases such as alpha-chain disease, chronic lymphocytic leukemia, macroglobulinemia of Waldenstrom, and Sjorgen's syndrome [97].

Table 3. NHL classification as modified by Rappaport in 1976 [97].

Nodular and/or diffuse	Diffuse
Poorly differentiated lymphocytic	Well differentiated lymphocytic (WDL)
Mixed	Intermediate lymphocytic
'Histiocytic'	Lymphoblastic
Burkitt's	Immunoblastic
Undifferentiated non-Burkitt's	Non-Hodgkin's lymphomas with a diffuse epithelioid histiocytic reaction (NHL of Lennert's type)
	Mycosis fungoides
	Unclassifiable

The modifications suggested by Rappaport [97] in 1976 are shown in Table 3. It is important to emphasize that these modifications were made prior to the initiation of the NCI sponsored study on the classifications of NHL [58]. At that time, several studies were in progress at the City of Hope National Medical Center aimed at further definition of many of these subtypes of NHL [91–96]. In 1980, for example, a report on the so-called 'Lennert's' lymphoma was published. The results indicated that the majority of non-Hodgkin's lymphomas exhibiting a diffuse epithelioid histiocytic reaction had morphologic features consistent with peripheral T-cell lymphoma [96]. These lymphomas manifested in elderly, symptomatic patients with generalized disease whose median survival was short [96]. Although it has not been stated explicitly by Rappaport [97], he believes (personal communication) that there should be a separate category for this lymphoma in the scheme of classification of NHL.

Within the framework of the topic suggested for this chapter by the Editor, it appears fair and appropriate to discuss only the most recent and evolved Rappaport [97] classification (Table 3) in reference to its pertinence for the 1980's. We will discuss this classification according to (1) the terminology, (2) the different morphologic subtypes, (3) the specific and distinct clinicopathologic entities, (4) the reproducibility of the classification and its value in the practice of pathology, and (5) the immunologic correlations. We also will compare the Rappaport classification with the Working Formulation [58] and to the Lukes-Collins classification [47].

3. Description of the Rappaport classification

3.1. Terminology

The major drawback of the current Rappaport classification is that its terminology is scientifically inaccurate. The reasons for this conclusion are as follows: (1) Since nodular lymphomas are derived from follicular center cells, the term 'follicular' is more appropriate than 'nodular' [17–20, 27, 28, 36, 47, 48]. (2) The term 'histiocytic' as employed for nodular lymphomas is incorrect in view of the fact that the cells are not 'histiocytes', but transformed large lymphoid cells [26, 28, 47, 48]. The designation 'mixed "histiocytic"–lymphocytic, nodular' is also not applicable. (3) The description 'differentiated' as applied to the lymphomas (well differentiated, poorly, differentiated, and undifferentiated) was derived from comparison of the morphology of the lymphoma cells with non-neoplastic, small, mature lymphocytes; however, it has been shown that most small, mature-appearing lymphocytes are not end-stage cells, but highly dynamic cells capable of dividing and of differentiating or transforming into other cell types [47, 77–80]. In light of these discoveries, the terms 'well differentiated', 'poorly differentiated', and 'undifferentiated' are not appropriate. (4) 'Undifferentiated' is additionally incorrect because most lymphomas so designated are B-cell tumors of follicular center cell origin [47, 49]. (5) The term 'diffuse "histiocytic"' is a misnomer, since most lymphomas so designated are of lymphoid rather than histiocytic origin. Rappaport had acknowledged this and suggested in 1976 that the term 'large cell' be used instead of 'histiocytic' [97].

Despite these shortcomings in terminology, the addition of new diagnostic categories appears justified. 'Intermediate lymphocytic' lymphoma, first introduced by Berard[9] and later adopted by Rappaport and the Pathology Panel for Clinical Studies [85] is appropriate for a diffuse lymphoma composed of lymphoid cells whose morphology is intermediate between that of the well-differentiated and that of the poorly differentiated lymphocytic lymphomas. This lymphoma is believed to arise from the small, mature-appearing lymphocytes of the mantle zones of follicles [82, 83].

The designation 'lymphoblastic' is used to describe lymphomas whose cells are morphologically indistinguishable from the immature cells of acute lymphoblastic leukemia (ALL) [81]. If the terms 'lymphoblasts' and 'prolymphocytes' are acceptable for ALL, then it is logical that they should be employed for a lymphoma that is morphologically identical to ALL [81, 95]. For this reason, the term 'lymphoblastic lymphoma' as applied in the current Rappaport classification is appropriate.

The 'Immunoblastic' category is restricted to large cell lymphomas that have plasmacytoid features and for those lymphomas that arise from pre-existing lympho- and immunoproliferative diseases [47, 97, 109–121]. The term 'non-Hodgkin's lymphoma with a diffuse epithelioid histiocytic reaction' is used since it defines a clinicopathologic entity, and since most lymphomas so designated have morphologic features of lymphomas derived from peripheral T-cells [96].

188

3.2. Morphologic subtypes

3.2.1. Nodular lymphomas. These have a characteristic back-to-back arrangement of follicles throughout the node (Fig. 1) [98]. In rare instances, however, florid reactive follicular hyperplasia may also impart such a pattern [99]. In these rare instances follicles usually are of intermediate or large size, and they characteristically exhibit a high phagocytic and mitotic activity [99]. Nodular (follicular) lymphomas, in contrast, characteristically have cells, both within and outside the follicles which are similar morphologically [98]. In the Lukes and Collins classification and the Working Formulation the term follicular is used instead of the term nodular.

Nodular and/or diffuse poorly differentiated lymphocytic lymphoma. 'Poorly differentiated lymphocytic' (PDL) lymphoma, in most instances, is associated with a purely follicular or a follicular and diffuse pattern. A totally diffuse pattern is uncommon with this subtype. The nodular PDL of Rappaport in the Lukes and Collins classification [47] has been identified as follicular, small

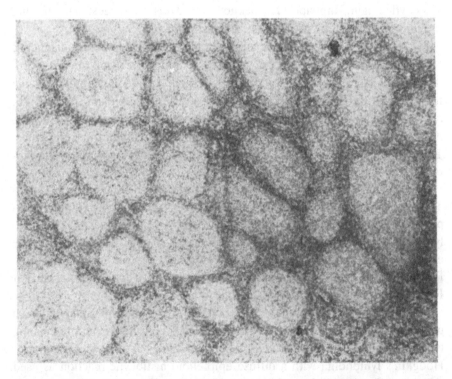

Figure 1. Throughout the lymph node, a back-to-back arrangement of follicles is noted. This pattern is characteristic of follicular lymphoma. In rare instances, similar pattern can be found in florid reactive follicular hyperplasia. (Lymph node – H&E x25.).

cleaved cell type and in the Working Formulation [58] it is called follicular, predominantly small cleaved cell type. For all practical purposes these three terms can be used interchangeably.

Figure 2 shows the typical morphologic features of PDL. There is a monotonous proliferation of small lymphoid cells having a clumped nuclear chromatin structure and showing marked variations in nuclear shape; nucleoli are absent. The tumor cells vary in size from six to 12 microns. Occasional transformed large lymphoid cells may be evident among these cells.

Nodular and/or diffuse mixed cell lymphoma. The mixed cell lymphoma often shows a follicular pattern of growth or a follicular and diffuse pattern. A purely diffuse pattern is uncommon. The follicular mixed cell type is synonymous to the follicular mixed cell type of the Working Formulation [58]. Lukes and

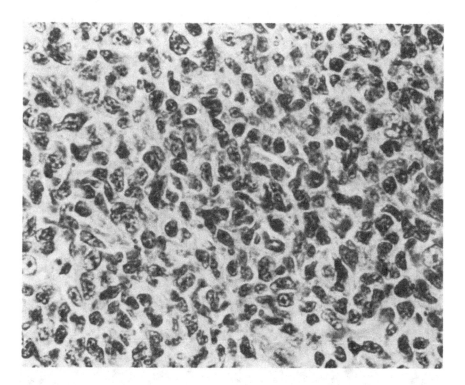

Figure 2. The characteristic morphology of poorly differentiated lymphocytic lymphoma. The neoplastic lymphoid cells are small; they have clumped nuclear chromatin without nucleoli, and they show variations in nuclear shape. These variations in the nuclear shape range from minimal to markedly irregular. Rarely, one can see multiple clefts in these small lymphoid cells. In the Working Formulation this would be classified as low grade lymphoma – predominantly small cleaved cell type. In the Lukes-Collins classification this would also be classified as small cleaved follicular center cell type. (Lymph node – H&E x730.).

Collins have indicated that the follicular mixed in most instances corresponds to their large cleaved cell type [47].

The term nodular and/or diffuse mixed implies that the diffuse form may represent progression of the follicular type. This statement implies that diffuse mixed type is of follicular center cell origin; however, it is well known that some diffuse mixed cell lymphomas do not have features of follicular center cells but rather those of periphernal T-cell lymphomas [58]. The clinicopathologic correlations and the immunological correlations are discussed under the headings of C and D.

In this lymphoma, a mixture of small and large lymphoid cells is present in varying proportions (Fig. 3). The small lymphoid cells have the morphologic features described above. The transformed large lymphoid cells vary in size from 20 to 30 microns and have vesicular nuclei containing one to several small nucleoli, many of which are located on the nuclear membranes.

Nodular and/or diffuse 'histiocytic'. The nodular histiocytic is morphologically

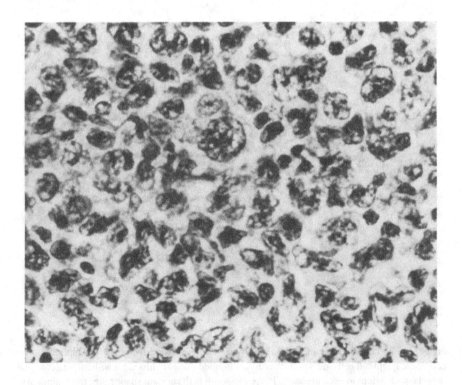

Figure 3. A mixed cell lymphoma showing a mixture of small and large lymphoid cells. These two populations have a common cellular origin. In the Working Formulation this would be classified as a mixed small cleaved and large cell type. In the Lukes-Collins classification this would probably be classified as large cleaved. (Lymph node – H&E x730.).

and immunologically a pure group and its diffuse counterpart is similar. In the Working Formulation, the corresponding terms for nodular and/or diffuse histiocytic are follicular and/or diffuse large cell (cleaved or noncleaved) [58]. In the Lukes-Collins classification, nodular histiocytic would be classified as large cleaved or large noncleaved [47]. The diffuse histiocytic can be sub-divided into five types – large cleaved, large noncleaved, B-immunoblastic, T-immunoblastic, and true histiocytic [47]. Although the diffuse 'histiocytic' is morphologically and immunologically a heterogeneous category, since Rap-paport has been using the terms immunoblastic, and 'non-Hodgkin's lym-phoma with a diffuse epithelioid histiocytic reaction', the category of diffuse histiocytic has a different meaning as currently utilized. In most instances, it is restricted for lymphomas that have features of follicular center cells. The lymphomas which have plasmacytoid features and those arising from pre-

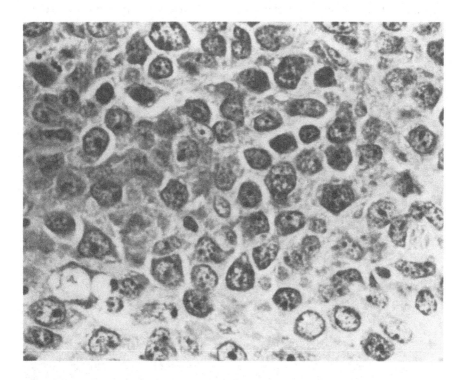

Figure 4. The cells of large-cell ('histiocytic') lymphomas have vesicular nuclei containing one to multiple nucleoli, many of which are placed on the nuclear membranes. These lymphomas were called 'histiocytic' by Rappaport in 1956 because the tumor cells were morphologically similar to the non-neoplastic benign histiocytes of the follicles. It has now been shown that these are not histiocytes, but transformed large lymphoid cells. In the Working Formulation this would be classified as intermediate grade lymphoma – large cell lymhoma of the noncleaved type; in the Lukes-Collins classification, as large noncleaved. (Lymph node – H&E ×730.).

existing lympho- and immunoproliferative diseases are classified as immunoblastic [47, 97, 109–121]. Whereas, the lymphomas which have features of peripheral T-cell lymphomas may be classified with the category of non-Hodgkin's lymphoma with a diffuse epithelioid histiocytic reaction. The morphologic criteria of the immunoblastic and non-Hodgkin's lymphoma with the diffuse epithelioid histiocytic reaction [96] are discussed under diffuse lymphomas.

A purely nodular (follicular) pattern is uncommon in 'histiocytic' lymphoma. When a nodular pattern is observed it is generally in association with diffuse areas. In most instances, however, a completely diffuse pattern is present. 'Histiocytic' lymphomas are composed of transformed large lymphoid cells which have round vesicular nuclei containing multiple small nucleoli (Fig. 4). Mitotic figures are readily identified. This type of lymphoma often contains a residual component of small lymphoid cells which have irregular nuclear contours ('cleaved' [47]). Histologic progression from a nodular to a diffuse pattern is common in this subtype.

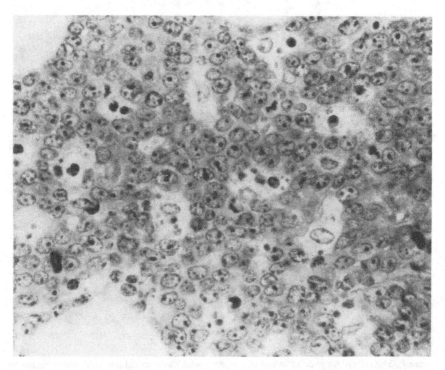

Figure 5. Undifferentiated lymphomas of the Burkitt's and the non-Burkitt's type can, in rare cases, have a nodular and/or diffuse pattern. The characteristic finding in Burkitt's lymphoma is the presence of multiple prominent nucleoli. In the Working Formulation this would be classified as a high-grade lymphoma – small noncleaved, Burkitt's type. In the Lukes-Collins classification this would be classified as small noncleaved Burkitt's type. (Lymph node – H&E ×730.).

Nodular and/or diffuse Burkitt's lymphoma. A nodular pattern [49] is rarely found in Burkitt's [8, 88, 100–103] lymphoma. This lymphoma was initially subclassified as undifferentiated, but we now know that it has its origin in transformed follicular center cells [49]. The hallmark of this lymphoma is the cellular uniformity and the presence of multiple prominent nucleoli (Fig. 5). The cytoplasm is often moderate and deeply pyroninophilic. The tumor cells are of an intermediate size (approximately equal to that of a benign histiocyte) and may range in size from 13 to 20 microns. At low magnification, the tumor often shows a characteristic starry-sky pattern and a high mitotic activity. In the Working Formulation [58] and in the Lukes-Collins classification, the Burkitt's lymphoma is called small noncleaved, Burkitt's type.

Nodular and/or diffuse undifferentiated non-Burkitt's lymphoma. This lymphoma lacks the cellular monotony of Burkitt's tumor [9, 103]. It shows greater variability in the size and the shape of the nuclei and nucleoli (Fig. 6). In the Working Formulation the non-Burkitt's type is identified as small noncleaved

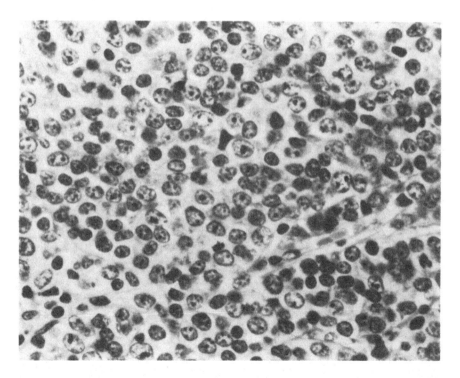

Figure 6. Undifferentiated non-Burkitt's lymphoma shows greater variability in the size and shape of the nuclei and nucleoli than is seen in Burkitt's lymphoma. In the Working Formulation this would be classified as a high-grade lymphoma – small noncleaved. In the Lukes-Collins classification this would be classified as small noncleaved non-Burkitt's type. (Lymph node – H&E ×730.).

[58]. In the Lukes and Collins classification it is called small noncleaved, non-Burkitt's type.

3.2.2. Diffuse lymphomas.

Well differentiated lymphocytic lymphoma. This lymphoma characteristically consists of a monotonous population of small, round, mature appearing lymphocytes with very low mitotic activity (Fig. 7) [7, 91]. However, at low magnification, there may be a vague nodularity which has been referred to as 'pseudofollicular proliferation centers' (Fig. 8) [104]. Typically, the proliferation centers contain loosely packed round cells which often are separated by clear spaces (Fig. 9). The 'pseudofollicular' areas may be populated by small lymphocytes only, or they may contain many transformed large lymphoid cells. Most large cells in this form of lymphoma have vesicular nuclei with a prominent, centrally placed nucleolus (Fig. 10). A few large cells, however, may have multiple small nucleoli [105]. Presumably, cell division takes place in these 'pseudofollicular centers'.

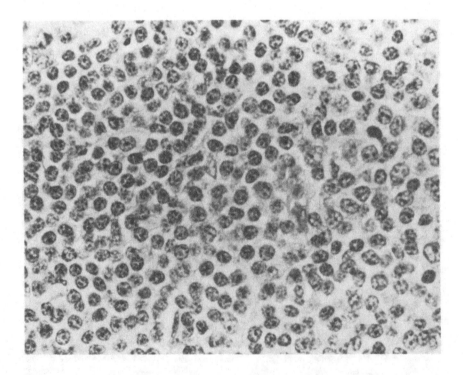

Figure 7. A monomorphic proliferation of small lymphoid cells is evident. The term 'well-differentiated lymphocytic lymphoma' was applied to this lymphoma because the tumor cells resembled non-neoplastic small, mature lymphocytes. In the Working Formulation this would be classified as a low-grade lymphoma – small lymphocytic type. In the Lukes-Collins classification this lymphoma would be classified as small lymphocyte type. (Lymph node – H&E ×730.).

It has been suggested that the presence of a 'pseudofollicular' pattern indicates a tissue manifestation of chronic lymphocytic leukemia (CLL). If 'pseudofollicular' centers are truly the sites of cell division, this concept would imply that the lymph node is a primary site for this lymphoma, and the observed lymphocytosis may well be the leukemic phase of the disease. Presumably, CLL is a primary bone marrow disease, and if it were to involve the lymph nodes secondarily (tissue manifestation of CLL), it should have a metastatic and not a 'pseudofollicular' pattern [105].

Well-differentiated lymphocytic lymphoma (WDL) may exist as a well-defined type of NHL not associated with CLL or a monoclonal gammopathy [91]. In our previous study, we found that 38% of the patients had neither monoclonal gammopathy nor CLL [91]. In 43.5% of the patients, an absolute lymphocytosis was evident, indicating a picture consistent with CLL [91]. In

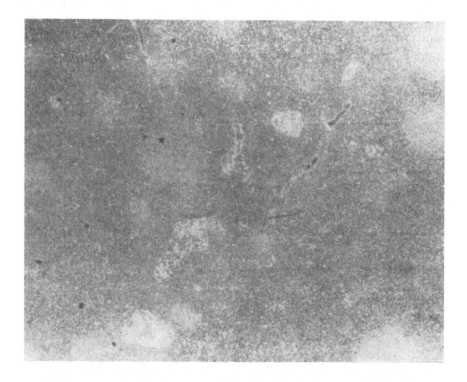

Figure 8. The characteristic of 'pseudofollicular proliferation growth centers' are: (1) They are always vague; (2) they are usually small; (3) they never have a mantle zone of mature-appearing lymphocytes surrounding them; (4) the cells within the pseudofollicles are loosely packed and show clear spaces among them; (5) these pseudofollicles may contain only small cells, only large cells, or a mixture of small and large cells; (6) regardless of their size, the cells are always round; (7) the majority of the transformed large lymphoid cells have a solitary, centrally placed, prominent eosinophilic nucleolus. Only few of the large cells show multiple, small nucleoli. (Lymph node – H&E x45.).

18.5% of the patients, a monoclonal gammopathy, usually the IgM type, was noted, together with plasmacytoid differentiation (Fig. 11) [91].

A totally nodular pattern is not found in this lymphoma [91]. In our previous study, we found a nodular and diffuse pattern in only two of 108 cases [91] and for all practical purposes, this lymphoma is diffuse. In the Working Formulation [58] this lymphoma is called small lymphocytic and in the Lukes-Collins classification, the WDL is called malignant lymphoma of small lymphocytes; and the WDL with plasmacytoid differentiation is identified as plasmacytoid lymphocyte in the Lukes-Collins classification [47].

Intermediate lymphocytic lymphoma. Intermediate lymphoma (IL) is believed to arise from the mature lymphocytes of the mantle zones of follicles (Fig. 12). At low magnification, one may observe a few small, atrophic follicles which are surrounded by thick, broad mantles [106]. These zones are often confluent suggesting that the lymphoma originates from the small lymphocytes of the mantle zones. The earliest phase of this type of lymphoma, in which this pattern is most striking, has been called 'mantle zone lymphoma' [107]. The majority of the neoplastic cells in IL have a nuclear shape intermediate

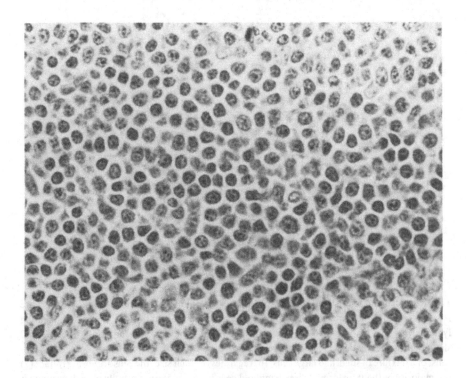

Figure 9. The cells within the 'pseudofollicles' are loosely packed and have clear spaces between them. (Lymph node – H&E x730.).

between that of the WDL and the PDL. In addition, a small portion of the cells have completely round nuclei as in WDL, and a small portion have irregular nuclei as in PDL [106]. Neither the Working Formulation nor the Lukes-Collins classification indicate any corresponding terms for this lymphoma.

Lymphoblastic lymphoma. Lymphoblastic lymphoma is characterized by immature lymphoid cells which are indistinguishable from the lymphoblasts and prolymphocytes of ALL [81]. Most tumor cells vary in size from 13 to 20 microns and have a delicate nuclear chromatin structure. Nucleoli are usually not observed, but if present, the nucleoli are very small and inconspicuous. On the basis of the nuclear shape, the cells may be divided into convoluted [87] and nonconvoluted types [81]. The convoluted type shows variations in the nuclear shape, with some nuclei having multiple clefts (Fig. 13), whereas the nonconvoluted type has round to ovoid nuclei. No convoluted nuclei nor any fine linear subdivisions are found in a round nucleus of the nonconvoluted subtype (Fig. 14) [108]. Regardless of the nuclear shape, the tumor cells exhibit

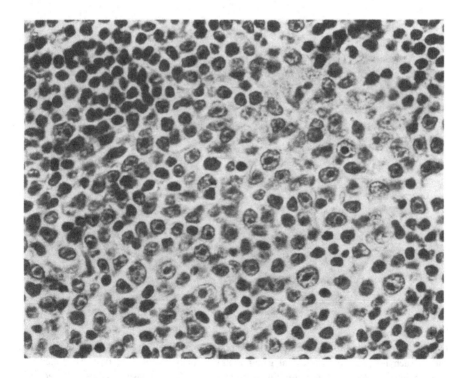

Figure 10. The 'pseudofollicles' may contain only small cells, only large cells, or a mixture of small and large cells. Regardless of their size, the cells are always round. However, the striking finding is that, when large cells are present, most of them have a solitary, prominent esosinophilic nucleolus. Only few of the large cells contain multiple small nucleoli. (Lymph node – H&E x730.).

a high mitotic activity.

The two most important morphologic features of this lymphoma are: (1) The small, intermediate, and larger tumor cells exhibit a similar fine nuclear chromatin structure, and all appear blastic; and (2) the large and the intermediate tumor cells do not show nucleoli, in contrast to peripheral T-cell lymphomas and B-cell tumors. We refer to the presence of nucleoli in the intermediate and larger cells as a transformation phenomenon, which is not evident in lymphoblastic lymphoma [81, 108].

Lymphoblastic lymphomas (convoluted and nonconvoluted) in the Rappaport classification, were previously included with the poorly differentiated lymphocytic, diffuse. Subsequent studies have shown that the lymphoblastic lymphoma is a distinct entity that requires a separate position in the scheme of the classification of non-Hodgkin's lymphomas. In the Working Formulation the lymphoblastic lymphomas (convoluted and nonconvoluted) are desig-

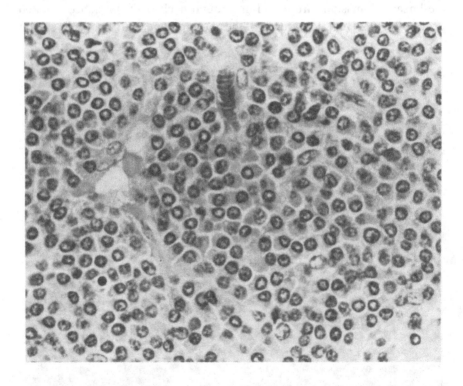

Figure 11. Well-differentiated lymphocytic lymphoma may show plasmacytoid differentiation, and in such instances a monoclonal gammopathy, usually of the IgM type, is found. The eosinophilic globular material present in large amounts in the cytoplasm has been referred to as 'Russell bodies'; when it extends to the nuclear surface, it has been called 'Dutcher bodies'. In the Working Formulation this would be classified as a low-grade lymphoma – small lymphocytic showing plasmacytoid features. In the Lukes-Collins classification it would be classified as plasmacytoid lymphocyte. (Lymph node – H&E ×730.).

nated by identical terms [58]. In the Lukes-Collins classification the term 'convoluted lymphocytic lymphoma' [87] is used which corresponds to the lymphoblastic convoluted but not with the lymphoblastic nonconvoluted.

Immunoblastic lymphoma. The immunoblastic lymphomas may or may not have plasmacytoid features [47, 97]. These lymphomas may arise *de novo* or from pre-existing lympho- and immunoproliferative diseases [47, 97]. The large-cell lymphomas that arise from macroglobulinemia of Waldenstrom, CLL, and alpha-chain disease [30, 94] often exhibit plasmacytoid differentiation, and the cells contain monoclonal, intracytoplasmic immunoglobulin (Fig. 15).

Lymphomas that arise in the background of angioimmunoblastic lymphadenopathy (AILD) contain many large cells [92]; however, many large cells do not exhibit plasmacytoid features [92]. Most lymphomas associated with AILD manifest a characteristic spectrum of cell size; many intermediate and large transformed lymphoid cells have abundant pale to clear cytoplasm [92]. The other characteristic feature of this lymphoma is the presence of

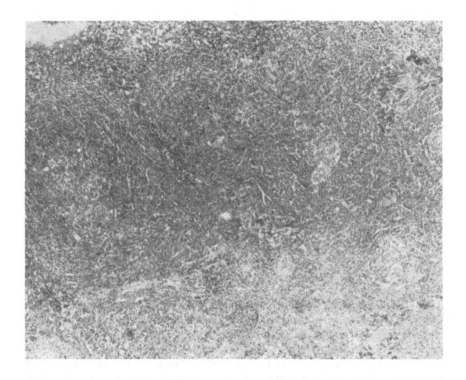

Figure 12. Intermediate lymphocytic lymphoma arises from the lymphocytes of the mantle zones surrounding the follicles. The mantle zones are composed of small lymphoid cells. Most neoplastic cells have slight nuclear irregularities. (Lymph node – H&E x45.).

200

clusters and/or islands of transformed large lymphoid cells [92].

The immunoblastic lymphomas which have morphologic features of peripheral T-cell lymphoma also contain cells of various sizes, with readily identifiable transitional forms (Figs 16, 17) [123–130]; clear cells also are frequent [123–137]. Cleaved cells and large cells with plasmacytoid features are not present. Mitotic activity is high, and at times the background shows a diffuse epithelioid histiocytic reaction [96]. In the Working Formulation, the immunoblastic lymphomas may be further subclassified into four types – plasmacytoid, polymorpous, clear cell, and epithelioid cell types [58]. The plasmacytoid type corresponds to the Lukes-Collins B-immunoblastic; and the polymorphous, clear cell and epithelioid cell types correspond to the T-immunoblastic or the peripheral T-cell lymphomas [58].

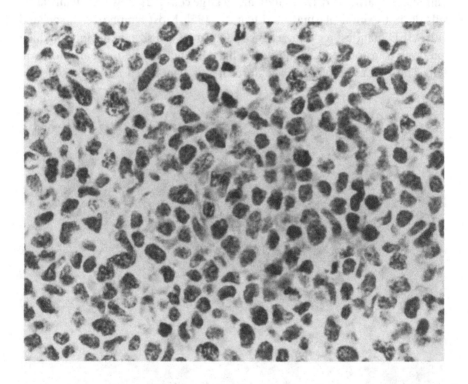

Figure 13. The characteristic feature of lymphoblastic lymphoma is the presence of a fine, delicate nuclear chromatin structure and high mitotic activity. In this convoluted type of lymphobhoblastic lymphoma, irregularities in the nuclear shape are readily identified. Although multiple clefts and indentations of the nuclei can be seen, they are not required for the designation of a lymphoblastic lymphoma. Moreover, the presence or absence of indentations and clefts is not associated with any significant difference in the patient's clinical history, response to therapy, or survival. In the Working Formulation this would be classified as a high-grade lymphoma – lymphoblastic, convoluted type. In the Lukes-Collins classification this would be classified as convoluted lymphocyte. (Lymph node – H&E ×730.).

Non-Hodgkin's lymphoma with a diffuse epithelioid histiocytic reaction (Lennert's lymphoma). Most non-Hodgkin's lymphomas which exhibit a diffuse epithelioid histiocytic reaction have the other morphologic features of a peripheral T-cell lymphoma (Fig. 18). These lymphomas are characterized by a proliferation of mixed cells with transitional forms [96]. In the Working Formulation, this lymphoma would be classified as either mixed cell type or immunoblastic-epithelioid cell type [58]. In the Lukes-Collins classification, this lymphoma has been identified as 'lymphoepithelioid cell' lymphoma.

3.3. Clinicopathologic correlations

3.3.1. Nodular and/or diffuse lymphomas. Nodular (follicular) lymphomas are the most common NHL in the United States [10–14, 58, 59, 138–140]. The

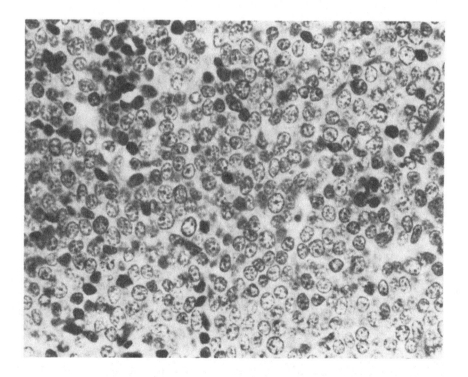

Figure 14. In lymphoblastic lymphomas, the nuclei of the small, intermediate, and large tumor cells have an identical blastic chromatin structure. The intermediate and large tumor cells do not contain any prominent nucleoli. In contrast, this feature is found in the peripheral T-cell lymphomas and in the other B-cell lymphomas. In the nonconvoluted type of lymphoblastic lymphoma, most of the nuclei are round to oval. In this type, no fine linear subdivisions are found in any round nuclei. In the Working Formulation this would be classified as a high-grade lymphoma – lymphoblastic, nonconvoluted type. In the Lukes-Collins classification it would probably be classified as 'undefined'. (Lymph node – H&E ×730.).

202

natural history of these lymphomas has been well documented [1, 10, 14, 58, 59, 138–150] and distinct clinicopathologic correlations with the different subtypes have been established. Nodular PDL is a favorable but slowly progressive, probably multicentric, disease in which remissions and relapses are the rule [10–14, 58, 59, 138–142]. On the other hand, nodular 'histiocytic' lymphoma is an aggressive lymphoma [1, 10, 58, 59, 149, 150]. With intensive combination chemotherapy, however, one can induce prolonged remissions and cure [149, 150].

The biological behavior of the nodular lymphomas of the mixed-cell type has been found to be variable [1, 10, 58, 59, 143–148]. Some studies have indicated that it behaves like PDL [10, 58, 142] and others have shown that it behaves similar to the 'histiocytic' type [1, 151]. Other studies, have found that the prognosis was intermediate between those for PDL and the 'histiocytic'

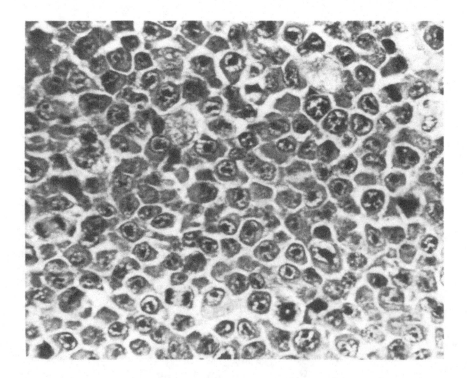

Figure 15. The large-cell lymphomas with plasmacytoid features have been referred to as B-immunoblastic lymphomas. They have moderate to abundant quantities of deeply staining cytoplasm and vesicular nuclei with one or several prominent nucleoli which are often centrally located. Sometimes, the nucleoli are small and peripherally located. The cytoplasmic features are more reliable than the nuclear for the identification of this lymphoma. In the Working Formulation this would be classified as a high-grade lymphoma – immunoblastic with plasmacytoid features. In the Lukes-Collins classification it would be classified as B-immunoblastic. (Lymph node – H&E ×730.).

type [59, 145–147]. In one study many patients had prolonged disease-free survival [143, 148]. The biologic behavior of this lymphoma is discussed elsewhere in this volume.

Bone marrow involvement occurs in most patients with nodular PDL, whereas it occurs in less than 10% of patients with the 'histiocytic' type [58, 152, 153]. The incidence of bone marrow involvement in mixed-cell lymphoma is intermediate between that in PDL and that in 'histiocytic' lymphoma [58, 143–146, 152, 153]. Most patients with nodular PDL have generalized lymphadenopathy and stage IV disease, whereas patients with the nodular 'histiocytic' type more often have localized disease [10–14, 58, 59, 138–153].

Although little information is available on the biologic behavior of nodular undifferentiated (Burkitt's and non-Burkitt's) lymphoma [49], the Working Formulation of NHL has labeled it as being the follicular, small noncleavedcell

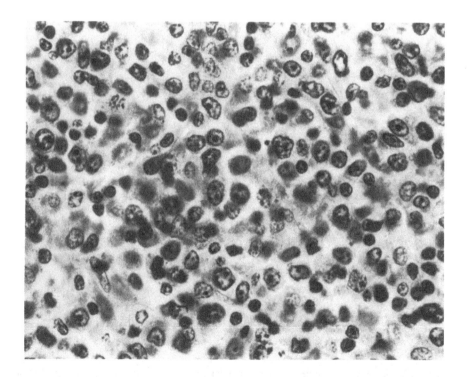

Figure 16. The lymphomas which show a spectrum of cell sizes and transitional forms, without any cleaved cells, have often been found to be of peripheral-T-cell origin. Many of the tumor cells have moderate to abundant quantities of pale to clear cytoplasm. These lymphomas may or may not show a diffuse epithelioid histiocytic reaction. In the Working Formulation this would be classified as an intermediate-grade lymphoma – diffuse mixed small cell and large cell type. In the Lukes-Collins classification this would be classified as T-Immunoblastic. (Lymph node – H&E x730.).

204

type and placed it among lymphomas of a high grade of malignancy [58]. Thus, undifferentiated nodular lymphoma is the most aggressive subtype [58].

There appear to be significant clinical differences between Burkitt's lymphoma and undifferentiated non-Burkitt's lymphoma which would justify separate categories for them in the classification of NHL [58, 103]. Burkitt's lymphoma commonly occurs in young children, predominately in boys. In the United States, this form characteristically presents as an abdominal mass with frequent small bowel involvement [88, 100–103]. The clinical staging system [101] for Burkitt's tumor is different from that for the other NHL, and many of these patients who were treated by the Ziegler protocol [101] have been cured. On the other hand, undifferentiated non-Burkitt's lymphoma commonly develops in elderly patients with frequent node involvement [103]. Clinically, undifferentiated non-Burkitt's lymphoma is perhaps, the most aggressive

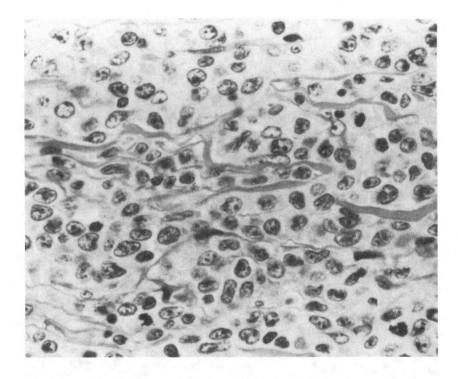

Figure 17. The characteristic finding in peripheral T-cell lymphomas is the spectrum of sizes of cells with transitional forms. The tumor cells often contain moderate to abundant cytoplasm and have well-defined cell borders. There are no large cells with plasmacytoid features. The tumor often exhibits a high mitotic activity and compartmentalization of tumor cells. In the Working Formulation this would be classified as a high-grade lymphoma – immunoblastic clear cell type. In the Lukes-Collins classification it would be classified as T-Immunoblastic or as a peripheral T-cell lymphoma by Waldron *et al.* [123] (Lymph node – H&E ×730.).

subtype among the non-Hodgkin's lymphomas, and associated with a short median survival [103].

Thus, there are significant differences among the subtypes of nodular lymphomas which justify their separation into different categories.

3.3.2. Diffuse lymphomas

Well-differentiated lymphocytic. Most patients with WDL are elderly and present with stage IV disease [10, 91]. The natural history is one of slow progression, and patients have a long median survival [10, 91]. When lymphocytosis is associated with this lymphoma, it is indistinguishable from CLL. The presence of lymphocytosis can be suspected on the basis of the presence of 'pseudofollicular proliferation growth centers' in the lymph node [104]. Plas-

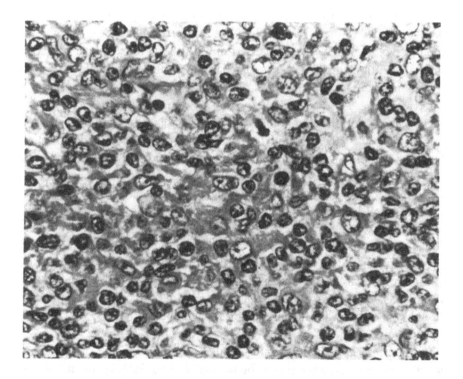

Figure 18. This lymphoma also shows a mixed cellular proliferation; however, the most striking finding is the presence of a diffuse epithelioid histiocytic reaction. The presence or absence of this feature is not associated with any significant difference in the patient's clinical history, response to therapy, or survival. The majority of these lymphomas resemble the peripheral T-cell lymphoma illustrated in Figures 16 and 17. In the Working Formulation this would be classified as an intermediate-grade lymphoma – diffuse mixed cell and large cell type within an epithelioid histiocytic reaction. In the Lukes-Collins classification this would be classified as malignant lymphoma of 'lymphoepithelioid lymphocyte'. (Lymph node – H&E x730.).

macytoid features in WDL is often associated with monoclonal gammopathy, usually of the IgM type [91]. In such instances, the patient may have signs and symptoms of macroglobulinemia of Waldenstrom. Thus, in WDL, subtle morphologic features enable one to make significant clinical correlations which help in the prediction of prognosis as well as in the design of treatment protocols.

Intermediate lymphocytic lymphoma. Most of these patients have stage IV disease; however, only a small portion have leukemia from the onset. An occasional patient may have monoclonal gammopathy. In one of our studies [106] the survival of the patients was similar to that observed for the diffuse PDL. If this survival data can be confirmed by others, then one may contemplate integrating this lymphoma with the diffuse PDL.

Diffuse mixed cell type. We have previously indicated that the mixed cell lymphomas have either a nodular or diffuse pattern, and under the heading of nodular lymphomas we have referred only to the nodular mixed cell type. Since the diffuse mixed cell category has some interesting features we are describing it here to emphasize and clarify some of the controversial aspects of this lymphoma.

This subcategory is morphologically, immunologically, and clinically heterogeneous. The recent study from the Repository Center and Pathology Panel for Lymphoma Clinical Studies indicated that the follicular center cell type of diffuse mixed-cell lymphoma was associated with a longer survival than was diffuse mixed-cell lymphoma having the morphologic features of peripheral T-cell lymphomas [127]. The latter subtype has a more aggressive natural history and behaves as a high-grade lymphoma [127]. In view of these clinical data, perhaps a modification should be considered – the diffuse mixed-cell category should be reserved only for lymphomas which have morphologic features of the follicular center cell type, whereas the diffuse mixed-cell lymphomas, which have morphologic features of peripheral T-cell lymphoma, should be included with the immunoblastic lymphomas [127].

Diffuse 'histiocytic' lymphoma and immunoblastic lymphoma. Nodular histiocytic has been discussed under the heading of nodular lymphomas and the diffuse counterpart of this lymphoma is morphologically and immunologically a pure category. However, because of the great interest and information that is available on this lymphoma, for the sake of clarity, we are discussing it here under the heading of diffuse lymphomas to highlight some of the controversies pertaining to this designation.

The so-called diffuse 'histiocytic' lymphoma (DHL) of the Rappaport classification is morphologically [58, 59–64, 66, 68], immunologically [67, 69–76], and clinically [51–58], heterogeneous. Morphologically, this lymphoma has been subdivided by Lukes and Collins into five different subtypes (large cleaved, large noncleaved, B-immunoblastic, T-immunoblastic, and true histiocytic [47]. Immunologically, the DHL can be divided into lymphomas of B-cell, T-cell, 'null'-cell, or true histiocytic origin [67, 69–76]. Clinically, about 40% of patients diagnosed as having DHL have been cured by aggressive combination chemotherapy [15, 51–58]. Therefore, for clinical purposes, several investigators have employed morphologic and/or immunologic criteria to subdivide these lymphomas to ascertain whether they could identify the group that is curable, and to formulate new and more effective protocols for noncurable patients [58, 59–64, 66–76]. The results of these studies are controversial, but the preponderance of evidence suggests that large-cell ('histiocytic') lymphomas that have features of follicular center cells have a relatively less aggressive clinical course than do the large-cell lymphomas of the immunoblastic type [58, 66, 67].

When Rappaport modified his classification in 1976, he included the category of immunoblastic lymphoma in the diffuse NHL, a term which had a morphologic and a conceptual definition [97]. Morphologically, the term 'immunoblastic' was employed for large-cell lymphomas with plasmayctoid features [97]. Conceptually, the term was employed for lymphomas that arise from pre-existing lympho- and immunoproliferative diseases [97]. The clinical information on lymphomas that arise from these pre-existing diseases [109–122] indicates that these lymphomas are aggressive, high-grade lymphomas. The introduction of the category of immunoblastic lymphoma connotes an aggressive natural history, a poor response to therapy, and a short median survival.

Diffuse lymphoblastic lymphoma. Although this lymphoma is common mainly in children and young adults, it can occur in adults [108]. However, mediastinal masses, leukemic conversion, and high mitotic activity are noted in a significantly higher percentage of young individuals than in older patients [108]. Lymphoblastic lymphoma is similar to ALL not only morphologically, but also clinically [81, 95–108]. The disease is aggressive, and it requires combination chemotherapy of the type used for ALL.

Non-Hodgkin's lymphoma with a diffuse epithelioid histiocytic reaction (Lennert's lymphoma). Most patients with this subtype are elderly symptomatic individuals who have stage IV disease [96]. The natural history of this disease is aggressive. Patients have a short median survival, indicating that this is a high-grade lymphoma [96]. Since the morphologic features are similar to those reported for the peripheral T-cell lymphomas [96], it may be appropriate to integrate this category with immunoblastic lymphomas.

Mycosis fungoides. This is a primary cutaneous lymphoma. Lymph node involvement is always secondary and represents a metastasis from the primary skin lesion.

3.4. Reproducibility

Rappaport has previously indicated that the requirements for an ideal histologic classification are that it should be (1) clinically useful, (2) scientifically accurate, (3) readily taught and easily learned and, (4) reproducible [97]. There is no question that the Rappaport classification is clinically very useful. However, in the last two decades it has become apparent that the terminology of the Rappaport classification is scientifically inaccurate and requires changes. Because of the relative simplicity of the Rappaport classification and the fact that it has existed for a long time, it is widely used in the practice of pathology and can be readily taught.

We ourselves believe that a classification is as good as its reproducibility. In several studies, the reproducibility of the Rappaport classification has been investigated and the results of these studies have shown conclusively that the single most highly reproducible feature is pattern (nodular *vs.* diffuse) recognition [58, 85, 139, 154–157]. Moreover, pattern can be recognized even when the technical quality of the sections is less than optimal. The importance of designating pattern is underscored by the fact that NHL with a nodular pattern comprise anywhere from 20 to 50% of all NHL [10, 13, 14, 58, 59, 140–151]. The vast data base available on nodular lymphomas has allowed meaningful clinicopathologic correlations to be established which have helped in the design and conduct of therapeutic trial [10, 138–151]. It would be most unfortunate if such valuable information were no longer to be a part of a classification system. Therefore, the pathologist should make every effort to designate pattern in every NHL, regardless of the classification used.

Many of the diffuse lymphoma categories (WDL, DH, lymphoblastic) are also reproducible. If an attempt is made to subdivide the diffuse histiocytic lymphomas morphologically into various subtypes, this creates significant problems in reproducibility, especially when the technical quality of the sections is less than optimal. Nonetheless, it appears that the Rappaport classification is probably the most reproducible of all the classifications currently available.

3.5. Immunologic correlations

3.5.1. Nodular lymphomas. It is now well recognized that all nodular lymphomas are follicular center cell lymphomas and, therefore, are of B-cell origin [17–21, 25, 28, 36, 47, 48]. The diffuse counterparts of lymphomas having a nodular pattern are also B-cell lymphomas, and their origin can often be predicted on the basis of morphology alone [25, 47]. Because nodular lymphomas or their diffuse counterparts comprise about 60–70% of all NHL, and because their phenotype (B-cell) can be predicted on the basis of their morphology, one can assume that a significant correlation exists between the morphologic types of the Rappaport classification and the immunologic findings.

3.5.2 Diffuse lymphomas

Well differentiated lymphocytic lymphoma. Most WDL's [7, 91, 158, 159] are of B-cell origin [160] as are lymphomas having plasmacytoid features [7, 91, 161].

Intermediate lymphocytic. Immunological correlation has shown that this lymphoma is a B-cell lymphoma and the intensity of surface immunoglobulin staining is intermediate between the well differentiated and the poorly differentiated lymphocytic lymphoma [82, 83].

Lymphoblastic lymphoma. Since most lymphoblastic lymphomas are of T-cell origin [162–167], there is a good correlation between morphology and immunology. Lymphoblastic lymphomas previously considered to be of the 'null' type have now been identified as pre-B, pre-T, or stem-cell types [167].

Histiocytic lymphoma. Although the old 'histiocytic' lymphoma was a heterogeneous category, the word 'histiocytic' as modified and currently employed is reserved only for large-cell lymphomas that have morphologic features of follicular center cells. In view of this, the category of 'histiocytic' lymphoma is a B-cell category.

Immunoblastic lymphoma. The immunoblastic category should be reserved for large-cell lymphomas which have plasmacytoid features. If a consensus can be achieved on this issue, then it follows that all immunoblastic lymphomas are of B-cell type. Most immunoblastic lymphomas that arise from pre-existing lymphoproliferative diseases such as WDL, macroglobulinemia of Waldenstrom, CLL, and alpha-chain disease are B-cell lymphomas and have plasmacytoid features [110–120].

It appears that the majority of lymphomas that arise from angioimmunoblastic lymphadenopathy have the morphologic features of peripheral T-cell lymphomas. We suggest that all lymphomas that have morphologic features of peripheral T-cell lymphoma be designated by an eponym such as

Waldron's lymphoma [123] or Suchi's lymphoma [133] or Kikuchi's lymphoma [134]. Since most of the non-Hodgkin's lymphomas which show a diffuse epithelioid histiocytic reaction also have the morphologic features of peripheral T-cell lymphomas, they should be identified by any of the eponyms suggested above.

4. Comparison of the Rappaport classification with the Working Formulation and the Lukes-Collins classification

4.2. Nodular lymphomas

The Rappaport classification, the Working Formulation (WF) [58], and the Lukes-Collins classification [47, 124] can be compared provided the Working Formulation and the Lukes-Collins classifications are rearranged according to pattern as in Table 4. In all three systems, lymphomas with a nodular (follicular) pattern are divided into four to five morphologic subtypes. These subtypes are very similar with respect to the morphologic criteria used and their capacity

Table 4. Comparison of the Rappaport classification with the working formulation and the Lukes-Collins classification.

Rappaport	Working Formulation	Lukes-Collins
Nodular and/or diffuse	Follicular and/or diffuse	Follicular and/or diffuse
1. Poorly differentiated lymphocytic	1. Predominantly small cleaved	1. Small cleaved
2. Mixed	2. Mixed, small cleaved, and large cell	2. Large cleaved
3. 'Histiocytic'	3. Predominantly large cell	3. Large noncleaved
4. Burkitt's	4. Small noncleaved-Burkitt's	4. Small noncleaved-Burkitt's
5. Non-Burkitt's	5. Small noncleaved	5. Small noncleaved-non-Burkitt's
Diffuse	Diffuse	Diffuse
6. Well-differentiated lymphocytic	6. Small lymphocytic	6. Small lymphocyte (B or T) – plasmacytoid lymphocyte
7. Intermediate lymphocytic	7. —	7. —
8. Lymphoblastic	8. Lymphoblastic	8. Convoluted lymphocyte
9. Immunoblastic	9. Immunoblastic-plasmacytoid	9. Immunoblastic (-B or T)
10. NHL with diffuse epithelioid histiocytic reaction (Lennert's)	10. Immunoblastic-clear -polymorphous -epithelioid	10. Lymphoepithelioid lymphocyte

to provide prognostic information. All are morphologically pure categories, and all include only B-cell lymphomas.

4.2. Diffuse lymphomas

Each of the subtypes in the 'diffuse' category, in all three systems conveys similar prognostic information. These systems could become even more comparable if some minor modifications were made (Table 5). We suggest that in the Rappaport classification [97], since the category of non-Hodgkin's lymphoma with diffuse epithelioid histiocytic reaction has morphologic features of peripheral T-cell lymphomas [96], it can be broadened to allow inclusion of all lymphomas which have morphologic features consistent with peripheral T-cell lymphoma. All such lymphomas could be identified by the eponym Waldron's lymphoma [123] , or Suchi's lymphoma [133] or Kikuchi's lymphoma [134]. Likewise, in the WF [58], the category of immunoblastic lymphoma with plasmacytoid features could be identified simply as immunoblastic; and the other three types of immunoblastic lymphoma, i.e. clear-cell, polymorphous,

Table 5. Comparison of classifications after introduction of minor modifications in all three systems.

Rappaport	Working Formulation	Lukes-Collins
Nodular and/or diffuse	Follicular and/or diffuse	Follicular and/or diffuse
1. Poorly differentiated lymphocytic	1. Predominantly small cleaved	1. Small cleaved
2. Mixed	2. (Large cleaved)	2. Large cleaved
3. 'Histiocytic'	3. (Large noncleaved)	3. Large noncleaved
4. Burkitt's	4. Small noncleaved-Burkitt's	4. Small noncleaved-Burkitt's
5. Non-Burkitt's	5. Small noncleaved (non-Burkitt's)	5. Small noncleaved-non-Burkitt's
Diffuse	Diffuse	Diffuse
6. Well differentiated lymphocytic	6. Small lymphocytic	6. Small lymphocytic – plasmacytoid lymphocyte
7. Intermediate lymphocytic	7. —	7. —
8. Lymphoblastic	8. Lymphoblastic	8. (Lymphoblastic)
9. Immunoblastic[a]	9. Immunoblastic[a]	9. Immunoblastic[a]
10. (Waldron's)[b]	10. (Waldron's)[b]	10. (Waldron's)[b]

[a] 'Immunoblastic' is used for lymphomas which have plasmacytoid features.

[b] 'Waldron's' lymphoma is an eponym suggested for lymphomas which have morphologic features of lymphomas derived from peripheral T-cells. It is used for all peripheral T-cell lymphomas. regardless of their size and cellular composition, and irrespective of the presence or absence of a diffuse epithelioid histiocytic reaction.

( ) Indicates changes suggested to achieve uniformity in all three systems.

and the epithelioid-cell type – could be integrated under a single heading, preferable an eponym. Although the Lukes-Collins classification has two categories – B-immunoblastic and T-immunoblastic, it might be perferable to reserve the term 'immunoblastic' for B-cell tumors, whereas the term 'T-immunoblastic' could be replaced by an eponym such as Waldron's lymphoma. We recommend, then, that all peripheral T-cell lymphomas be identified by one eponym such as Waldron's lymphoma.

Thus, if the three systems of classification were modified slightly (Table 5), they would be remarkably similar, if not identical. In most instances, the pathologic categories are morphologically pure groups with immunologic correlations. Moreover, most represent distinct clinicopathologic entities.

The immunologic methods that recently became available have provided very valuable information for an understanding of the biology and histogenesis of malignant lymphomas. It is therefore imperative studies be performed, using not only immunology, but also cytogenetics, cell kinetics and gene immunoregulation. However, it should be emphasized that such comprehensive research should be carried out only by those centers that have the necessary expertise and financial resources.

For the daily practice of pathology, on the other hand, a classification is required that consists of morphologically pure categories which have distinct clinical correlations and would thus help in prognosis and the design of therapeutic protocols. One needs to consider what one would gain by changing the terminology of the Rappaport classification. The mere change of name from 'PDL' to 'small cleaved', or, for that matter, changes for all the other subtypes, do not help in (1) the understanding of the biology of these tumors, (2) the prognosis, and (3) the development of treatment protocols for these lymphomas. The advantages of changes in the terms of the Rappaport classification are that utilization of histogenetic terms makes a classification scientifically accurate, enhances its understanding, and facilitates teaching. The classification of Rappaport is certainly very valid for the 1980's as long as one is aware of the scientific inaccuracies of the terminology. This Rappaport classification in its present form consists of pure morphologic groups, and most represent distinct clinicopathologic entities.

The Lukes-Collins classification has been modified 18 times (Table 6), and in no instance have the reasons for the modifications been given [47, 124, 168–175]. The latest version is intended to be an immunologic one, as indicated by its title (Table 7) [175]. An immunologic classification, however, cannot be used in the everyday practice of pathology. If Lukes and Collins want their classification to be used routinely, they could easily rearrange it based on morphologic, rather than immunologic criteria. We hope that they will subdivide the NHL on the basis of pattern, because pattern recognition is a highly reproducible morphologic parameter.

In summary, it is apparent that all three systems shown in Tables 4 and 5 have almost identical numbers of categories, and that each category represents a distinct clinicopathologic entity. The only significant difference among them is the terminology employed for the different subtypes. Although it is generally known that NHL are tumors of B or T lymphocytes, the statement by

Table 6. Modifications made by Lukes in the Lukes-Collins classifications.

1. In 1973, follicular lymphomas were subdivided into three categories: cleaved, noncleaved, and mixed [168]. In 1974, this subclassification was modified, and the mixed cell category was eliminated [47].
2. In 1974, the subdivision of follicular center cell tumors was modified – the cleaved-cell ype was subdivided into small- and large-cell subtypes; the noncleaved-cell type was also subdivided into small- and large-cell subtypes [47].
3. In 1973, Lukes and Collins stated that Burkitt's lymphoma always had a diffuse pattern [168]; in 1974, however, they stated that it could have a follicular and/or a diffuse pattern [47].
4. In 1974, the Lukes-Collins classification listed Hodgkin's disease with a question mark [47]. In 1975, Hodgkin's disease was no longer listed as a T-cell lymphoma [169, 170].
5. In 1974, the Lukes-Collins classification listed immunoblastic sarcoma (T-cell) with a question mark [47]. In 1975, the same category was listed as T-cell lymphoma, and, the question mark was deleted [170].
6. In 1977, under T-cell lymphomas, the categories of small lymphocyte and Lennert's lymphoma were added [171].
7. In 1977, under B-cell lymphomas, the category of hairy-cell leukemia was introduced [171].
8. In 1977, under B-cell lymphomas, the small lymphocyte was listed; however, in previous publications after 'small lymphocyte' the term CLL was included in parentheses [171].
9. In 1977, the terms 'small transformed' and 'large transformed' were introduced, and the designation 'noncleaved' for these lymphomas was placed in parentheses [171].
10. In 1978, Lukes deleted the category of Lennert's lymphoma from the T-cell lymphomas and instead introduced the category the 'lymphoepithelioid cell lymphoma' [172].
11. In 1978, Hodgkin's disease was placed under the category of 'cell of uncertain origin' [173].
12. In 1979, Lukes deleted the terms 'small and large transformed' and retained the terms 'small noncleaved' and 'large noncleaved' without placing them in parentheses [174].
13. In 1982, the small noncleaved lymphomas were subdivided into Burkitt's and non-Burkitt's types [175].
14. In 1982, the term 'FCC' was placed after each of the terms 'small cleaved', 'large cleaved', 'small noncleaved', 'large noncleaved' [175].
15. In 1982, a new term, 'cerebriform lymphocyte', was introduced, and 'mycosis fungoides' and 'Sezary syndrome', previously identified as such, were now listed in parentheses [175].
16. In 1982, Lukes *et al.* introduced a new term, 'lymphoepithelioid lymphocyte', as one of the types of T-cell lymphoma [175]. No explanation was provided as to how one can recognize a lympho cyte which is 'lymphoepithelioid' [175].
17. In most publications, the title of the Lukes-Collins classification was 'Classification of Malignant Lymphomas'. However, in the most recent communication, their classification is called 'Immunological Classification of Malignant Lymphomas' [175]. This clearly indicates that immunologic indentification of lymphoid cells is a prerequisite for their classification.
18. In 1977, Waldron *et al.*, from Collins's laboratory, for the first time described the morphologic features of the peripheral T-cell lymphomas [123]. However, no explanation was provided as to why the term peripheral T-lymphoma was employed instead of 'T-immunoplastic'.

Table 7. The latest version of the Lukes-Collins classification.

Immunologic classification of malignant lymphomas [175]

Ucell (undefined)
B-cell types
  Small lymphocyte (B)
  Plasmacytoid lymphocyte
  Follicular center cell (FCC) types
    (Follicular, follicuar and diffuse, and diffuse with or without sclerosis)
    Small cleaved FCC
    Large cleaved FCC
    Small noncleaved FCC
      Burkitt
      Non-Burkitt
    Large noncleaved FCC
  Immunoblastic sarcoma (B)

T-cell types
  Small lymphocyte (T)
  Convoluted lymphocyte
  Cerebriform lymphocyte
    (Mycosis fungoides and Sezary's syndrome)
  Lymphoepithelioid lymphocyte
  Immunoblastic sarcoma (T)

Histiocytic type

---

[175] Reproduced from Malignant Lymphomas 1982: 309–350.

Lukes that the immunologic designations B- and T-cells are important is not necessarily true. The mere omission of the terms B and T from the Working Formulation does not imply obsolescence. Adding these designations (B or T) either before or after each of the morphologic subtypes does not improve or detract from our understanding of the classifications of the NHL because they (B or T) do not convey the prognostic information that is available when morphologic terms are employed.

Acknowledgements

This study was supported in part by Grant Nos. 5T32-CA-09308, 5R01-CA-26422, 5U10-18044 and CA-16434 awarded by the National Cancer Institute, DHEW, and by Hematopathology Tutorials, Inc.

    The author thanks Dr. Jerome S. Burke for critical comments, Mrs. Maryalice Miller for secretarial assistance, Ms. Rosalie Barazandeh and Miss Pamela Edwards for typing manuscript, and Mrs. Elisabeth Lanzl for editorial assistance.

References

1. Rappaport H, Winter WJ, Hicks EB: Follicular lymphoma. A re-evaluation of its position in the scheme of malignant lymphoma, based on a survey of 253 cases. Cancer 9:792–821, 1956.
2. Hodgkin T: On some morbid appearances of the absorbent glands and spleen. Trane Med Chir Soc Lond 17:68–114, 1832.
3. Virchow RLK: Die Krankhaftern Geschwuelste 2:728–738 Berlin: Hirschwald, 1863.
4. Roulet F: Das primare Retothelsarkom der Lymphknoten. Virchows Arch [Pathol Anat] 277:15–47, 1930.
5. Roulet F: Oeitere Beitrage zur Kenntnis des Retothelsarkoms der Lymphknoten und anderer Lymphoiden-Organe. Virchows Arch [Pathol Anat] 286:702–732, 1932.
6. Baehr G: The clinical and pathological picture of follicular lymphoblastoma. Trans Assoc Am Phys 47:330–338, 1932.
7. Rappaport H: Tumors of the hematopoietic system. In: Atlas of tumor pathology, Section III, Fasicle 8. Washington D.C. Armed Forces Institute of Pathology, pp. 97–161, 1966.
8. Berard CW, O'Conor GT, Thomas LB, Torloni H: Histopathological definition of Burkitt's tumor. Bull WHO 40:601–607, 1969.
9. Berard CW: Chapter 15 Reticuloendothelial System: An overview of neoplasia. In: International Academy of pathology Monograph No. 16: The Reticuloendothelial System, JW Rebuck, CW Berard, MR Abell (eds.), Baltimore: Williams and Wilkins, 1975, pp. 301–317.
10. Jones SE, Fuks Z, Bull M, Kadin ME, Dorfman RF, Kaplan HS, Rosenberg SA, Kim H: Non-Hodgkin's lymphomas IV. Clinicopathologic correlation in 405 cases. Cancer 31:806–823, 1973.
11. Schein PS, Chabner BA, Canellos GP, Young RC, Berard C, DeVita VT: Potential for prolonged disease-free survival following combination chemotherapy of non-Hodgkin's lymphoma. Blood 43:181–189, 1974.
12. Bloomfield CD, Goldman A, Dick F, Brunning RD, Kennedy BJ: Multivariate analysis of prognostic factors in the non-Hodgkin's malignant lymphoma. Blood 43:181–189, 1974.
13. Patchefsky AS, Brodovsky HS, Menduke H, Southard M, Brooks J, Nicklas D, Hoch WS: Non-Hodgkin's Lymphomas: A clinicopathologic study of 293 cases. Cancer 34:1173–1186, 1974.
14. Brown TC, Peters MV, Bergsagel DE, Reid J: A retrospective analysis of the clinical results in relation to the Rappaport histological classification. Br J Cancer (Suppl. 11) 31:174–186, 1975.
15. DeVita VT Jr, Canellos GP, Chabner B, Schein P, Hubbard SP, Young RC: Advanced diffuse histiocytic lymphoma, a potentially curable disease. Lancet 1:248–250, 1975.
16. Schein PS, DeVita VT, Hubbard S, Chabner BA, Canellos GP, Berard C, Young RC: Bleomycin, adriamycin, cyclophosphamide, vincristine, and prednisone (BACOP) combination chemotherapy in the treatment of advanced diffuse histiocytic lymphoma. Ann Intern Med 85:417–422, 1976.
17. Lennert K, Niedorf HR: Nachweis von desmosomal verknupften reticulumzellen im follikularen lymphom (Brill Symmers). Virchows Archiv 4:148–150, 1969.
18. Kojima M, Imai Y, Mori N: A concept of follicular lymphoma. A proposal for the existence of a neoplasm originating from the germinal center. In: Malignant Diseases of the Hematopoietic System. GANN Monograph on Cancer Research No. 15, K. Akazaki, H. Rappaport, CW Berard, JM Bennett, E. Ishikawa (eds.), Tokyo: University of Tokyo Press, 1973, pp. 195–207.
19. Glick AD, Leech JH, Waldron JA, Flexner JM, Horn RG, Collins RD: Malignant lympho-

mas of follicular center cell origin in man. II Ultrastructural and cytochemical studies. J Natl Cancer Inst 54:23–27, 1975.

20. Levine GD, Dorfman RF: Nodular lymphoma: An ultrastructural study of its relationship to germinal centers and a correlation of light and electron microscopic findings. Cancer 35:148–164, 1975.

21. Dorfman RF: Enzyme histochemistry of normal, hyperplastic, and neoplastic lymphoreticular tissues. In: Symposium on Lymphoreticular Tumours in Africa, Roulet, FC (ed.), Paris, Basel, Switzerland, New York, S. Karger 1964, pp. 304–326.

22. Aisenberg AC, Bloch KJ: Immunoglobulins on the surface of neoplastic lymphocytes. New Eng J Med 287:272–276, 1972.

23. Preud'homme JL, Seligmann M: Surface bound immunoglobulins as a cell marker in human lymphoproliferative diseases. Blood 40:777–794, 1972.

24. Braylan RC, Rappaport H: Tissue immunoglobulins in nodular lymphomas as compared with reactive follicular hyperplasias. Blood 42:579–589, 1973.

25. Braylan RC, Jaffe ES, Berard CW: Malignant lymphomas: Current classification and new observations. In: Pathology Annual, Sommers, SC (ed.), New York: Appleton-Century-Crofts, 1975, pp. 213–217.

26. Brouet JC, Labaume S, Seligmann M: Evaluation of T and B lymphocyte membrane markers in human non-Hodgkin malignant lymphomata. Br J Cancer (Suppl. 11) 31:121–127, 1975.

27. Dorfman RF: The non-Hodgkin's lymphomas. In: The Reticuloendothelial System. IAP Monograph No. 16, JW Rebuck, CW Berard, MR Abell (eds.), Baltimore: Williams and Wilkins, 1975, pp. 262–281.

28. Leech JH, Glick AD, Waldron JA, Flexner JM, Horn RG, Collins RD: Malignant lymphomas of follicular center cell origin in man. I. Immunologic studies. J Natl Cancer Inst 54:11–21, 1975.

29. Taylor CR: An immunohistological study of follicular lymphoma, reticulum cell sarcoma and Hodgkin's disease. Eur J Cancer 12:61–75, 1976.

30. Pangalis GA, Rappaport H: Common clonal origin of lymphoplasmacytic proliferation and immunoblastic lymphoma in intestinal α-chain disease. Lancet 1977; 2:880.

31. Warnke R, Pederson M, Williams C, Levy R: A study of lymphoproliferative diseases comparing immunofluorescence with immunohistochemistry. Am J Clin Pathol 70:867–875, 1978.

32. Issacson P, Wright DH: Anomalous staining patterns in immunohistologic studies of malignant lymphoma. J Histochem Cytochem 27:1197–1199, 1979.

33. Banks PM: Diagnostic applications of an immunoperoxidase method in hematopathology. J Histochem Cytochem 27:1192–1194, 1979.

34. Pangalis GA, Nathwani BN, Rappaport H: Detection of cytoplasmic immunoglobulin in well-differentiated lymphoproliferative diseases by the immunoperoxidase method. Cancer 45:1334–1339, 1980.

35. Tubbs RR, Sheibani K, Sebek BA, Weiss RA: Immunohistochemistry versus immunofluorescence for non-Hodgkin's lymphomas. Am J Clin Pathol 73:144–145, 1980.

36. Jaffe ES, Shevach EM, Frank MM, Berard CW, Green I: Nodular lymphoma – Evidence for origin from follicular B lymphocytes. N Engl J Med 290:813–819, 1974.

37. Cossman J, Jaffe ES: Distribution of complement receptor subtypes in non-Hodgkin's lymphomas of B-cell origin. Blood 58:20–26, 1981.

38. Warnke R, Levy R: Detection of T and B cell antigens with hybridoma monoclonal antibodies: a biotin-avidin-horseradish peroxidase method. J Histochem Cytochem 28:771–776, 1980.

39. Lampson L, Levy R: Two populations of Ia-like molecules on a human B cell line. J Immunol 125:293–299, 1980.

40. Engleman EG, Warnke R, Fox RI, Dilley J, Benike CJ, Levy R: Studies of a human T lymphocyte antigen recognized by a monoclonal antibody. Proc Natl Acad Sci USA 78:1791–1795, 1981.

41. Poppema S, Bhan AK, Reinherz EL, McCluskey RT, Schlossman SF: Distribution of T cell subsets in human lymph nodes. J Exp Med 153:30–41, 1981.

42. Payne BC, Kim H, Pangalis GA, Rothman A, Rappaport H: A method for the ultrastructural demonstration of non-specific esterase in human blood and lymphoid tissue. Histochem J 12:71–86, 1980.

43. Kim H, Pangalis GA, Payne BC, Kadin ME, Rappaport H: Ultrastructural identification of neoplastic histiocytes-monocytes. An application of a newly developed cytochemical technique. Am J Pathol 106:204–223, 1982.

44. Braylan RC, Fowlkes BJ, Jaffe ES, Sanders SK, Berard CW, Herman CJ: Cell volumes and DNA distributions of normal and neoplastic human lymphoid cells. Cancer 41:201–209, 1978.

45. Shackney SE, Skramstad KS: A dynamic interpretation of multiparameter studies in the lymphomas. Am J Clin Pathol 72:756–764, 1979.

46. Diamond LW, Braylan RC: Flow analysis of DNA content and cell size in non-Hodgkin's lymphoma. Cancer Res 40:703–712, 1980.

47. Lukes RJ, Collins RD: Immunologic characterization of human malignant lymphomas. Cancer 34:1488–1503, 1974.

48. Lennert K, Mohri N, Stein H, Kaiserling E: The histopathology of malignant lymphoma. Br J Haematol (Suppl.) 31:193–203, 1975.

49. Mann RB, Jaffe ES, Braylan RC, Nanba K, Frank MM, Ziegler JL, Berard CW: Non-endemic Burkitt's lymphoma: A B-cell tumor related to germinal centers. N Engl J Med 295:685–691, 1976.

50. Mann RB, Jaffe ES, Berard CW: Malignant lymphomas: a conceptual understanding of morphologic diversity. Am J Pathol 94:105–192, 1979.

51. Berd D, Cornog J, DeConti RC, Levitt M, Bertino JR: Long term remission in diffuse histiocytic lymphoma treated with combination sequential chemotherapy. Cancer 35:1050–1054, 1975.

52. Bitran JD, Kinzie J, Sweet DL, Variakojis D, Griem ML, Golomb HM, Miller JB, Oetzel N, Ultmann JE: Survival of patients with localized histiocytic lymphoma. Cancer 39:342–346, 1977.

53. Fisher RI, DeVita VT, Johnson BL, Simon R, Young RC: Prognostic factors for advanced diffuse histiocytic lymphoma following treatment with combination chemotherapy. Am J Med 63:177–182, 1977.

54. Elias L, Portlock CS, Rosenberg SA: Combination chemotherapy of diffuse histiocytic lymphoma with cyclophosphamide, adriamycin, vincristine and prednisone (CHOP). Cancer 42:1705–1710, 1978.

55. Skarin A, Canellos G, Rosenthal D, Moloney W, Frei E: Therapy of unfavorable histology and non-Hodgkin's lymphoma (NHL) with high dose methotrexate and citrovorum factor rescue (MTX/CF), bleomycin, (B), adriamycin, (A), cyclophosphamide (C), oncovin (o), and decadron (D) (M-BACOD). (Abstr) Am Assoc Cancer Res/Am Soc Clin Oncol Proc 19:400, 1978.

56. Jones SE, Grozea PN, Metz EN, Haut A, Stephens RL, Morrison FS, Butler JJ, Byrne GE Jr, Moon TE, Fisher R, Haskins CL, Coltman CA Jr: Superiority of adriamycin-containing combination chemotherapy in the treatment of diffuse lymphoma. Cancer 43:417–425, 1979.

57. Sweet DL, Golomb HM, Ultmann JE, Miller B, Stein RS, Lester EP, Mintz U, Bitran JD, Streuli RA, Daly K, Roth NO: Cyclophosphamide, vincristine, methotrexate with leuco-

vorin rescue, and cytarabine (COMLA) combination sequential chemotherapy for advanced diffuse histiocytic lymphoma. Ann Int Med 92:785–790, 1980.

58. National Cancer Institute sponsored study of classifications of non-Hodgkin's lymphoma. Summary and description of a working formulation for clinical usage. The non-Hodgkin's lymphoma pathologic classification project. Cancer 49:2112–2135, 1982.

59. Nathwani BN, Kim H, Rappaport H, Solomon J, Fox M: Non-Hodgkin's lymphoma: A clinicopathological study comparing two classifications. Cancer 41:303–325, 1978.

60. Strauchen JA, Young RC, DeVita VT, Anderson T, Fantone JC, Berard CW: Clinical relevance of the histopathological subclassification of diffuse 'histiocytic' lymphoma. N Engl J Med 299:1382–1387, 1978.

61. Berard CW, Jaffe ES, Braylan RC, Mann RB, Nanba K: Immunologic aspects and pathology of the malignant lymphomas. Cancer 42:911–921, 1978.

62. Armitage JO, Dick FR, Platz CE, Corder MP, Leimert JT: Clinical usefulness and reproducibility of histologic subclassification of advanced diffuse histiocytic lymphoma. Am J Med 67:929–934, 1979.

63. Fisher RI, Hubbard SM, DeVita VT, Berard CW, Wesley R, Cossman J, Young RC: Factors predicting long-term survival in diffuse mixed, histiocytic or undifferentiated lymphoma. Blood 58:45–51, 1981.

64. Whitcomb CC, Cousar JB, Flint A, Crissman JD, Bartolucci AA, Durant JR, Gams RA, Collins RD, Byrne GE Jr: Subcategories of histiocytic lymphoma: Associations with survival and reproducibility of classification. The Southeastern Cancer Study Group Experience. Cancer 48:2464–2474, 1981.

65. Foucar K, Armitage JO, Dick F: The clinical and pathologic features of diffuse mixed non-Hodgkin's lymphoma. (Abstr) Blood 58 (Suppl. 1):158a, 1981.

66. Newcomer LN, Nerenberg MI, Cadman EC, Waldron JA Jr, Farber LR, Bertino JR: The usefullness of the Lukes-Collins classification in identifying subsets of diffuse histiocytic lymphoma responsive to chemotherapy. Cancer 50:439–443, 1982.

67. Warnke RA, Strauchen JA, Burke JS, Hoppe RT, Campbell BA, Dorfman RF: Morphologic types of diffuse large-cell lymphoma. Cancer 50:690–695, 1982.

68. Nathwani BN, Dixon DO, Jones SE, Hartsock RJ, Rebuck JW, Byrne GE Jr, Sheehan WW, Kim H, Coltman CA Jr, Rappaport H: The clinical significance of the morphological subdivision of diffuse 'histiocytic' lymphoma: A study of 162 patients treated by the Southwest Oncology Group. Blood 60:1068–1074, 1982.

69. Brouet JC, Preud'Homme JL, Flandrin G, Chelloul N, Seligmann M: Membrane markers in histiocytic lymphoma (reticulum cell sarcomas). J Natl Cancer Inst 56:631–633, 1976.

70. Bloomfield CD, Kersey JH, Brunning RD, Gajl-Peczlaska KJ: Prognostic significance of lymphocyte surface markers in adult non-Hodgkin's malignant lymphoma. Lancet 2:1330–1333, 1976.

71. Epstein AL, Levy R, Kim H, Henle W, Henle G, Kaplan HS: Biology of the human malignant lymphomas. IV. Functional characterization of ten diffuse histiocytic lymphoma cell lines. Cancer 42:2379–2391, 1978.

72. Bloomfield CD, Gajl-Peczalska KJ, Frizzera G, Kersey JH, Goldman, AI: Clinical utility of lymphocyte surface markers combined with the Lukes-Collins histologic classification in adult lymphoma. N Engl J Med 301:512–518, 1979.

73. Frizzera G, Gajl-Peczalska KJ, Bloomfield CD, Kersey JH: Predictability of immunologic phenotype of malignant lymphomas by conventional morphology: a study of 60 cases. Cancer 43:1216–1224, 1979.

74. Jaffe ES, Strauchen JA, Berard CW: Predictability of immunologic phenotype by morphologic criteria in diffuse aggressive non-Hodgkin's lymphomas. Am J Clin Pathol 77:46–49, 1982.

75. Warnke R, Miller R, Grogan T, Pederson M, Dilley J, Levy R: Immunologic phenotype in 30 patients with diffuse large cell lymphoma. N Engl J Med 303:293–300, 1980.
76. Rudders RA, Ahl ET, DeLellis RA: Surface marker and histopathologic correlation with long-term survival in advanced large cell non-Hodgkin's lymphoma. Cancer 47:1329–1335, 1981.
77. Nowell PC: Phytohemagglutinin: An initiator of mitosis in cultures of normal human leukocytes. Cancer Res 20:462–466, 1960.
78. Biberfield P: Morphogenesis in blood lymphocytes stimulated with phytohaemagglutinin (PH): A light and electron microscopic study. Acta Pathol Microbiol Scand (A) (Suppl.) 223:1–70, 1971.
79. Cottier H, Turk J, Sobin L: A proposal for a standardized system of reporting human lymph node morphology in relation to immunological function. Bull WHO 47:375–417, 1972.
80. Dorfman RF: Classification of non-Hodgkin's lymphomas. Lancet 1:1295, 1974.
81. Nathwani BN, Kim H, Rappaport H: Malignant lymphoma, lymphoblastic. Cancer 38:964–983, 1976.
82. Jaffe ES, Braylan RC, Frank MM, Green I, Berard CW: Functional markers: A new perspective on malignant lymphomas. Cancer Treat Rep 61:953–962, 1977.
83. Nanba K, Jaffe ES, Braylan RC, Soban EJ, Berard CW: Alkaline phosphatase positive malignant lymphomas: A subtype of B-cell lymphomas. Am J Clin Pathol 68:535–542, 1977.
84. DeVita VT, Rappaport H, Frei E, III: Announcement of formation of: The Lymphoma Task Force and Pathology Reference Center. Cancer 2:1087–1088, 1968.
85. Kim H, Zelman RJ, Fox MA, Bennet JM, Berard CW, Butler JJ, Byrne GE Jr, Dorfman RF, Hartsock RJ, Lukes RJ, Mann RB, Neiman RS, Rebuck JW, Sheehan WW, Variakojis D, Wilson JF, Rappaport H: Pathology Panel for lymphoma Clinical Studies: A comprehensive analysis of cases accumulated since its incention. J Natl Cancer Inst 68:43–67, 1982.
86. Frizzera G, Moran EM, Rappaport H: Angio-immunoblastic lymphadenopathy with dysproteinaemia. Lancet 1:1070–1073, 1974.
87. Barcos MP, Lukes RJ: Malignant lymphoma of convoluted lymphocytes – A new entity of possible T-cell type. In: Conflicts in childhood cancer. An evaluation of current management, Vol. 4, Sinks LF, Godden JO (eds.), New York: Alan R. Liss, 1975, pp. 147–178.
88. Banks PM, Arsenau JC, Gralnick HR, Canellos GP, DeVita Jr VT, Berard CW: American Burkitt's lymphoma: A clinicopathologic study of 30 cases. II. Pathologic correlations. Am J Med 58:322–329, 1975.
89. Kim H, Jacobs C, Warnke RA, Dorfman RF: Malignant lymphoma with a high content of epithelioid histiocytes: A distinct clinicopathologic entity and a form of so-called 'Lennert's lymphoma'. Cancer 41:620–635, 1978.
90. Burke JS, Butler JJ: Malignant lymphoma with a high content of epitheliod histiocytes (Lennert's lymphoma). Am J Clin Pathol 66:1–9, 1976.
91. Pangalis GA, Nathwani BN, Rappaport H: Malignant lymphoma, well differentiated lymphocytic: Its relationship with vchronic lymphocytic leukemia and macroglobulinemia of Waldenstrom. Cancer 39:999–1010, 1977.
92. Nathwani BN, Rappaport H, Moran EM, Pangalis GA, Kim H: Malignant lymphoma arising in angio-immunoblastic lymphadenopathy. Cancer 41:578–606, 1978.
93 Pangalis GA, Moran EM, Rappaport H: Blood and bone marrow findings in angioimmunoblastic lymphadenopathy. Blood 51:71–83, 1978.
94. Rappaport H, Pangalis GA, Nathwani BN: The evolution of immunoblastic lymphomas in morphologically non-neoplastic immunoproliferative diseases. In: Cold Springs Harbor Conferences on Cell Proliferation, Vol 5. Differentiation of normal and neoplastic hematopoietic cells, Clarkson B, Marks PA, Tills JA (eds.), 1978, pp. 877–897.
95. Pangalis GA, Nathwani BN, Rappaport H, Rosen RB: Acute lymphoblastic leukemia: The

220

significance of nuclear convolutions. Cancer 43:551–557, 1979.

96. Kim H, Nathwani BN, Rappaport H: So-called 'Lennert's lymphoma': Is it a clinicopathologic entity? Cancer 45:1379–1399, 1980.
97. Rappaport H: Non-Hodgkin's lymphoma: Roundtable discussion of histopathologic classifications. Cancer Treat Rep 61:1037–1042, 1977.
98. Nathwani BN, Winberg CD, Diamond LW, Bearman RM, Kim H: Morphologic criteria for the differentiation of follicular lymphoma from florid reactive follicular hyperplasia: a study of 80 cases. Cancer 48:1974–1806, 1981.
99. Osborne BM, Butler JJ, Variakojis D, Kott, M: Reactive Lymph node hyperplasia with giant follicles. Am J Clin Pathol 78:693–499, 1982.
100. Arseneau JC, Canellos GP, Banks PM, Berard CW, Gralnick HR, DeVita VT Jr: American Burkitt's lymphoma: A clinicopathologic study of 30 cases. I. Clinical factors relating to prolonged survival. Am J Med 58:314–321, 1975.
101. Ziegler JL: Treatment results of 54 American patients with Burkitt's lymphoma are similar to the African experience. N Engl J Med 297:75–80, 1977.
102. Ziegler JL, Magrath IT, Olweny CLM: Long survival of Burkitt's lymphoma in Uganda: A 10-year study. In: Seventieth Annual Meeting of the American Association for Cancer Research of the American Society of Clinical Oncologists. 1979, pp. 20:430.
103. Milauskas MB, Berard CW, Young RC, Garvin AJ, Edwards BK, DeVita Jr VT: Undifferentiated non-Hodgkin's lymphomas (Burkitt's and non-Burkitt's types). The relevance of making this histologic distinction. Cancer 2115–2121, 1982.
104. Lennert K, Mohri N: Histopathology and diagnosis of non-Hodgkin's lmphomas. In: Malignant lymphomas other than Hodgkin's disease. New York: Springer-Verlag. 1978, pp. 111–469.
105. Nathwani BN, Winberg CD: Non-Hodgkin's lymphomas: An appraisal of the Working Formulation of Non-Hodgkin's lymphomas for clinical usage. In: Malignant Lymphomas. A Pathology Annual Monograph. SC Sommers, PP Rosen (eds.) New York, Appleton-Century-Crofts, 1983, pp. 1–64.
106. Weisenburger DD, Nathwani BN, Diamond LW, Winberg CD, Rappaport H: Malignant lymphoma, intermediate lymphocyte type: A clinicopathologic study of 42 cases. Cancer 48:1415–1425, 1982.
107. Weisenburger DD, Kim H, Rappaport H: Mantle-zone lymphoma: A follicular variant of intermediate lymphocytic lymphoma. Cancer 49:1429–1438, 1982.
108. Nathwani BN, Diamond LW, Winberg CD, Kim H, Bearman RM, Glick JH, Jones SE, Gams RA, Nissen NI, Rappaport H: Lymphoblastic lymphoma: A clinicopathologic study of 95 patients. Cancer 48:2347–2357, 1981.
109. Brouet JC, Labaume S, Seligmann M: Evaluation of T and B lymphocyte membrane markers in human non-Hodgkin's malignant lymphomas. Br J Cancer (Suppl.) 31:121–127, 1975.
110. Long JC, Aisenberg AC: Richter's syndrome: A terminal complication of chronic lymphocytic leukemia with distinct clinicopathologic features. Am J Clin Pathol 63:786–795, 1975.
111. Richter MN: Generalized reticular cell sarcoma of lymph nodes associated with lymphatic leukemia. Am J Pathol 4:285–292, 1928.
112. Kjeldsberg CR, Marty J: Prolymphocytic transformation of chronic lymphocytic leukemia. Cancer 48:2447–2457, 1981.
113. Brouet JC, Mason DY, Danom F, Preud'home JL, Seligmann M, Reyes F, Navab F, Galian F, Rene E, Rambaud JC: Alpha-chain disease: Evidence for common clonal origin of intestinal immunoblastic lymphoma and plasmacytic proliferation. Lancet 1:861, 1977.
114. Galian A, Lecestre MJ, Scotto J, Bognel C, Matuchansky C, Rambaud JC: Pathological study of alpha-chain disease with special emphasis on evolution. Cancer 39:2081–2101, 1977.
115. Ramot B, Levanon M, Hahn Y, Lahat N, Moroz C: The mutual clonal origin of the

lymphoplasmacytic and lymphoma cell in alpha-heavy chain disease. Clin Exp Immunol 27:440–445, 1977.

116. Anderson LG, Talal N: The spectrum of benign to malignant lymphoproliferation in Sjogren's syndrome. Clin Exp Immunol 10:199–221, 1972.

117. Talal N, Bunim JJ: The development of malignant lymphoma in the course of Sjorgen's syndrome. Clin Exp Immunol 10:199–221, 1972.

118. Talal N, Sokoloff L, Barth WF: Extra-salivary lymphoid abnormalities in Sjorgen's syndrome (reticulum cell sarcoma, 'pseudolymphoma', macroglobulinemia). Am J Med 43:50–65, 1967.

119. Zulman J, Jaffe R, Talal N: Evidence that the malignant lymphoma of Sjogren's syndrome is a monoclonal B-cell neoplasm. N Engl J Med 299:1215–1220, 1978.

120. Matas AJ, Hertel BF, Rosai J, Simmons RL, Najarian JS: Post-transplant malignant lymphoma: Distinctive morphologic features related to its pathogenesis. Am J Med 61:716–720, 1976.

121. Frizzera G, Hanto DW, Gajl-Peczalska KJ, Rosai J, McKenna RW, Sibley RK, Holahan KP, Lindequist LL: Polymorphic diffuse β-cell hyperplasias and lymphomas in renal transplant recipients. Cancer Res 41:4262–4279, 1981.

122. Lukes RJ, Tindle BH: Immunoblastic lymphadenopathy. A hyperimmune entity resembling Hodgkin's disease. N Engl J Med 292:1–8, 1975.

123. Waldron JA, Leech JH, Glick A, Flexner JM, Collins RD: Malignant lymphoma of peripheral T-lymphocyte origin: Immunologic, pathologic and clinical features in six patients. Cancer 40:1604–1617, 1977.

124. Lukes RJ, Parker JW: The pathology of lymphoreticular neoplasms. In: The immunopathology of lymphoreticular neoplasms, Twomey JJ, Good RA (eds.), New York: Plenum Publishing, 1978, pp. 239–279.

125. Nathwani BN: A critical analysis of the classification of non-Hodgkin's lymphoma. Cancer 44:347–384, 1979.

126. Nathwani BN, Winberg CD, Rappaport H, Zelman RJ: Malignant lymphoma, T-immunoblastic. A clinicopathologic and immunologic study of 41 patients. Blood 54 (Suppl. 1): 201a, 1979 (Abstr).

127. Nathwani BN, Metter GE, Gams RA, Bartolucci AA, Hartsock RJ, Neiman RS, Byrne GE Jr, Barcos M, Kim H, Rappaport H: Malignant lymphoma, mixed cell type, diffuse. Blood 62:200–208, 1983.

128. Schneider DR, Taylor CR, Parker JW, Cramer AS, Meyer PR, Lukes RJ: Immunoblastic sarcoma of T- and B-cell types: A morphologic comparison. Lab Invest 46:73a, 1982 (Abstr).

129. Levine AM, Taylor CR, Schneider DR, Koehler SC, Forman SJ, Lichtenstein A, Lukes RJ, Feinstein DI. Immunoblastic sarcoma of T-cell versus B-cell origin: I. Clinical features. Blood 58:52–61, 1981.

130. Palutke M, Tabaczka P, Weise RW, Axelrod A, Palacas C, Margolis H, Khilanani P, Ratanatharathorn M, Piligian J, Pollard R, Husain M: T-cell lymphomas of large cell type. Cancer 46:87–101, 1980.

131. Suchi T: Atypical lymph node hyperplasia with fatal outcome – A report on the histopathological, immunological, and clinical investigations of the cases. Recent adv in RES Res 14:13–34, 1974.

132. Suchi T: 'Atypical hyperplasia' of lymph nodes with poor prognosis – Immunoological characterization of the proliferating cells. Recent Adv in RES Research 18:124–133, 1978.

133. Suchi T, Tajima K: Peripheral T-cell malignancy as a problem in Lymphoma classification. Jpn J Clin Oncol 9 (Suppl. 1), 443–450, 1979.

134. Kikuchi M, Mitsui T, Matsui N, Sato E, Tokunaga M, Hasui K, Ichimaru M, Kinoshita K,

222

Kamihira S: T-cell malignancies in adults: Histopathological studies of lymph nodes in 110 patients. Jpn J Clin Oncol 9 (Suppl. 1), 407–422, 1979.

135. Watanabe S, Nakajima T, Shimosato Y, Shimoyama M, Minato K: T-cell malignancies: Subclassification and interrelationship. Jpn J Clin Oncol 9 (Suppl. 1), 423–442, 1979.

136. Shimoyama M, Minato K, Saito H, Takenaka T, Watanabe S, Nagatani T, Maruto M: Immunoblastic lymphadenopathy (IBL)-like T-cell lymphoma. Jpn J Clin Oncol 9 (Suppl. 1):347–356, 1979.

137. Watanabe S, Shimosato Y, Shimoyama M, Minato K, Suzuki M, Abe M, Nagatani T: Adult T-cell lymphoma with hypergammaglobulinemia. Cancer 46:2472–2483, 1980.

138. Portlock CS, Rosenberg SA: Chemotherapy of the non-Hodgkin's lymphomas: The Stanford experience. Cancer Treat Rep 61: 1049–1055, 1977.

139. Ezdinli EZ, Costello W, Wasser LP, Lenhard RE, Berard CW, Hartsock J, Bennett JM, Carbone PP: Eastern Cooperative Oncology Group experience with the Rappaport classification of non-Hodgkin's lymphomas. Cancer 43:544–550, 1979.

140. Glick JH: Chemotherapy of Hodgkin's lymphomas. In: Lymphomas 1 including Hodgkin's disease Bennet JM (ed.), The Hague, Boston, London: Martinus Nijhoff Publishers, 1981, pp. 343–446.

141. Ezdinli EZ, Costello W, Lenhard Jr RE, Bakemeier R, Bennett JM, Berard CW, Carbonne PP: Survival of nodular versus diffuse pattern lymphocytic poorly differentiated lymphoma. Cancer 41:1990–1996, 1978.

142. Rudders RA, Kaddis M, DeLellis RA, Casey Jr H: Nodular non-Hodgkin's lymphoma (NHL). Factors influencing prognosis and indications for aggressive treatment. Cancer 43:1643–1651, 1979.

143. Anderson T, Bender BA, Fisher RI, DeVita VT, Chabner BA, Berard CW, Norton L, Young RC: Combination chemotherapy in non-Hodgkin's lymphoma: Results of long-term follow-up. Cancer Treat Rep 61:1057–1066, 1977.

144. Bitran JC, Golomb HM, Ultman JE, Sweet Jr DL, Lester EP, Stein RS, Miller JB, Moran EM, Kinnealey, Vardiman JE, Kinzie J, Roth NO: Non-Hodgkin's lymphoma, poorly differentiated lymphocytic and mixed cell types: Results of sequential staging proc, Berardresponse to therapy, and survival of 100 patients. Cancer 42:88–95, 1978.

145. Ezdinli EZ, Costello WB, Icli F, Lenhard RE, Johnson GJ, Silverstein M, Berard CW, Bennett JM, Carbone PP: Nodular mixed lymphocytic-histiocytic lymphoma: Response and survival. Cancer 45:261–267, 1980.

146. Glick JH, Barnes JM, Ezdinli EZ, Berard CW, Orlow EL, Bennett JM: Nodular mixed lymphoma: Results of randomized trial failing to confirm prolonged disease-free survival with COPP chemotherapy. Blood 58:920–925, 1981.

147. Colby TV, Hoppe RT, Burke JS: Nodular lymphoma: Clinicopathologic correlations of parafollicular small lymphocytes and degree of nodularity. Cancer 45:2364–2367, 1980.

148. Longo D, Hubbard S, Wesley M, Jaffe E, Chabner B, DeVita VT, Young R: Prolonged initial remission in patients with nodular mixed lymphoma. Proc Am Soc Oncol 22:521, 1981.

149. Osborne CK, Norton L, Young RC, Garvin AJ, Simon RM, Berard CW, Hubbard S, DeVita VT: Nodular histiocytic lymphoma: An aggressive nodular lymphoma with potential for prolonged disease-free survival. Blood 56:98–102, 1980.

150. Glick JH, McFadden E, Costello W, Ezdinli EZ, Berard CW, Bennett JM: Nodular histiocytic lymphoma: Factors influencing prognosis and implications for aggressive chemotherapy. Cancer 49:840–845, 1982.

151. Fuller LM, Banker FL, Butler JJ, Gamble JF, Sullivan MP: The natural history of non-Hodgkin's lymphomata stages I and II. Br J Cancer (Suppl. 11) 31:270–285, 1975.

152. Rosenberg SA, Dorfman RF, Kaplan HS: The value of sequential bone marrow biopsy and

laparotomy and splenectomy in a series of 127 consecutive untreated patients with non-Hodgkin's lymphoma. Br J Cancer (Suppl. 11) 31:221–227, 1975.

153. Stein RS, Ultmann JE, Byrne Jr GE, Moran EM, Golomb HM, Oetzel N: Bone marrow involvement in non-Hodgkin's lymphoma. Implications for staging and therapy. Cancer 37:629–636, 1976.

154. Jones SE, Butler JJ, Byrne GE, Coltman CA, Moon TE: Histopathologic review of lymphoma cases from the Southwest Oncology Group. Cancer 39:1071–1076, 1977.

155. Byrne GE: Rappaport classification of non-Hodgkin's lymphoma: histologic features and clinical significance. Cancer Treat Rep 61:935–944, 1977.

156. Coltman CA, Gams RA, Glick JH, Jenkin RD: Lymphoma. In: Cancer research. Impact of the cooperative groups, Hoogstraten B (ed.), New York: Masson Publishing USA, Inc., 1980, pp. 39–84.

157. Velez-Garcia E, Durant J, Gams R, Bartolucci A: Results of a uniform histopathologic review system of lymphoma cases: A ten-year study from the Southeastern Cancer Study Group. Cancer 52:675–679, 1983.

158. Icli F, Ezdinli EZ, Costello W, Berard CW, Bennett JM, Carbone PP: Diffuse well-differentiated lymphocytic lymphoma (DLWD). Response and survival. Cancer 42:1936–1942, 1978.

159. Evans HL, Butler JJ, Youness EL: Malignant lymphoma, small lymphocytic type. Cancer 41:1440–1455, 1978.

160. Braylan RC, Jaffe ES, Burbach JW, Frank MM, Johnson RC, Berard CW: Similarities of surface characteristics of neoplastic well-differentiated lymphocytes from solid tissues and from peripheral blood. Cancer Res 36:1619–1625, 1976.

161. Kim H, Heller P. Rappaport H: Monoclonal gammopathies associated with lymphoproliferative disorders: A morphologic study. Am J Clin Pathol 59:282–294, 1973.

162. Stein H, Petersen N, Gaedicke G, Lennert K, Landbeck G: Lymphoblastic lymphoma of convoluted or acid phosphatase type – A tumor of T precursor cells. Int J Cancer 17:292–295, 1976.

163. Jaffe ES, Braylan RC, Frank MM, Green L, Berard CW: Heterogeneity of immunologic markers and surface morphology in childhood lymphoblastic lymphoma. Blood 48:213–222, 1976.

164. Koziner B, Fillippa DA, Mertelsmann R, Gupta S, Clarkson B, Good RA, Siegal FP: Characterization of malignant lymphomas in leukemic phase by multiple differentiation markers of mononuclear cells. Correlation with clinical features and conventional morphology. Am J Med 63:556–567, 1977.

165. Bloomfield CD, Frizzera G, Gail-Peczalska KJ, Brunning RD, Kersey J: Malignant lymphoma, lymphoblastic (MLLB) in the adult. (Abstr) Proc Am Soc Clin Oncol 19:378, 1978.

166. Long JC, McCaffrey RP, Aisenberg AC, Marks SM, Kung PC: Terminal deoxynucleotidyl transferase positive lymphoblastic lymphoma. A study of 15 cases. Cancer 44:2127–2139, 1979.

167. Cossman J, Chused TM, Bollum F, Jaffe ES: Diversity of Immunologic phenotype of lymphoblastic lymphoma. Cancer Res (in press).

168. Lukes RJ, Collins RD: New observations on follicular lymphoma. In: Malignant diseases of the hematopoietic system. GANN Monograph on Cancer research, no. 15, Akazaki K, Rappaport H, Berard CW, Bennett JM, Ishikawa E (eds.), Tokyo: University of Tokyo Press, 1973, pp. 209–215.

169. Lukes RJ, Collins RD: A functional classification of malignant lymphomas. In: The reticuloendothelial system, IAP Monograph No. 16, Rebuck JW, Berard CW, Abell MR (eds.), Baltimore: Williams and Wilkins, 1975, pp. 213–242.

170. Lukes RJ, Collins RD: New approaches to the classification of the lymphomata. Br J Cancer (Suppl. 11) 31:1–28, 1975.
171. Lukes RJ, Collins RD: Lukes-Collins classification and its significance. Cancer Treat Rep 61:971–979, 1977.
172. Lukes RJ: Functional classification of malignant lymphoma of Lukes and Collins. Recent Results Cancer Res 64:19–30, 1978.
173. Lukes RJ, Lincoln TL, Parker JW, Alavaikko MJ: Cold Spring Harbor Conferences on Cell Proliferation. In: Differentiation of normal neoplastic hematopoietic cells. Clarkson B, Marks PA, Tills JE (eds.) An immunologic approach to classification of malignant lymphomas: A cytokinetic model of lymphoid neoplasia. USA Vol. 5. 1978, pp. 935–952.
174. Lukes RJ: The immunologic approach to the pathology of malignant lymphomas. Am J Clin Pathol 72:657–669, 1979.
175. Lukes RJ, Taylor CR, Parker JW: In: Malignant lymphoma: Immunological surface marker studies in the histopathological diagnosis of non-Hodgkin's lymphomas based on multiparameter studies of 790 cases. Bristol Meyer: Academic Press, 1982, pp. 310–347.

10. Nodular mixed cell lymphoma: Is there a potential for a prolonged disease free survival and cure?

TOM ANDERSON

1. Introduction

The malignant lymphomas represent a significant contribution to the morbidity and mortality of malignant diseases in the United States. It was estimated in 1982 that 23 000 new cases of malignant lymphoma will be diagnosed, and 12 600 deaths will occur. By disease site, malignant lymphoma is one of the ten most common malignancies, and one of the eight most common fatal malignancies. Although this mortality rate is high (over 50%), the mortality rate appears to be decreasing with the introduction of more effective modalities of treatment for the malignant lymphomas at their various stages of disease. This more effective therapy represents the incorporation of better histopathological classification systems, better supportive medical care systems, and the introduction of new and improved treatment programs. In addition, the development of systematic staging procedures to identify otherwise occult disease has been an important addition to our management of these patients. These techniques have not only allowed for more appropriate application of initial therapy, but have identified sites of otherwise occult disease that need to be re-evaluated at the time of completion of therapy.

The above developments have occurred at a variety of institutions worldwide, and represent the ongoing dynamic expansion of oncological knowledge. Prior to the introduction of effective therapy, a better histopathological classification system was not needed. However, with the development of radiotherapy and subsequent single agent and combination chemotherapy, the desireability of an improved pathological classification system with better prognostic significance became apparent. The first step in improvement of such histopathological classifications was made by Rappaport in the original Armed Foces Institute of Pathology fascicle [1] which subsequently became widely applied after the publication of data by Jones, *et al.* regarding the staging and efficacy of radiotherapy and single agent chemotherapy [2, 3]. With the reports of the efficacy of combination chemotherapy regimens, the desireability of better prognostic staging systems became widely appreciated.

Bennett JM (ed), Controversies in the Management of Lymphomas. ISBN 0-89838-586-5.
© *Martinus Nijhoff Publishers, Boston. Printed in the Netherlands.*

During this period of time the development of a large number of histological and cytological classification systems for malignant lymphomas arose, and has led to a variety of efforts to validate these new systems. This has recently culminated in the report of the Non-Hodgkin's Lymphoma Pathologic Classification Project [4]. This report compares the six major pathological classification systems in use worldwide, and proposes a working formulation of ten major subtypes of disease utilizing morphological criteria alone.

With the rapid development of a variety of treatment programs, together with the application of the newer pathological classification systems, it is not surprising that a number of apparent discrepancies exist in the literature. One intriguing subset of malignant lymphomas is the nodular mixed histiocytic lymphocytic lymphoma of Rappaport. As originally defined, this is 'a malignant tumor of reticular tissue that is characterized by proliferations of neoplastic histiocytes and lymphocytes, without appreciable predominance of either cell type' [1]. It was noted in the original description that these lymphomas rarely retain their original mixed cellular elements but with progression of disease usually evolve into a histiocytic or poorly differentiated lymphocytic type. It was also noted that there may be composite lymphomas in this category with varying degrees of histiocytic or lymphocytic components. It was originally thought by Rappaport to be rare [1].

It is now recognized that the term histiocytic in the Rappaport system is a misnomer, and that what was originally thought to be the morphologic equivalent of a malignant histiocyte is now recognized as a relatively undifferentiated transformed lymphocyte usually of B cell origin. This recent information arises from the knowledge generated in the area of immunology, and is reflected in the various classification systems with various more immunologically correct terminologies such as 'follicular cells, mixed small and large' (British non-Hodgkin's Lymphoma Investigation Classification System), 'follicular mixed, small and large lymphoid' (Dorfman classification) [4–6]. In some of the newer classification systems the mixed category does not exist per se; in the Lukes–Collins system, patients in this category would be divided between the follicular center cell small cleaved, and the follicular center cell large cleaved subcategories. In the Kiel system they would be listed as centroblastic–centrocytic (small) categories, and in the WHO system as prolymphocytic–lymphoblastic types. All of the above categories refer to the nodular or follicular patterns of growth [4].

Just as there are a variety of histopathological and/or cytological classification systems, a variety of treatment programs have evolved at various institutions worldwide. As early as 1972 it was recognized that the nodular lymphomas in general had a relatively high response rate to single agent chemotherapy and/or the careful application of radiotherapy in a variety of treatment field and dose schedules [3]. Utilizing the models of carefully designed combination chemotherapy programs successfully applied in acute lymphocytic leukemia of childhood and advanced stage Hodgkin's disease, a number of institutions developed comprehensive combination chemotherapy programs for the malignant lymphomas including the nodular subtypes. During the past decade a variety of combination chemotherapy programs were shown to be efficacious in inducing remissions in the nodular lymphomas, and in prolonging survival. However, followup in several of these trials suggested that these remissions might not be durable, that the morbidity of aggressive therapy in older patients with malignant lymphomas appeared to be greater than in the younger patients with Hodgkin's disease, and the observation that some patients with nodular lymphomas appeared to have an indolent disease course regardless of how aggressively they were treated, all raised the possibility that a re-evaluation should occur regarding the approach to patients with nodular lymphomas. Nodular mixed lymphoma has in particular been a controversial subgroup of patients as this re-evaluation has occurred.

As early as 1972 it was reported that patients with advanced stage nodular mixed lymphoma responded well to a variety of sequential single agent chemotherapy programs. Jones *et al.* reported a 31% complete clinical remission in 16 patients treated with cyclophosphamide or chlorambucil, with an additional 50% of patients having a partial response [3]. Median duration of response was over 17 months on this continuous alkylating agent regimen, with responses lasting from 2 to over 66 months. This observed response rate fell intermediately between the nodular poorly differentiated lymphocytic and nodular histiocytic lymphoma patients treated similarly, and the actuarial survival of such patients also was observed to be intermediate between these two groups of patients. This was one of the first clearcut demonstrations that effective therapy serves as an important biological probe as to the behavior of the malignant lymphomas [3].

In 1977, Anderson *et al.* reported the results of combination chemotherapy in a series of patients with advanced stage nodular mixed lymphoma [7]. In this study 24/31 patients (77%) achieved a complete remission; at the time of that report only four patients had relapsed, all within the first three years after achieving a complete remission, producing an apparent level remission duration curve and survival curve for patients achieving a complete remission. This was in contrast to patients with nodular poorly differentiated lymphocytic lymphoma who had a similarly high complete response rate (67%), but a relatively steady relapse rate thereafter with no apparent long term disease free survival curve.

Subsequent results from other series have in general corroborated the ability of combination chemotherapy to achieve complete remissions in nodular mixed lymphoma but disagreement exists as to what proportion of patients appear to have long term disease free survival. The exact magnitude of this proportion of patients, the difference between these patients and other patients with nodular or other nonaggressive forms of lymphoma, are currently being investigated by a number of institutions.

2. Pathological classification issue

Confounding the issue is the reproducibility and consistency of pathological classification systems. In the original study of reproducibility of pathological classification reported by the University of Chicago, reproducibility of classification of mixed lymphocytic histiocytic subtypes of malignant lymphoma was achieved in only 69%, while in a subsequent Southwest Oncology Group study, the reproducibility was only 50% [7]. This lack of reproducibility or inaccuracy is of profound significance when interpreting the clinical data presented in the subsequent section [4]. The current information would suggest that nodular poorly differentiated lymphocytic lymphoma, a disease at the more indolent end of the spectrum from nodular mixed lymphoma is a kinetically relatively inactive disease which can be effectively palliated by a variety of means, and which tends to have a relatively constant relapse rate after comprehensive treatment programs with induction chemotherapy but no maintenance program. Such a relapse pattern suggests a small growth fraction to this tumor, and perhaps inadequate treatment in terms of the duration of such therapy. However, given the age of the patients with this disease, and the therapeutic index of most treatment modalities, this disease is currently considered to be noncurable and to have a constant finite relapse rate from remission induction. At the other end of the spectrum from nodular mixed lymphoma is nodular large cell or histiocytic lymphoma. This disease appears to be a wolf in sheep's clothing. It probably has a relatively high growth fraction, and clinically is an aggressive disease requiring therapy analogous to its diffuse counterpart. Clinical trials have suggested that with aggressive combination chemotherapy for advanced disease a finite subset of such patients may well be curable. Thus nodular mixed lymphoma sits between two divergent poles, NPDL patients represent an indolent recurring disease, NHL representing an aggressive disease requiring aggressive therapy.In a population of patients with nodular lymphomas, it is clear that there are various assignments to the various categories dependent upon the perceptions of the pathologist reading the biopsies. Thus in the original AFIP fascicle Rappaport [1] refers to approximately equal numbers of histiocytes and lymphocytes required to identify a patient as nodular mixed lymphoma. Other authors have tried to set rigid guidelines, assigning to this category those patients who have no less than 30% and no greater than 70% of the malignant appearing cells of a mixed category. In essence, however, pathology, like many fields of clinical

medicine, is a pattern-recognition phenomenon, and the judgment of pathologists will vary from case to case. Thus when one reviews the new working
formulation for lymphomas, it is clear that different pathologists assign cases
to different categories. In the current comprehensive review of the same case
materials [4], the British National Lymphoma Investigation Classification
characterized 356 patients as follicular lymphoma with 292 patients (82%)
having the predominantly small variant, and 62 patients (18%) as follicular
lymphoma, follicular cells mixed small and large. This system has no category
equivalent to nodular large cell or histiocytic lymphoma. In this system 82% of
the 356 patients thought to have a follicular (nodular) lymphoma would be
thought to be at the most indolent end of the spectrum of nodular lymphomas.
In the Dorfman classification [4] 351 of the cases were felt to be follicular
(nodular); 230 patients (65.5%) had follicular small lymphoid lymphoma, 74
patients (21.1%) were felt to have a follicular mixed small and large lymphoid
lymphoma comparable to the Rappaport nodular (follicular) mixed lymphoma category and 47 patients (13.3%) had follicular large lymphoid lymphomas. Concurrently, using the Rappaport system [4], only 329 patients were
considered to have a nodular (follicular) lymphoma; 216 patients (65.7%) had
NPDL, 93 patients (28.3%) were felt to have nodular (follicular) mixed
lymphoma, and only 20 patients (6.1%) had nodular histiocytic lymphomas. In
comparing the Dorfman and Rappaport classifications in this review, both
systems characterized roughly equal numbers of nodular (follicular) lymphoma patients, and almost equal numbers or proportions of nodular (follicular) small lymphoid lymphoma patients. The difference was between the
proportions of nodular (follicular) mixed and nodular (follicular) large lymphoid lymphomas with Dorfman classifying twice as many patients as follicular
large lymphoid lymphoma (13.4% *vs.* 6.1%) and correspondingly fewer patients comparable to the NML category of Rappaport (21.1% *vs.* 28.3%).
Thus, depending upon which pathologist is classifying one's patient material,
the category of nodular mixed lymphoma may contain a variable proportion of
patients with the more aggressive end of the nodular (follicular) lymphoma
spectrum, and probably a smaller but finite proportion of patients with the
more indolent end of the spectrum of disease.

The result of the working formulation pathology review highlights the
diversity and complexity of histopathological classification systems [4, 6]. It is
doubtful that new morphological systems will significantly advance the insights
taught us by these insightful pathologists, but that further classification of
lymphomas will have to be achieved on the basis of functional marker studies
which assess the immunological degree of development of the lymphocytes
involved in the particular malignant process, and/or kinetic analyses to define
the aggressiveness of the tumor. Many institutions are currently pursuing
functional marker studies, but it will be some time until it is clear whether or

not such currently available technology can add significantly to the prognostic characteristics of the current morphologically based systems.

3. Justification for non-aggressive therapy for nodular mixed lymphoma

The argument against using aggressive induction therapy for nodular mixed lymphomas rests upon basically two issues. The first is that durable complete remissions cannot be achieved, the second that the therapeutic index of the treatment utilized does not justify aggressive treatment for patients with indolent lymphomas. The first point is a complex one because of the implications of the pathology classification systems discussed above. Depending upon the pathology classification applied, the nodular mixed lymphoma category will include a variable spectrum of relatively indolent, moderately aggressive, and aggressive lymphomas. Thus, even with comparable therapy between institutions, variable response rates and durations of response may well be observed. As noted, as early as 1972 the Stanford group, with Dorfman directing their lymphoma pathology group, discovered that there appeared to be a difference in the response rate and response durations of patients with nodular mixed lymphoma *versus* the other nodular or follicular categories when comparable chemotherapy was utilized [3]. However, with this therapy, which was relatively nonaggressive, the survival curves for the nodular mixed lymphomas appeared to be inferior to the nodular poorly differentiated lymphocytic lymphomas, at least with a moderate followup time. What was not answered in this study was whether beyond five years a subgroup of patients with nodular mixed lymphoma might have a more durable response than those with nodular poorly differentiated lymphocytic lymphoma. The early 70's characterized the development of an ongoing debate in the literature regarding whether the indolent lymphomas benefited more from aggressive than nonaggressive therapy. Analysis of such data has led to the question regarding the nodular mixed lymphoma subcategory. In 1977, a review of the NCI series by Anderson *et al.* [7] reported the observation that with combination chemotherapy, together with careful restaging of patients before defining complete remissions and discontinuation of therapy, 77% of patients with advanced nodular mixed lymphoma had achieved a complete remission and that only 4 patients had relapsed, none beyond three years after discontinuation of therapy. These results were achieved with an acceptable morbidity rate from standard combination chemotherapy regimens derived from the experience in treating Hodking's disease. Conversely, a series of reports from the Stanford group indicated that patients with 'indolent' lymphomas did not appear to benefit significantly from more aggressive combination chemotherapy plus or minus total lymphoid irradiation (TLI) or whole body irradiation (WBI) radiotherapy programs when compared to what was designed to be a palliative single alkylating agent regimen [9–13]. These reports were unable to verify a prolonged disease free survival in any histological category of the 'indolent lymphomas', including the nodular mixed lymphoma subgroup. However, in the original prospective randomized study only 8 patients with nodular mixed lymphoma were treated, one in the CVP group, 4 in the CVP/TLI group, and 3 in the single alkylating agent group [9, 10]. Obviously the numbers are too small to make a meaningful comparison. In the subsequent prospective randomized trial from Stanford, the program was altered to compare CVP *versus* whole body irradiation *versus* single alkylating therapy [13]. The nodular mixed lymphoma group of patients include 4, 3, and 4, respectively. Numbers are again too small to make comparison; as pointed out by the authors themselves, there is statistically only a 50% chance that the currently reported study would pick up a true difference as great as 2.5-fold between the treatment arms.

The second important observation to come from the Stanford group has been the report regarding the ultraconservative approach to management of indolent lymphomas [10]. Noting the apparent lack of durable remissions and significant toxicity from the original CVP/TLI arm of the prospective randomized study, the Stanford group began a more careful evaluation of management of the indolent lymphomas in which no initial therapy was utilized; using the chronic lymphocytic leukemia analogy, it was felt that patients could be managed conservatively and treated only when their disease clinically progressed. These results were then evaluated, compared to patients entering the two sequential prospective randomized trials alluded to above. Of the 44 patients with deferred initial therapy, 8 had nodular mixed lymphoma. When initially reported in 1979, several striking observations were made [10]. For the entire group of indolent lymphoma patients the median time to requiring therapy was approximately 3 years. For diffuse well differentiated lymphocytic lymphoma the median time to requiring therapy had not yet been reached [10]. For nodular poorly differentiated lymphocytic lymphoma, therapy was required on the average within three years [10]. The nodular mixed lymphoma group seemed to have a more aggressive disease, with the median time to therapy approximately 10 months [10]. All NML patients required therapy within approximately five years; this difference in time to treatment was statistically significant, $p < 0.02$. There have been no statistically significant differences in actuarial survival; however, at 5 years the survival for the nodular mixed lymphoma group is only 43% as opposed to 80% for the NPDL group, $p > 0.09$, and 4 of the 8 nodular mixed lymphoma patients have expired [10]. Of the 25 patients in this study subsequently treated after initial observation, 13 were treated with single alkylating agent chemotherapy, with combined chemotherapy, 4 with local field radiotherapy and 2 with whole body irradiation. The report does not detail therapy given by histological subtype.

Bitran *et al.* also reported their inability to document prolonged disease free survival in this group of patients when treated with COPP *vs.* palliative regimens; again, however, only 12 patients in the entire series had NML and it is not clear what proportion of NML patients received aggressive therapy [19].

The second point to argue for conservative therapy for the nodular mixed lymphoma group is that the toxicity of combination chemotherapy or combined modality treatments has been excessive. This appeared to be a significant consideration in the original prospective randomized trials from Stanford utilizing CVP plus total lymphoid irradiation. In addition to a comparable incidence of bacterial and herpetic infections, the CVP-TLI arm of this study included a 20% incidence of persistent cytopenias whereas none were observed in the other treatment arms [9]. In the NCI study looking at 199 consecutive patients with all subtypes of malignant lymphoma treated with combination chemotherapy the induction chemotherapy mortality was approximately 4% [7]. Two of these deaths were within the first few weeks of initiation of the therapy in patients with poor performance status and far advanced disease. If the toxicity data is analyzed utilizing the technique of many current studies, the morbidity and mortality rates would be significantly lower. In the NCI study the incidence of morbidity requiring hospitalizations including bacterial infection, herpetic infections, thrombocytopenic hemorrhages and hemorrhagic cystitis, was approximately 11%.

In the followup prospective randomized trials from Stanford utilizing CVP versus whole body irradiation versus single alkylating agent chemotherapy, the combination chemotherapy arm appeared to have a higher incidence of hospitalization for infection and fever, and a higher incidence of cystitis [12]. Persistent cytopenias are seen predominantly in the whole body irradiation arm, a fragment program designed to be palliative [12].

One of the important considerations in terms of assessing complications of therapy has been the question regarding the long term development of second malignancies induced by the therapy for the initial disease process. Long term followup from a variety of Hodgkin's disease studies has demonstrated an increased incidence of second malignancies, particularly acute nonlymphocytic leukemia in patients receiving chemotherapy and/or radiotherapy. Because of the similar treatment approaches in the malignant lymphomas, such questions obviously are relevant. To date there has not been a clearly defined increased risk in such patients. In the NCI study of Anderson *et al.*, 4/199 patients were identified as having a second neoplasm [7]; 2 of the 4 were expected (carcinoma of the lung in a patient with a history of cigarette smoking, development of a leiomyosarcoma at the site of a previously resected leiomyoma). One patient who had received single alkylating agent therapy for

8 years for a nodular lymphoma was treated with induction combination chemotherapy at the time of conversion of her lymphoma to a diffuse large cell type. One month after completing six cycles of BACOP combination chemotherapy, the patient developed acute nonlymphocytic leukemia and died one month later. A fourth patient in complete remission after six cycles of C-MOPP chemotherapy developed a fatal duodenal carcinoma [7]. In the most recent prospective randomized trials from Stanford, one of 17 patients treated in the single alkylating agent arm of the study has developed acute nonlymphocytic leukemia [12].

The data regarding the leukemogenic risk of chronic alkylating agent therapy has become significant. Lerner reported that 3 of 13 patients with carcinoma of the breast treated with chronic chlorambucil developed acute nonlymphoytic leukemia [15]. A recent report from Scandinavia reports that 6 of 51 patients treated with phenylalanine mustard for ovarian carcinoma have similarly developed acute nonlymphocytic leukemia [16]. The prospective randomized trial of the P, vera study group appears to have identified that chronic alkylating agent chemotherapy while symptomatically nontoxic, and relatively effective, appears to carry an increased risk of induction of leukemia in this patient population who may or may not have an identified predisposition to leukemic conversion of their underlying myeloproliferative disease [17]. Finally, the update from Greene et al. of the NCI study looking at palliative radiotherapy suggests that patients receiving repeated doses of radiotherapy including involved field and whole body irradiation appear to have an increased risk of acute nonlymphocytic leukemia [18]. Thus treatment regimens which are acutely relatively nontoxic may carry a significant risk to survival in patients who otherwise may have a prolonged survival due to effective therapy and/or the natural history of their disease.

4. Evidence that nodular mixed lymphoma has a different biological course than nodular poorly differentiated lymphocytic lymphoma

As early as 1972, using nonaggressive single akylating agent chemotherapy programs, Jones et al. reported initial data from Stanford suggesting that nodular mixed lymphoma patients had a different clinical course than nodular poorly differentiated lymphocytic lymphoma patients [3]. In this instance they had a slightly lower complete remission rate and decreased survival; their survival curve in fact was intermediate between the NPDL and NHL patients reported. It is important to note that these patients were not treated as aggressively with single agent therapy as was utilized in the subsequent prospective randomized trials discussed above. Anderson et al. reviewed the NCI results utilizing combination chemotherapy in 1976 [7]. As part of an ongoing series of trials in malignant lymphomas, 199 consecutive patients were treated with combination chemotherapy. As reported, all patients underwent extensive staging procedures utilized during the period involved with these studies, and with rare exception all patients who achieved a complete clinical remission had documentation of that remission by extensive restaging procedures utilizing repeat bone marrow aspirates and biopsies, repeat percutaneous liver biopsies, repeat peritoneoscopy with multiple liver biopsies, etc. These procedures were utilized to augment clinical restaging techniques such as repeat lymphangiograms, etc. During the early portion of this study, patients were classified as having lymphosarcoma or reticulum cell sarcoma. Based upon this histological classification system, patients with the diagnosis of lymphosarcoma were treated with cyclophosphamide, vincristine, prednisone with the dose schedule previously reported. Patients with the diagnosis of reticulum cell sarcoma were treated with the C-MOPP regimen derived from the MOPP program utilized in Hodgkin's disease, details of which ave also been reported. With the integration of the Rappaport histological classification system, the entity of nodular mixed lymphoma was identified. It was decided that such patients would be treated based upon the worst prognostic element of their biopsy, namely the large cell lymphocyte ('histiocyte'), and thus the predominance of patients were treated with the original C-MOPP regimen; a few patients were treated with the BACOP regimen subsequently utilized for the diffuse large cell lymphoma patients.

In the report by Anderson *et al.*, 24/31 patients (77%) achieved a complete remission documented by restaging prodedures [7]. Four of these 24 patients subsequently relapsed, 2–39 months after discontinuation of therapy. At the time of this report, the median duration of remission had not been reached with 79% of patients still in complete remission with followup as long as 90 months or longer; the median survival of the entire group of patients had not been reached, with 69% of all patients still alive with followup up to 101 months or longer. This was in contrast to concurrently treated NPDL patients who had a 67% complete remission rate, but a median duration of remission of only 16 months or more; median survival of the entire group of NPDL patients was 83 months, and of the complete responder patients 95 months.

Subsequent studies from other institutions tend to confirm that the nodular mixed lymphoma patients treated at other institutions have a different disease course than comparably treated NPDL patients. Cabanillas, Rodriguez, and Bodey reported on the results of combination chemotherapy in patients with nodular mixed lymphomas [19]. Complete remission rates in these patients were 55% utilizing the CVP regimen, and 67% in the subsequent patients treated with a variety of adriamycin containing regimens. All patients received induction chemotherapy with one year of maintenance therapy. In their study, late relapses were seen in patients classified as NPDL, but not in nodular mixed or nodular histiocytic lymphoma patients. Longo *et al.* updated the NCI series in 1981 [20], noting that the median duration of complete remission for advanced stage nodular mixed lymphoma patients treated with combination chemotherapy had still not been reached with average followup of over 6 years. Sixty-three percent of all patients were still in complete remission. Several late relapsers were identified, but the remission duration curve remains strikingly different from the analogous curves for concurrently treated patients with NPDL. In this series patients treated with C-MOPP appeared to do significantly better than those patients treated with CVP. Of importance in this followup study was the observation of several late relapses, but there clearly has not been a significant continued relapse rate analogous to the NPDL patients. Of equal importance is the observation that with the change in the pathologists responsible for analyzing the data, some patients were reclassified [20]; some patients previously classified as nodular mixed lymphoma were excluded on rereview, and some patients previously classified as NPDL were now included in the nodular mixed lymphoma category. It is not clear whether the several isolated late relapses were always considered nodular mixed lymphoma by both the original and subsequent pathologists, or whether they are reclassified as nodular mixed lymphoma only by the new pathologist. Lister *et al.* [21] reported in 1978 that patients with nodular mixed lymphoma had a statistically significant different relapse-free survival curve than patients with NPDL. In this study 65% of nodular mixed lymphoma patients had a durable remission after induction with CVP or chlorambucil treatment compared to about 20% of NPDL patients. Ezdinli *et al.* summarized four different ECOG prospective trials in 1980; 80 patients with NML were treated on four different combination chemotherapy regimens [22]. This study verified the relative indolent nature of 249 comparably treated NPDL patients regardless of their treatment; it also verified that nodular mixed lymphoma patients had an inherently more aggressive disease, but that durable complete remissions could be achieved which had a significant impact on the survival of the patient population. Bishop *et al.* and Morovic *et al.* also reported data suggesting a prolonged disease free survival [23, 24]. Herrman *et al.* in 1982 have reported their results of a large series of patients treated at Roswell Park Memorial Institute [25]. These patients were classified using a modification of the Lukes–Collins system; in the classic Lukes–Collins system there is no subgroup combining both small and large cleaved or noncleaved cells. The report by Herrmann *et al.* modifies the Lukes–Collins system such that there are only two major categories of follicular (nodular) lymphoma, one designated cleaved follicular, small and large, the other designated mixed (cleaved and noncleaved) follicular. It is probable that the nodular mixed lymphoma patients of Rappaport would have been predominantly categorized in the latter category, but probably not exclusively. The complete remission rate for these two subgroups of patients were reported at 76 and 79%, and duration of remissions reported at 34 and 41 months, respectively. Finally, Glick *et al.* compared the survival curves of patients with nodular histiocytic lymphomas treated on recent ECOG protocols and noted that the nodular mixed lymphoma and nodular histiocytic lymphoma patients had comparable survival patterns which were different from NPDL patients followed for approximately 3–5 years [26].

In summary, it appears that in most series reported, patients which fit into the category of nodular mixed lymphoma appear to have a good complete remission rate when treated with aggressive chemotherapy and have a prolonged disease free survival compared to patients with nodular poorly differentiated lymphocytic lymphoma treated with comparable regimens. While occasional relapses have occurred, the disease free survival curves are clearly different from NPDL data from the same institutions. The major exceptions are the Stanford and Chicago experiences, but it must be pointed out that only small numbers of patients with this histology have been treated in any one treatment arm, and the Stanford data suggests that these patients have a biologically different disease in that when they are approached conservatively they require therapy significantly sooner than other 'indolent' lymphomas. It is clear that this group of patients appears to have an intermediate prognosis and can only be considered indolent because of it's striking response to chemotherapy rather than the inherently nonaggressive nature of the disease itself.

Finally, the major difficulty in analyzing the data on efficacy of treatment of nodular mixed lymphomas refers to the lack of consensus in histopathological classification. Again, the data from Stanford suggests that their pathology department has a lower proportion of patients classified as nodular mixed lymphoma (in the Dorfman system technically classified as follicular mixed, small and large lymphoid with and without sclerosis), and a relatively higher proportion of patients classified as nodular histiocytic lymphoma (in the Dorfman system follicular large lymphoid) [4]. Thus it is not clear but what many of the patients who would be classified as nodular mixed lymphoma by other pathologists may be included in the more unfavorable nodular histiocytic lymphoma group at Stanford. This latter group is recognized by all investigative institutions as a nonindolent aggressive disease requiring aggressive therapy designed to induce complete remissions.

With the acceptability of the morbidity and mortality of standard combination chemotherapy for malignant lymphomas, the potential long term complications of apparently nonaggressive nontoxic prolonged exposure to alkylating agents, and the difficulty in consistently identifying patients as having an indolent lymphoma, it is recommended that unless medical contraindications dictate otherwise that advanced stage patients with nodular mixed lym-

237

phomas be treated with aggressive chemotherapy designed to induce complete remission and ultimate prolonged disease free survival.

References

1. Rappaport H: Tumors of the hematopoietic system. *In* Atlas of tumor pathology, Section 3, Fascicle 8. Washington D.C., US Armed Forces Institute of Pathology, 1966.
2. Jones SE, Fuks Z, Bull M, *et al.*: Non-Hodgkin's lymphomas. IV. Clinicopathological correlation in 405 cases. Cancer 31:806–823, 1973.
3. Jones SE, Rosenberg SA, Kaplan HS, Cadin ME, Dorfman RF: Non-Hodgkin's lymphomas. II. Single agent chemotherapy. Cancer 30:31–38, 1972.
4. The Non-Hodgkin's lymphoma pathology classification project. National Cancer Institute sponsored study of classifications of non-Hodgkin's lymphomas. Summary and description of a working formulation for clinical usage. Cancer 49:2112–2135, 1982.
5. Stein RS, Cousar J, Flexner JN, Collins RD: Correlations between immunologic markers and histologic classifications; clinical implications. Semin Oncol 7:244–254, 1980.
6. Garvin AJ, Simon R, Young RC, DeVita VT, Berard CW: The Rappaport classification of non-Hodgkin's lymphoma: A closer look using proposed classifications. Semin Oncol 7:234–243, 1980.
7. Anderson T, Bender RA, Fisher RI, DeVita VT, Chabner BA, Berard CW, Norton L, Young RC: Combination chemotherapy in non-Hodgkin's lymphoma; results of long term followup. Cancer Treat Rep 61:1057–1066, 1977.
8. Byrne GE: Rappaport classification of non-Hodgkin's lymphoma: histologic features and clinical significance. Cancer Treat Rep 61:935–944, 1977.
9. Portlock CS, Rosenberg SA, Glatstein E, Kaplan HS: Treatment of advanced non-Hodgkin's lymphomas with favorable histologies; Preliminary results of a prospective trial. Blood 47:747–756, 1976.
10. Portlock CS, Rosenberg SA: No initial therapy for stage III and IV non-Hodgkin's lymphomas of favorable histologic types. Ann Int Med 90:10–12, 1979.
11. Portlock CS: Management of indolent non-Hodgkin's lymphomas. Semin Oncol 7:292–301, 1980.
12. Hoppe RT, Kushlan P, Kaplan HS, Rosenberg SA, Brown BW: The treatment of advanced stage favorable histology non-Hodgkin's lymphoma; A preliminary report of a randomized trial comparing single agent chemotherapy, combination chemotherapy and whole body irradiation. Blood 58:592–598, 1981.
13. Portlock CS: Deferral of initial therapy for advanced indolent lymphomas. Cancer Treat Rep 66:417–419, 1982.
14. Bitran JD, Golomb HM, Ultmann JE, Sweet DL *et al.*: Non-Hodgkin's lymphoma, poorly differentiated lymphocytic and mixed cell types. Cancer 42:88–95, 1978.
15. Lerner H: Second malignancies diagnosed in breast cancer patients receiving adjuvant chemotherapy at the Pennsylvania Hospital. Proc Am Soc Clin Onc 18:340, 1977.
16. Einhorn N, Eklund G, Franzer S, *et al.*: Late side effects of chemotherapy in ovarian carcinoma. Cancer 49:2234–2241, 1982.
17. Berk PD, Goldberg JD, Silverstein MN, *et al.*: Increased incidence of acute leukemia in polycythemia vera associated with chlorambucil therapy. New Eng J Med 304:441–447, 1981.
18. Greene MH, Young RC, Glatstein EJ, Simon RN, Merril JN, DeVita VT: Acute non-lymphocytic leukemia (ANL) following treatment of non-Hodgkin's lymphoma (NHL). Proc Am Assn Clin Oncol 22:515, 1981.

238

19. Cabanillas F, Rodriguez V, Bodey GP: The impact of intensive chemotherapy on the duration of remission and survival of patients (PTS) with nodular malignant lymphoma (HML). Proc Am Soc Clin Oncol 19:310, 1978.
20. Longo D, Hubbard S, Wesley M, Jaffe E, Chabner B, DeVita VT, Young RC: Prolonged initial remissions in patients with nodular mixed lymphoma. Proc Am Soc Clin Oncol 22:521, 1981.
21. Lister TA, Cullen MH, Beard MEJ, Brearly RL, Whitehouse JMA, Wrigley PFN, Stansfeld AG, Sutcliffe SBJ, Malpas JS, Crowther D: Comparison of combined and single agent chemotherapy in non-Hodgkin's lymphoma of favorable histologic type. Br Med J 1:533–537, 1978.
22. Ezdinli EZ, Costello WG, Icli F, Lenhard RE, Johnson GJ, Silverstein M, Berard CW, Bennett JM, Carbone PP: Nodular mixed lumphocytic–histiocytic lymphoma. Response and survival. Cancer 45:261–267, 1980.
23. Bishop JF, Wiernik PH, Kaplan RS, Wesley M, Diggs CH, Sutherland JC, Markus SD: High dose cyclophosphamide, vincristine, and prednisone plus or minus adriamycin (CAVP vs. CVP) in advanced poorly differentiated lymphocytic and lymphocytic–histiocytic non-Hidgkin's lymphoma (NHL); A randomized trial. Proc Am Soc Clin Oncol 22:518, 1981.
24. Morovic D, Armitage J, Foucar K, Dick F, Burnas CP: Nodular mixed lymphoma – A curable disease? Proc Am Soc Clin Oncol 1:164, 1982.
25. Herrmann R, Barcos M, Stutzman L, Walsh D, Freeman A, Skokal J, Henderson ES: The influence of histologic type on the incidence and duration of response in non-Hodgkin's lymphoma. Cancer 49:314–322, 1982.
26. Glick JM, McFadden E, Costello W, Ezdiuli E, et al.: Nodular histiocytic lymphoma. Factors influencing prognosis and implications for aggressive chemotherapy. Cancer 49:840–845, 1982.

11. Nodular mixed lymphoma: Failure to demonstrate prolonged disease free survival and cure

JOHN H. GLICK and ERICA L. ORLOW

1. Introduction

The natural history of nodular mixed lymphocytic–histiocytic (NM) lymphoma is not well defined because of its relative rarity and lack of precise histopathologic definition. Using the Rappaport classification, approximately 10–20% of all non-Hodgkin's lymphomas will be classified as having nodular mixed histology [1–3]. Historically, nodular mixed lymphoma has been classified as a favorable pathologic subtype with the other nodular lymphomas. In a retrospective review of previously untreated patients with non-Hodgkin's lymphoma referred to Stanford University between 1960 and 1971, Jones *et al.* [1] observed that the actuarial survival of NM patients was similar to that of nodular lymphocytic poorly differentiated lymphoma (NLPD). Median survival for both histologic subtypes was 7 years and a pattern of continuous late relapse was noted. More recently, the non-Hodgkin's Lymphoma Pathologic Classification Project reported that 8% of the 1153 patients could be classified as having NM histology which was re-named follicular mixed lymphoma [4]. This histologic subtype was placed in the low-grade category of the Working Formulation on the basis of a 5.1 year median survival.

Controversy also exists as to whether combination chemotherapy can produce prolonged disease-free survival equivalent to cure for the NM subtype. Rosenberg [5] has perceptively observed that controversy in this field is complicated by the following factors: (1) lack of precise histopathologic definition, leading to problems with reproducibility of data; (2) precision of initial staging, and more importantly, the variability in restaging procedures to determine remission status of patients in complete response; (3) over-emphasis on disease-free survival, whereas overall survival with adequate followup is of major importance; (4) lack of prospectively controlled clinical trials; (5) failure to accurately weigh the toxicity of aggressive chemotherapy regimens. This chapter will review the importance of the above factors in attempting to answer the question: Are patients with advanced stages of nodular mixed lymphoma curable with aggressive combination chemotherapy?

Bennett JM (ed), Controversies in the Management of Lymphomas. ISBN 0-89838-586-5.
© *Martinus Nijhoff Publishers, Boston. Printed in the Netherlands.*

2. The histopathologic maze

Rappaport [6] initially defined nodular mixed lymphoma as composed of intermixtures of atypical histiocytes and poorly differentiated lymphocytes. This definition was widely adopted during the 1960's and 1970's by both the cooperative groups and by larger single institutions with expertise in malignant lymphomas. However, two cooperative groups soon reported a lack of concordance in 40% of NM cases when the institutional diagnosis was compared to the diagnosis rendered by a panel of referee hematopathologists [7, 8]. To their credit, the cooperative groups promptly began reporting the results of their clinical trials in non-Hodgkin's lymphomas based on the referee pathologic review by the Panel for Lymphoma Clinical Trials.

Recently, Berard reported his precise criteria for the histopathologic diagnosis of nodular mixed lymphoma [9]. These criteria were used consistently by him over the past 15 years both at the National Cancer Institute and as the regional referee pathologist for the Eastern Cooperative Oncology Group (ECOG) cases submitted to the Panel for Lymphoma Clinical Trials. Dr. Berard's criteria are described in detail below to emphasize the importance of expert pathologic review in interpreting data from retrospective or prospective clinical trials.

Cases in which any portion of the histologic material had an unequivocally nodular (follicular) pattern were included. They were designated as nodular when such a pattern was present in at least 75% of the surface area of the sections of lymphoma (uninvolved areas were excluded from consideration). Cases were designated as nodular and diffuse when (1) a focus of definitive nodularity, however small, was present in an otherwise diffuse lymphoma, or (2) more than 25% of the malignant proliferation was diffuse in a lymphoma with a definite nodular pattern elsewhere. The cytologic designation of mixed lymphocytic-histiocytic type was based on the numerical frequency of large malignant cells in areas of neoplastic cellular composition (either neoplastic nodules or areas of diffuse infiltration by malignant cells). To qualify as mixed lymphocytic–histiocytic type, a case had to contain an average of 5–15 large neoplastic cells per high power field (10X oculars, 40X objective lens) in a majority of microscopic fields. At least 20 such fields were evaluated in each case. The large cells had to be easily discernible (without prolonged searching and fine focusing) and usually had oval to round vesicular nuclei with 2–3 prominent nucleoli, often apposed to the nuclear membrane (neoplastic 'histiocytes' of the Rappaport classification). Cases with an average of fewer than 5 large neoplastic cells per high power field were designated as nodular lymphocytic poorly differentiated. Cases with an average of more than 15 large neoplastic cells per high power field were designated as nodular histiocytic. In all types of nodular (follicular) lymphoma, the small neoplastic cells had compact chromatin, inconspicuous nucleoli, and irregularly indented or clefted nuclei (neoplastic lymphocytes of the Rappaport classification) [9]. These criteria are highly reproducible, yielding an excellent concordance rate with other members of the Pathology Panel for Lymphoma Clinical Trials [10].

More recently, the National Cancer Institute sponsored a study of six major classifications of non-Hodgkin's lymphoma [4]. This retrospective review included 1175 cases from four institutions, three in the United States and one in Italy. The reproducibility and clinical relevance of the six classifications were tested by six 'expert' pathologists, each a proponent of a major classification, and by six very experienced pathologists not identified with one of the major classifications. Immunologic methods were not employed in the study design. Among the 1153 evaluable patients, the maximum followup was 9.2 years, with a mean of 5.4 years for patients who were alive at the time of the analysis, and a mean of 3.3 years for the total group, including dead patients.

In each of the six classifications within the same cytologic subtype, those patients with follicular or nodular patterns had a more favorable survival than those with diffuse patterns. Multivariate analysis in 554 patients with follicular center cell (nodular) lymphomas demonstrated a significantly improved survival predicted by the follicular pattern as an independent variable from cell type ($p < 0.00001$). However, the cell type (large cleaved versus small cleaved, large non-cleaved versus small cleaved, small non-cleaved versus small cleaved) was also of significant importance ($p < 0.0001$) (4).

As a result of this project, the investigators involved developed A Working Formulation of Non-Hodgkin's Lymphoma for Clinical Usage [4]. The nodular mixed lymphocytic-histiocytic subtype of Rappaport was re-named malignant lymphoma, follicular, mixed small cleaved and large cell type. This mixed cell category encompassed those cases of follicular lymphoma in which there was no clear preponderance of one cell type (small or large) over the other. The large cells which may have cleaved or non-cleaved nuclei were frequently two to three times the diameter of normal lymphocytes and have vesicular nuclei. In the non-cleaved type, one to three nucleoli are often apposed to the nuclear membrane. Related terms in the Kiel classification corresponded to the centroblastic-centrocytic (small) follicular; and in the Lukes-Collins classification to the small-cleaved FCC, follicular and also to the large-cleaved FCC, follicular.

In the Working Formulation, the follicular mixed cell type was diagnosed in 89 cases or 7.7% of the total. Median age was 56 years, and 28% of the patients were stage III while 46% were stage IV. Median survival of all cases was 5.1 years. A complete response rate of 65% was reported in this subtype, with a median time to relapse of 5.2 years. A pattern of continuous late relapse was noted on the disease-free survival curves, although the numbers at risk beyond

5 years are small. Because of the relatively long median survival, the follicular mixed subtype was placed in the 'low-grade' category. However, it should be noted that the median survival of the follicular mixed cell patients (5.1 years) was less than the 7.2 year median survival for the follicular, small cleaved cell type (corresponding to NLPD) reported by the same investigators [4].

It must be remembered that the Working Formulation of Non-Hodgkin's Lymphomas is based on a retrospective review and has not been evaluated in prospective clinical trials. Thus, it will be some years before the clinical significance of this classification is confirmed by ongoing randomized trials. In addition, recent advances in the immunologic classification of the non-Hodgkin's lymphomas may be of critical importance in our functional classification of patients with histologically favorable patterns.

In this paper for the purpose of discussing different chemotherapy trials in advanced nodular mixed lymphoma, the Rappaport system and nomenclature are utilized based on the commonly accepted clinical practice in the late 1960's and 1970's. Comparison between the National Cancer Institute and Eastern Cooperative Oncology Group nodular mixed patients is facilitated by the fact that the same hematopathologist (Costan W. Berard) reviewed the pathologic material at the NCI and for ECOG during this time period.

3. Chemotherapy trials for advanced stages of nodular mixed lymphoma

3.1. The National Cancer Institute experience

Anderson et al. [11], reporting for the NCI, first suggested that patients with disseminated NM were potentially curable. This conclusion was initially based on a series of 31 previously untreated NM patients with stage III or IV disease treated with combination chemotherapy. Twenty-four of these patients received the C-MOPP regimen. This consists of substituting cyclophosphamide for nitrogen mustard in the MOPP combination. The other seven patients were treated with CVP or BACOP, because initially their biopsies were reported as another histologic subtype but were eventually reclassified as NM. A complete response (CR) was achieved in 77% of these 31 patients, and more specifically, 71% of the C-MOPP treated patients obtained CR. Only one patient in this series received maintenance chemotherapy after achieving a complete remission. Since only 4/31 patients had relapsed at the time of their report in 1977, the median duration of remission had not been reached. Seventy-nine percent of patients were still in their original CR at that time, but only 10 patients were at risk beyond 2.5 years. No late relapses were reported with short followup. On the basis of this preliminary publication, the nodular mixed subtype was widely held to be a potentially curable malignancy. However, the apparent plateau in the relapse-free survival curve should have been regarded with caution because of the limited followup at the time of the initial publication.

A recent update of the NCI data has been presented by Longo *et al.* [12] with a median followup of five years. After re-classification of the NCI histologic material utilizing the same pathologic criteria described above by Berard, followup data were available on only 22 patients with nodular mixed lymphoma treated with C-MOPP. Of the 17 patients who achieved a complete response with C-MOPP, 7 had now relapsed. Although the disease-free survival of this subgroup was 59%, one patient relapsed at seven years. Since occult or minimal disease may be well tolerated and slowly growing in these patients, the possibility exists that further relapses may occur with additional followup. Longo *et al.* observed that the median duration of complete response was longer with four-drug therapy than with the three-drug cyclophosphamide–vincristine–prednisone (CVP) regimen.

A more recent publication by Anderson *et al.* [13] retrospectively reviewed the treatment results in 473 consecutively staged and treated non-Hodgkin's patients at the NCI over a 22-year period from 1953 to 1975. Seventy-six patients with NM lymphoma were reported, representing 16% of all patients with non-Hodgkin's lymphoma. Thirty-nine percent of their patients were stage III and 38% stage IV. Patients with stage III and IV disease were treated with chemotherapy, and after 1968, these patients received combination chemotherapy (either C-MOPP, CVP, or BACOP). It is interesting to note that the actuarial survival curves comparing NM treated prior to January, 1968 with patients treated since then show no substantial or significant improvement in survival between the two admission periods ($p = 0.39$). Moreover, the actuarial survival curves for the 57 patients treated after January, 1968 show a pattern of continuous failure and death with no plateau being demonstrated.

An additional observation of potential importance is their comparison of the survival data for patients with different histologic types of nodular lymphoma. Anderson *et al.* [13] reported that of 88 patients with NLPD, 40 have died with an observed median survival of 78 months, compared to a 55 month median survival for NM patients ($p<0.03$, two-sided generalized Wilcoxon test). This suggests that patients with the NM subtype may not belong in the same favorable or low-grade prognostic category as patients with NLPD.

3.2. The Eastern Cooperative Oncology Group experience

Ezdinli *et al.* [14] retrospectively reviewed 80 patients with nodular mixed lymphoma whose pathology was confirmed by the Panel for Lymphoma

Clinical Trials, and who were entered onto four different ECOG protocols over a six-year period. All patients had stage III and IV disease, and most were previously untreated with chemotherapy. This retrospective study defined complete remission primarily on clinical grounds since pathologic restaging was not mandatory. Ezdinli *et al.* compared these 80 patients with NM to 249 patients with NLPD who were treated on the same protocols. Ninety percent of the previously untreated NLPD patients, but only 59% of the comparable group of NM survived two years (p<0.001). Patients with NM in whom the pattern was reported as both nodular and diffuse had a significantly shorter two-year survival than did patients with a pure nodular pattern. In addition, patients with NM who achieved a complete response survived significantly longer than did partial responders, suggesting a role for a more aggressive therapeutic strategy with the goal of improving CR rates.

In 1974 ECOG initiated a prospective controlled trial in which patients with stage III and IV nodular mixed lymphoma were randomized to either COPP (similar to the NCI C-MOPP regimen), BCNU + CVP (BCVP), or to moderate chemotherapy with cyclophosphamide-prednisone (CP). The schema of this protocol EST 2474 is illustrated in Figure 1. The details of the specific chemotherapy regimens are described in Table 1. The objective of this study was to confirm whether intensive chemotherapy with COPP or BCVP could achieve prolonged disease-free survival as had been reported with C-MOPP. The details of the study, diagnostic methods, staging designations, and preliminary results have been previously described [9]. Fifty-two patients with stage III or IV disease were entered. All patients classified as stage IV had histologic confirmation of extra-nodal disease or radiologic evidence of lung involvement. This study was based on central pathologic review by the Panel for Lymphoma Clinical Trials.

The standard ECOG response criteria have also been previously reported

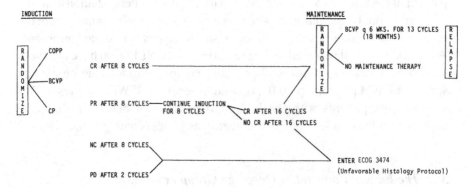

Figure 1. ECOG 2474 – treatment of stage III and IV nodular lymphomas. CR = complete response; PR = partial response; NC = no change; PD = progressive disease. For definitions of COPP, BCVP, and CP chemotherapy regimens, see Table 1.

Table 1. Chemotherapy regimens used in ECOG 2474.

COPP regimen
Cyclophosphamide 600 mg/m^2 IV days 1 and 8
Vincristine 1.2 mg/m^2 IV days 1 and 8 (max 2.0 mg)
Procarbazine 100 mg/m^2/day po × 14 days
Prednisone 100 mg/m^2/day po × 5 days
   Repeat cycles every 28 days
BCVP regimen
BCNU 60 mg/m^2 IV day 1
Cyclophosphamide 1000 mg/m^2 IV day 1
Vincristine 1.2 mg/m^2 IV day 1 (max 2.0 mg)
Prednisone 100 mg/m^2/day po × 5 days
   Repeat cycles every 21 days
CP Regimen
Cyclophosphamide 600 mg/m^2 IV days 1 and 8
Prednisone 100 mg/m^2/day po × 5 days
   Repeat cycles every 28 days

[9, 14]. The definition of a re-staged complete response required a repeat bone marrow and/or liver biopsy examination if these organs were involved prior to treatment (repeat lymphangiogram was not a protocol requirement). In those cases in which this re-biopsy information was not available, the designation of a clinical complete response (CCR) was used. Complete response (CR) denotes restaged complete responses plus CCR.

Survival was calculated from the date of randomization. Differences in discrete or frequency data were calculated using Fisher's exact test [15]. Tests for differences in time data, such as duration of remission and survival were made using the log-rank test [16]. Survival curves were drawn using life table methods [17], unless fewer than 16 failures occurred in any group, when the Kaplan-Meier method was used [18]. Medians were determined from the survival curves. All patients were followed for at least 4.0 years, with a median follow-up time of 4.5 years. Survivors currently have a median follow-up time of 6 years.

The patient characteristics for the 52 NM patients are described in Table 2. Specific attention is directed at the 18 patients treated with COPP. The median age for this group was 53 (range 20–68). Utilizing ECOG performance status, only 1 patient was partially bedridden at the time of entry on study; the remaining 17 COPP patients were ambulatory. Four patients had received prior local radiotherapy and then relapsed. The histologic pattern was nodular in 14, while 4 had both nodular and diffuse architecture.

Table 3 summarizes response as a function of the chemotherapy regimen. Of the 52 patients, 62% achieved a CR. Of the 32 achieving a CR, 28 were pathologically restaged. The differences in CR rates among the induction

Table 2. Patient characteristics.

		COPP (18)	BCVP (14)	CP (20)
Age	> 50	7	9	15
	< 50	11	5	5
Sex	Male	11	6	10
	Female	7	8	10
ECOG performance status				
	0	9	10	15
	1	8	3	4
	2–3	1	1	1
Prior radiotherapy		4	0	4
Stage	III	9	5	14
	IV	9	9	6
Symptoms	A	14	6	18
	B	4	8	2
Histologic pattern				
Nodular		14	12	14
Nodular and diffuse		4	2	6

Table 3. Response to treatment.

	COPP (18)	BCVP (14)	CP (20)
Complete response (CR)	11 (61%)	8 (57%)	13 (65%)
Restaged CR	9	7	12
Clinical CR	2	1	1
Partial response (PR)	6	5	6
No response	1	1	1
Grade 3–4 hematologic toxicity*	4 (22%)	6 (43%)	0

* Hematologic toxicity: Grade 3, severe (WBC 1000– < 2000; platelets 25 000– < 50 000); grade 4, life threatening (associated with major infection or bleeding).

regimens are not significant. Sixty-one percent of the COPP patients achieved CR, with 9/11 being pathologically restaged. Six partial responses on COPP were noted, and 1 additional patient had no response to this regimen.

The response duration for complete responders is seen in Fig. 2. Although COPP patients had a shorter median disease-free interval of 16.5 months, this difference is not significant when compared to BCVP and CP ($p = 0.30$). Of the 9 pathologically restaged complete responders on the COPP arm, 7 have relapsed; 1/2 clinical CR has also relapsed. Of the 3 complete responders continuing in remission, 2 have died with no evidence of recurrent disease (the duration of each of their responses has been censored at time of death). There is no difference in the response duration for COPP patients between

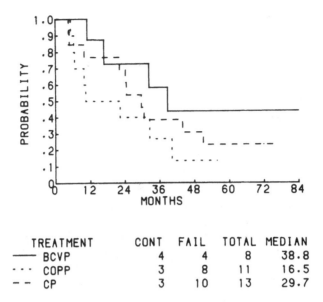

TREATMENT	CONT	FAIL	TOTAL	MEDIAN
—— BCVP	4	4	8	38.8
··· COPP	3	8	11	16.5
– – CP	3	10	13	29.7

Figure 2. Response duration for complete responders by type of induction chemotherapy.

CR + CCR compared to PR (p = 0.92), probably because of the small numbers involved.

Only complete responders were eligible for randomization to the maintenance phase (BCVP chemotherapy versus observation). Of the 32 complete responders on induction, 29 were eligible for maintenance (2 relapsed from CR and 1 died in CR prior to randomization). Of these 29 patients, 6 were not randomized (4 patient refusals, 1 physician refusal, and 1 improper direct assignment to observation). Of the 23 randomized, only 7 patients actually received BVCP maintenance, primarily because of physician or patient refusal to accept further chemotherapy once the induction phase was completed. Although there are no significant differences in either disease-free survival or overall survival by maintenance regimen at present, the numbers are extremely small and the results preliminary because of the relatively short followup. It should be noted that only one COPP complete responder actually received BCVP maintenance; the rest were observed after completing the induction phase.

Median survival for the entire group of 52 patients is 64 months, with 27/52 still alive. Fig. 3 compares survival by type of induction regimen for all patients entered on that arm. Median survival for the COPP patients is 46 months and for the CP patients 64 months, but there is no significant difference when compared to BCVP (p = 0.70). There is no significant difference in the survival of complete responders between the three regimens (p = 0.21).

The survival of the 18 NM patients treated with COPP was compared to the

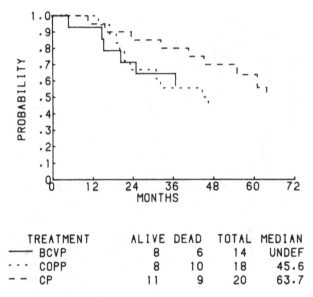

TREATMENT	ALIVE	DEAD	TOTAL	MEDIAN
—— BCVP	8	6	14	UNDEF
· · · COPP	8	10	18	45.6
— — CP	11	9	20	63.7

Figure 3. Overall survival by induction regimen.

survival of 46 patients with nodular lymphocytic poorly differentiated lymphoma (NLPD) also treated with COPP and entered on the same protocol. Fig. 4 illustrates that there is no significant difference to date in the survival for these two histologic subtypes when treated with COPP ($p = 0.39$). Although this difference is not statistically significant, NLPD patients had a median survival of 78 months compared to 46 months for the NM patients treated with COPP.

The best tolerated regimen was CP with no patients experiencing Grade 3 or 4 hematologic toxicity as defined in Table 3. This is less than the 22% Grade 3–4 hematologic toxicity observed with COPP and significantly less than the 43% with BCVP ($p<0.006$). Two cases of Grade 4 hematology toxicity were noted, one on COPP, and one on BCVP. The COPP patient had gram-negative sepsis with a WBC of $600/\mu l$ and platelets of $6000/\mu l$. The patient on BCVP developed a rectal abscess, fever, and a WBC of $300/\mu l$, requiring hospitalization for drainage of the abscess. Severe nausea with vomiting was observed in 17% of COPP patients, while only 1 patient experienced severe neurologic toxicity on this combination.

The COPP regimen in this ECOG trial was virtually identical to the NCI C-MOPP combination. Only minor differences exist between the NCI and the ECOG regimens. The dose of cyclophosphamide was 650 mg/m² IV on days 1 and 8 in the NCI regimen and 600 mg/m² in the ECOG combination. In addition, the dose of vincristine was 1.4 mg/m² in the NCI version and 1.2 mg/m² in the ECOG regimen. However, there was a maximum of 2.0 mg

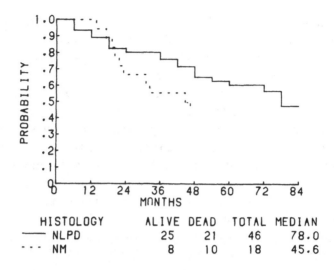

Figure 4. Survival curves of patients treated with COPP on ECOG protocol EST 2474 by histologic subtype. There is no significant difference between NM (nodular mixed) and NLPD (nodular lymphocytic poorly differentiated) histologies (p = 0.39).

vincristine administered per dose in the ECOG regimen, and this 2.0 mg dose was adopted as the standard by most investigators in this trial. Finally, the NCI group administered prednisone 40 mg/m^2 on days 1–14 of each cycle. ECOG initially recommended the same prednisone dose and 4/18 of the COPP patients received this schedule. Early in the ECOG trial, however, the dose of prednisone was changed to 100 mg/m^2 per day on days 1–5. The dose of procarbazine was identical in both the NCI and ECOG combinations. Most importantly, patients in the ECOG COPP group received 84% of the calculated ideal doses of 600 mg/m^2 cyclophosphamide and 78% of the ideal dosage of procarbazine. Thus, all 18 patients treated with COPP received an adequate trial of this regimen with excellent adherence to both the calculated dosages and scheduling on the every 28-day cycle. Grade 3–4 hematologic toxicity was experienced by 22% of the COPP patients, further demonstrating that adequate doses of chemotherapy were administered.

This ECOG study reports the only prospectively controlled trial utilizing COPP in nodular mixed lymphoma. A complete remission rate of 61% with COPP was observed, and this is not significantly different from the 71% CR rate reported by Anderson *et al.* [11]. However, the median response duration of the complete responders on COPP in the ECOG series has been reached and is 16.5 months. These data do not confirm the NCI results of prolonged disease-free survival with C-MOPP.

Bitran *et al.* [19] also evaluated COPP in a small series of 12 patients with NM lymphoma and 17 with NLPD. Their 41% CR rate and median survival of 4 ycars in these patients was disappointing. For patients achieving CR, the actuarial disease-free survival was 60% at 4 years with a downward sloping curve suggesting future relapses. The concluded that intensive COPP chemotherapy offered little benefit in the treatment of nodular mixed lymphoma.

The ECOG protocol 2474 not only compared the COPP regimen, but also investigated the equally intense and more toxic BCVP combination, to an intentionally moderate chemotherapy program of cyclophosphamide-prednisone. No significant differences in complete response rates, disease-free or overall survival were noted among the three regimens. A pattern of continuous late relapse was observed with all three chemotherapy programs. Although 10 of the 32 complete responders remain in complete remission, the limited followup of approximately five years is too short to assume permanent disease control equivalent to cure for this population. Thus, the apparent plateau in the disease-free survival curves in Fig. 2 must also be viewed with caution because of the small numbers at risk beyond 60 months. Clearly late relapses are expected. If these patients were thoroughly restaged at the present time, occult or minimal disease would undoubtedly be detected in some of the apparent complete responders.

3.3. The Stanford trials

Jones et al. [20] reported the Stanford data using single-agent cyclophosphamide or chlorambucil in 16 patients with advanced NM lymphoma prior to 1971. A complete response rate of 31% was reported with a median disease-free survival of over 17 months. The overall survival at 2 years was 47% for all NM patients.

Since 1971, the prospective Stanford trials have used the Rappaport classification and rigorous staging with bipedal lymphangiograms, bone marrow biopsy for staging and restaging, and, until recently, exploratory laparotomy for patients with less than stage IV disease. The initial J6 program at Stanford compared single-agent chemotherapy to the CVP regimen as originally described by Bagley et al. [21], to split course CVP plus total lymphoid irradiation. The J8 trial was initiated in 1974, and replaced the program of combined CVP and total lymphoid irradiation with whole body irradiation. The details of these studies have been previously described [22, 23]. There were no differences in relapse-free or overall survival between any of the treatment arms. Of the 112 protocol patients entered in these two studies, only 21 patients had the NM histology. The vast majority of cases (81 patients) were classified as having NLPD, while 10 patients had DLWD. For the purposes of this discussion, it is noteworthy that there was no difference in overall survival or disease-free survival among the three histologic subtypes NM, NLPD, and DLWD [5, 22]. The disease-free survival for the 21 NM patients was 26% at six years, and a pattern of continuous late relapse was observed.

In addition to these protocol cases, a group of 44 patients with advanced favorable histologies of non-Hodgkin's lymphoma have been followed. These patients were ineligible or refused to participate in the randomized J6 or J8 protocols. They were managed with an individualized program of no initial active therapy, but were treated as necessary for progressive or symptomatic disease [24]. In a small group of eight NM patients who were initially observed with no treatment, little was gained by withholding treatment. The median time to requiring treatment was eight months, and all but one patient required therapy within two years.

3.4. The role of combination chemotherapy regimens including adriamycin

An investigation of the adriamycin-containing combinations CHOP and HOP was conducted by the Southwest Oncology Group (SWOG). McKelvey *et al.* [25] first reported the SWOG results in 20 patients with NM lymphoma. They noted a 78% CR rate with CHOP as compared to 64% CR with HOP. The disease-free survival of complete responders was only 71% at one year. Although the overall survival for all 20 patients was 88% at one year, a sharp fall-off in the actuarial survival curves at two years was noted. These data have not been updated, and the short-followup does not permit a meaningful conclusion about the durability of these complete remissions.

Cabanillas and Freireich [26] also described a series of 14 patients with NM lymphoma, some of whom received adriamycin-containing combination chemotherapy, but the numbers of patients on each regimen were not stated. Patients not receiving adriamycin were generally treated with cyclophosphamide-vincristine-prednisone. Eleven of these 14 patients achieved a complete response (79%). Although the median followup was not reported, an analysis of the disease-free survival curves indicated that the median followup was less than five years. However, only one of the 11 complete responders has thus far relapsed.

Jones *et al.* [27] recently reported the results of a controlled randomized trial comparing CHOP-Bleomycin to CHOP-BCG immunotherapy to COP-Bleomycin. Forty-two patients with NM histology were described. Ninety-two percent of the 13 NM patients on the CHOP-BCG arm achieved CR, compared to 74% of 19 patients achieving CR on CHOP-Bleomycin, compared to 70% CR in 10 patients on the COP-Bleomycin arm. These differences were not statistically significant. These authors did not specifically report disease-free survival for the nodular mixed patients according to the initial induction chemotherapy regimen. Although the duration of median followup was not stated, the investigators did report no further relapses after 18 months for patients with NM in complete remission. Nodular mixed patients who received CHOP-BCG survived somewhat better, but not significantly so, than those receiving the other two regimens. Further followup of these NM patients is clearly required before concluding that the addition of adriamycin with or without BCG or bleomycin is superior to a non-adriamycin containing regimen in achieving improved overall survival.

4. Discussion

The nodular histologic subtypes of non-Hodgkin's lymphoma are thought to respond well to non-aggressive chemotherapy with long survival despite a pattern of continuous relapse. However, it is now recognized that not all nodular subtypes fit into one favorable prognostic category. Both the Eastern Cooperative Oncology Group [28] and the National Cancer Institute [29] recently reviewed their experience with nodular histiocytic (NH) lymphoma and reported the potential for prolonged disease-free survival with aggressive combination chemoherapy programs designed to achieve complete remission.

Conversely, no study reported to date has been able to demonstrate a plateau in the disease-free survival curve for patients with advanced stages of nodular lymphocytic poorly differentiated lymphoma. A variety of approaches has been utilized in the treatment of these patients, including single alkylating agents, aggressive combination chemotherapy, whole-body irradiation, and combined modality therapy. Although any one of these treatment options are extremely effective in achieving a high rate of complete response, prolonged relapse-free survival is a goal that has generally eluded this group of patients. Several investigators [11,, 26, 30] have argued that patients with nodular lymphomas who achieve a complete remission survive longer than those who do not. Rosenberg [5] has countered this argument by emphasizing that prognostic factors, such as systemic symptoms, bulk of disease, site of stage IV disease, occult histologic conversion, may actually be resonsible for the lower complete response rate and are probably responsible for the observed poorer survival. However, multivariate analysis in the studies by Ezdinli et al. [30] and Cabanillas et al. [26] have shown that achievement of a complete remission has a strikingly favorable effect on the duration of survival, independent of other major prognostic factors. This was true not only for patients with NLPD, but also for the nodular mixed subtype [14, 30]. Thus, the goal of treatment for stage III and IV NM patients should be the achievement of a restaged complete remission.

What then is the optimal treatment for patients with advanced stages of nodular mixed lymphoma? The C-MOPP regimen was thought to produce the best results, with an apparent plateau in the disease-free survival curve. However, the NCI data with the C-MOPP program have demonstrated the potential for late relapse even at 7 years. Since occult disease may be well tolerated and slowly growing in these patients, the real probability exists that further relapses will occur with additional followup. It is also disappointing that when Anderson *et al.* [11] first reported these data in 1977, 24 NM patients with stage III and IV had been treated with the C-MOPP regimen. Four and one-half years later, Longo *et al. [12]* updated these data, but now only 22 patients with NM lymphoma had been treated with C-MOPP. The question must be raised: If the C-MOPP program was so successful at the NCI, why did these investigators not treat any additional patients with this regimen over a four-year period?

Neither the small study of Bitran *et al.* [19], nor the randomized prospective ECOG trial described in this chapter have been able to confirm the potential for prolonged disease-free survival with the COPP regimen. No significant differences in either complete response rate, disease-free or overall survival were noted when the non-toxic cyclophosphamide–prednisone regimen was compared with the more aggressive and toxic BCVP and COPP regimens by ECOG. The case for conservative management is particularly pertinent in the older patient with advanced nodular mixed lymphoma who is asymptomatic and who has no immediate threat because of the location and size of lymph node masses or organ involvement. Portlock and Rosenberg [24] did not recommend deferring initial treatment for this histology. In their small group of NM patients who were initially observed, little was gained by withholding initial treatment.

If there is little evidence that non-adriamycin combination regimens produce prolonged disease-free survival in randomized trials, what is the role of adriamycin in this histology? Although the complete response rates reported by Jones *et al.* [27] in the controlled trial from the Southwest Oncology Group ranged from 74–92% on the two CHOP arms, the numbers of patients were small. Moreover, there was no significant difference in the complete response rate when compared to the non-adriamycin COP–Bleomycin arm. Although they did not report prolonged followup, no further relapses after 18 months were observed for patients with NM in complete remission. However, at the time of their most recent report, there did not appear to be a survival advantage for either of the adriamycin-containing regimens. Further followup of these NM patients, and additional controlled trials utilizing adriamycin in other combination chemotherapy programs are required. Controlled trials are clearly indicated in an attempt to find more effective induction chemotherapy regimens with the goal of not only improving the complete response rate and disease-free survival, but most importantly, to improve overall survival for this histology.

There is little evidence to date that aggressive combination chemotherapy has significantly altered the overall survival for nodular mixed patients. Anderson *et al.* [13], reporting the retrospective NCI data, noted that the actuarial survival of patients treated in the palliative chemotherapy era prior to January 1968, was not significantly different than that seen in the past decade, during which time aggressive combination chemotherapy was utilized. Although the proposed Working Formulation of non-Hodgkin's Lymphoma for Clinical Usage re-named the nodular mixed subtype of Rappaport follicular, mixed small cleaved and large cell type, their decision to place these patients into the 'low-grade' category must be questioned. Even the data of these investigators [4] demonstrated a median survival of 5.1 years for the follicular mixed subgroup compared with the longer median survival of 7.2 years for the follicular small cleaved cell type (NLPD). Both Anderson *et al.* [13] and Ezdinli *et al.* [14, 30] have reported significantly better survival in patients with NLPD compared to the nodular mixed type. These studies suggest that patients with NM histology may not belong in the same favorable or low-grade prognostic category as patients with NLPD. Future controlled clinical trials should recognize this important difference in survival between NLPD and NM and either stratify for histologic subtype, or design separate protocols for nodular mixed patients with prospective histologic review.

Acknowledgements

The authors acknowledge the permission of the editor and publisher to include partial material from our previous manuscript in Blood 58:920–925, 1981. The secretarial assistance of Deborah Cleary is gratefully acknowledged.

This study was supported in part by USPHS grants no. CA-15488 and CA-23318.

Appendix: abbreviations and acronyms of drug combinations

BACOP:	bleomycin, adriamycin, cyclophosphamide, vincristine, and prednisone
BCG:	Bacillus Calmette-Guérin
BCVP:	BCNU, cyclophosphamide, vincristine, and prednisone
CHOP:	cyclophosphamide, adriamycin, vincristine, and prednisone
CP:	cyclophosphamide and prednisone
COP-Bleomycin:	cyclophosphamide, vincristine, prednisone and bleomycin
COPP and C-MOPP:	cyclophosphamide, vincristine, procarbazine, and prednisone
CVP (COP):	cyclophosphamide, vincristine, and prednisone
HOP:	adriamycin, vincristine, and prednisone
MOPP:	nitrogen mustard, vincristine, procarbazine, and prednisone

References

1. Jones SE, Fuks Z, Bull M, Kadin ME, Dorfman RF, Kaplan HS, Rosenberg SA, Kim H: Non-Hodgkin's lymphomas IV: Clinico-pathologic correlation in 405 cases. Cancer 31:806–823, 1973.
2. Patchefsky AS, Brodovsky HS, Menduke H: Non-Hodgkin's lymphomas: A clinicopathologic study of 293 cases. Cancer 34:1173–1186, 1974.
3. Anderson T, Chabner BA, Young RC, Berard CW, Garvin AJ, Simon RM, and DeVita VT: Malignant lymphoma. I. The histology and staging of 473 patients at the National Cancer Institute. 50:2699–2707, 1982.
4. The Non-Hodgkin's Lymphoma Pathologic Classification Project: National Cancer Institute sponsored study of classifications of non-Hodgkin's lymphomas: Summary and description of a working formulation for clinical usage. Cancer 49:2112–2135, 1982.
5. Rosenberg SA: Is intensive treatment of favorable non-Hodgkin's lymphoma necessary? In: Controversies in oncology, Wiernik P (ed.), New York, John Wiley & Sons 1982, pp. 45–60.
6. Rappaport H: Tumors of the hematopoietic system. In: Atlas of tumor pathology, Section III, Fasicle 8. Washington, DC, US Armed Forces Institute of Pathology 1966, p. 101.
7. Jones SE, Butler JJ, Byrne GE Jr, Coltman CA Jr, Moon TE: Histopathology review of lymphoma cases from the Southwest Oncology Group. Cancer 39:1071–1076, 1977.
8. Ezdinli EZ, Costello W, Wasser LP, Lenhard RE, Berard CW, Hartsock R, Bennett JM, Carbone PP: Eastern Cooperative Oncology Group experience with the Rappaport classification of non-Hodgkin's lymphomas. Cancer 43:544–550, 1979.
9. Glick JH, Barnes JM, Ezdinli EZ, Berard CW, Orlow EL, Bennett JM: Nodular mixed lymphoma: Results of a randomized trial failing to confirm prolonged disease-free survival with COPP chemotherapy. Blood 58:920–925, 1981.
10. Berard CW: Personal communication, 1981.
11. Anderson T, Bender RA, Fisher RI, DeVita VT, Chabner BA, Berard CW, Norton L, Young RC: Combination chemotherapy in non-Hodgkin's lymphoma: Results of a long-term followup. Cancer Treat Rep 61:1057–1066, 1977.
12. Longo D, Hubbard S, Wesley M, Jaffe E, Chabner B, DeVita V, Young R: Prolonged initial remission in patients with nodular mixed lymphoma. Proc Am Soc Clin Oncol 22:521, 1981.
13. Anderson T, DeVita VT, Simon RM, Berard CW, Canellos GP, Garvin AJ, Young RC: Malignant lymphoma. II. Prognostic factors and response to treatment of 473 patients at the National Cancer Institute. Cancer 50:2708–2721, 1982.
14. Ezdinli EZ, Costello WB, Icli F, Lenhard RE, Johnson GJ, Silverstein M, Berard CW, Bennett JM, Carbone PP: Nodular mixed lymphocytic–histiocytic lymphoma: Response and survival. Cancer 45:261–267, 1980.
15. Cox DR: Analysis of binary data. Methuen, London, 1970.
16. Peto R, Peto J: A symptomically efficient rank invariant test procedures. J R Stat Soc A 35:185–206, 1972.
17. Cox DR: Regression models and life tables. J R Stat Soc B 34:187–202, 1972.
18. Kaplan EL, Meier P: Nonparametric estimation from incomplete observations. J Am Stat Assoc 53:457–481, 1958.
19. Bitran JC, Golomb HM, Ultmann JE, Sweet DL, Lester EP, Stein RS, Miller JB, Moran EM, Kinnealey AE, Vardiman JE, Kinzie J, Roth NO: Non-Hodgkin's lymphoma, poorly differentiated lymphocytic and mixed cell types: Results of sequential staging procedures, response to therapy, and survival of 100 patients. Cancer 42:88–95, 1978.
20. Jones SE, Rosenberg SA, Kaplan HS, Kadin ME, Dorfman RF: Non-Hodgkin's lymphomas: Single agent chemotherapy. Cancer 30:31–38, 1972.
21. Bagley CM, DeVita VT, Berard CW, Canellos GP: Advanced lymphosarcoma: Intensive cy-

clical combination chemotherapy with cyclophosphamide, vincristine, and prednisone. Ann Intern Med 76:227–234, 1972.

22. Portlock CS: Management of the indolent non-Hodgkin's lymphomas. Semin Oncol 7:292–301, 1980.

23. Hoppe RT, Kushlan P, Kaplan HS, Rosenberg SA, Brown BW: The treatment of advanced stage favorable histology non-Hodgkin's lymphoma: A preliminary report of a randomized trial comparing single agent chemotherapy, combination chemotherapy, and whole body irradiation. Blood 58:592–598, 1981.

24. Portlock CS, Rosenberg SA: No initial therapy for stage III and IV non-Hodgkin's lymphomas of favorable histologic types. Ann Intern Med 90:10–13, 1979.

25. McKelvey EM, Gottlieb JA, Wilson HE, Haut A, Talley RW, Stephens R, Lane M, Gamble JF, Jones SE, Grozea ON, Gutterman J, Coltman C, Moon TE: Hydroxyldaunomycin (adriamycin) combination chemotherapy in malignant lymphoma. Cancer 38:1484–1493, 1976.

26. Cabanillas F, Freireich EJ: Intensive treatment of nodular non-Hodgkin's lymphoma. In: Controversies in oncology, Wiernik P (ed.), New York: John Wiley & Sons 1982, pp. 31–43.

27. Jones SE, Grozea PN, Metz EN, Haut A, Stephens RL, Morrison FS, Talley R, Butler JJ, Byrne GE, Hartsock R, Dixon D, Salmon SE: Improved complete remission rates and survival for patients with large cell lymphoma treated with chemoimmunotherapy. A Southwest Oncology Group Study. Cancer 51:1083–1090, 1983.

28. Glick JH, McFadden E, Costello W, Ezdinli E, Berard CW, Bennett JM: Nodular histiocytic lymphoma: Factors influencing prognosis and indications for aggressive chemotherapy. Cancer 49:840–845, 1982.

29. Osborne CK, Norton L, Young RC, Garvin AJ, Simon RM, Berard DW, Hubbard S, DeVita VT: Nodular histiocytic lymphoma: An aggressive nodular lymphoma with potential for prolonged disease-free survival. Blood 56:98–102, 1980.

30. Ezdinli EZ, Costello W, Glick JH: Nodular non-Hodgkin's lymphomas: Effect of histological pattern and response on survival. Proc Am Soc Clin Oncol 22:516, 1981.

12. The role of treatment deferral in the management of patients with advanced, indolent non-Hodgkin's lymphomas

CAROL S. PORTLOCK

1. Introduction

The management of patients with stages III and IV indolent non-Hodgkin's lymphomas remains controversial. As initially reported by Jones et al. [1] in 1973, the median survival for patients with 'favorable' histology lymphomas (Table 1) was more than 8 years, in contrast to a median survival of less than one year for those with 'unfavorable' histologic subtypes.[1] With the use of intensive combination chemotherapy over the intervening decade, there has been dramatic improvement in the prognosis of patients with aggressive lymphomas [4], whereas there has been a virtual standstill in the development of more effective therapy for those with indolent histologies. Although complete remissions can be achieved in the majority of patients with advanced stage lymphomas of either indolent or aggressive histologic subtypes, it is only those with aggressive subtypes who experience prolonged remission durations. And with observations extending well beyond 10 years, confidence is high that such patients may be cured. The impact of this paradox is illustrated in Figs. 1 and 2 [5]. In spite of intensive therapy, patients with advanced indolent histologies experience a pattern of continuous late relapse following induction of complete remission; whereas the disease-free survival curve of complete responders with aggressive histologies reveals few relapses, all occurring within the first two years, and none subsequently. Although median disease-free survival is only 1–2 years for patients with indolent lymphomas, patients continue to live for long periods with active disease. Nevertheless, since cure is not achieved, patients succumb to the disease as illustrated by a downward-sloping survival curve. With follow-up beyond 10 years, one can see divergence of the survival curves: those complete responders with aggressive histologies remaining alive and cured; and complete responders, with indolent histologies dying of progressive lymphoma.

---

[1] Nodular (NHL) and diffuse histiocytic lymphomas (DHL), diffuse mixed lymphocytic and histiocytic lymphoma (DML), diffuse undifferentiated lymphoma (DUL).

Bennett JM (ed), Controversies in the Management of Lymphomas. ISBN 0-89838-586-5.
© *Martinus Nijhoff Publishers, Boston. Printed in the Netherlands.*

Management decisions for patients with advanced aggressive lymphomas relate to the kinds of intensive therapy employed and the goal of treatment is cure. For patients with advanced indolent lymphomas, the management choices are less well-defined and the goal of cure remains elusive.

Table 1. Non-Hodgkin's lymphomas: pathologic classification of indolent histologies.

Rappaport classification [2]
1. DLWD : Diffuse lymphocytic well differentiated lymphoma
2. NLPD : Nodular lymphocytic poorly differentiated lymphoma
3. NML : Nodular mixed lymphocytic and histiocytic lymphoma

International Working Formulation [3]
1. Malignant lymphoma, small lymphocytic
    a. Consistent with chronic lymphocytic leukemia
    b. Plasmacytoid
2. Malignant lymphoma, follicular: predominantly small cleaved cell
    a. Diffuse areas
    b. Sclerosis
3. Malignant lymphoma, follicular: mixed, small cleaved and large cell
    a. Diffuse areas
    b. Sclerosis

---

2. Treatment options

The vast majority of patients with indolent lymphoma have stage III or IV disease. Pathologic stage III is most often identified in NML (25–50% of patients) and less commonly found in NLPD (10–30%) and DLWD (<5%). More than 95% of patients with DLWD, 60–80% of those with NLPD and 40–70% of patients with NML are pathologic stage IV [6, 7, 8].

3. Stages I and II

Although rare, patients with pathologic stage I and II disease must be distinguished from those with more advanced presentations. Representing less than 10% of all patients with indolent histologies, it is this subgroup of patients whose disese-free survival following therapy may be prolonged. In a prospective trial comparing 4400 rads involved field irradiation *vs.* total lymphoid irradiation, the Stanford group has reported a relapse-free survival of >80% at 10 years among 20 PS I and II patients treated [19]. There were only 3 deaths during the 10-year period and statistically significant differences were not observed according to the extent of irradiation employed. A second study by

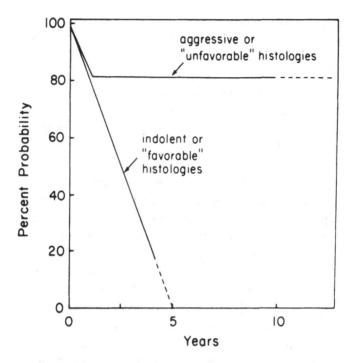

Figure 1. Remission duration of complete responders with stages III and IV non-Hodgkin's lymphomas (adapted from Portlock [5] by permission).

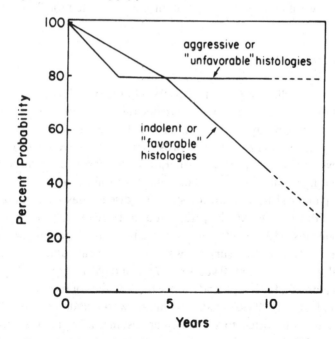

Figure 2. Actuarial survival of complete responders with stages III and IV non-Hodgkin's lymphomas (adapted from Portlock [5] by permission).

Monfardini *et al.* [10] compared regional radiation therapy (RT) alone (11 patients) with RT followed by combination chemotherapy (15 patients) in PS I and II patients with nodular lymphoma. Five year relapse-free survival was 55% for RT and 63% for RT + CT (p = 0.60) and survival was 62% and 93%, respectively (p = 0.10). Although based on very limited patient numbers and relatively short follow-up, it would appear that regional irradiation is the treatment of choice for patients with PS I and II indolent lymphomas. And in contrast to those with PS III and IV, relapse-free survival, may be of long duration.

On the other hand, in clinical stage I and II patients, regional irradiation usually does not result in durable remissions. Jones *et al.* [11] have reported a median relapse-free survival of 5 years for CS I (NLPD and NML) and of 3.5 years for CS II (NLPD and NML). In spite of good local control with 3000–4000 rads to the involved regions, the majority of patients relapsed in unirradiated lymph nodes and extranodal sites. The median actuarial survival was approximately 6 years for both CS I and II. These findings have been confirmed by Chen *et al.* [12] utilizing extended field irradiation for CS I, relapse-free survival was 88% and actuarial survival 100% at 5 years; and for CS II, 67% were relapse-free at 2 years and all were alive at 5 years. Since occult intra-abdominal disease may be present in the majority of patients with CS I and II presentations, it is not surprising that the results of regional irradiation would be less favorable than those reported for PS I and II.

4. Stages III and IV

As discussed earlier, in patients with PS III and IV indolent lymphomas, the shape of the relapse-free survival curve does not yet suggest cure, regardless of the treatment employed. A summary of this data, according to kind of therapy, is listed in Table 2. Few prospective trials have been conducted to answer whether one approach is superior to another, and conclusions are also hampered by small patient numbers and short follow-up.

Total lymphoid irradiation for stage III disease has been utilized in two studies. Glatstein *et al.* [13] reported a retrospective experience with 3500–4000 rads TLI (mantle and inverted Y) in 51 patients with nodular lymphoma. Relapse-free survival was 43% at 5 years and 33% at 10 years; actuarial survival at 5 and 10 years was 75% and 65%, respectively. In 64% of patients unirradiated lymph nodes were the sole sites of relapse. Nevertheless, wider field TLI (2000–3000 rads), including whole abdomen and Waldeyer's ring, has been reported to yield similar results in 29 patients with nodular lymphoma [14]. Disease-free survival was 61% and actuarial survival 78% at 5 years. Relapses occurred both within the treated volume (3 patients), at the

Table 2. Results of treatment for stages III and IV indolent lymphomas.

Treatment	No. of patients	Complete response (%)	Remission duration (median in months)	Actuarial survival (median in months)	References
Total lymphoid irradiation (stage III only)	80	–	48–60+	60+ -120+	[13, 14]
Whole body irradiation	152	71–85	12–30	26+ –96+	[15, 19]
Single alkylating agent	81	13–65	12–36	30–96+	[17, 20, 21, 22]
Combination chemotherapy	446	37–89	6.5+ –90+	8.3+ –101+	[17, 20, 29]
Combined modality	36	70–75	15+ –48	24+ –96+	[17, 19, 22]

margins of the fields (4 patients), and as part of generalized progression (6 patients).

Whole body irradiation, a 'systemic' form of radiation therapy, has been employed in both stages III and IV [15–19]. Total doses of 150 rads are delivered in 15 rad fractions twice per week. This is often supplemented by involved field treatment (1000–2000 rads) to areas of bulk disease. Complete remissions are documented in 70–85% of patients. However, remissions are usually not durable and median relapse-free survivals of 12–30 months have been reported by several groups. In spite of early relapse, actuarial survival is prolonged with median survivals of 26+–96+ months.

Studies of systemic chemotherapy have yielded similar results. Complete response rates generally range from 40–80%, median remission durations 12–36 months, and the majority of patients survive more than 5 years.

The Stanford group has performed two prospective trials [17] comparing systemic therapies: (1) in 63 patients with stage IV indolent histologies, the three arms were daily single alkylating agent *vs.* combination chemotherapy (CVP)[2] *vs.* combined modality therapy (CVP – total lymphoid irradiation – CVP); and (2) in 51 patients with stages III and IV indolent histologies, daily single alkylating agent *vs.* CVP *vs.* whole body irradiation. Pathologically documented complete responses were reported in 65% *vs.* 83% *vs.* 70% in the first trial and 64% *vs.* 81% *vs.* 71% in the second. Median relapse-free survival was 36 *vs.* 36 *vs.* 48 months in the first trial, 36 *vs.* 36 *vs.* 12 months in the

---

[2] Cyclophosphamide, vincristine, prednisone.

second. None of these differences was statistically significant, nor were those for actuarial survival (>65% at 6 years for the first trial and >80% at 4 years for the second). In two other prospective trials [20, 21] single alkylating agent therapy has been compared to CVP and neither study has reported significant differences between the treatment groups.

Aside from CVP, the experience with other combination chemotherapy is limited. The National Cancer Institute has reported a complete response rate of 77% in 31 patients with NML, 24 of whom received C-MOPP[3] [23]. Notable in this study was that the remission duration was dramatically prolonged (79% disease-free at 90+ months) suggesting potential cure. As discussed in more detail elsewhere in this series, subsequent follow-up, however, has revealed a median remission duration of 6 years [30] and such late relapses suggest that C-MOPP is not a curative regimen. Furthermore, other groups have been unable to achieve a similar prolongation of relapse-free survival using C-MOPP in NML (60% at 4 years [24] and 50% at 16.5 months [25]). Nonetheless, the NCI data do suggest that C-MOPP may provide superior relapse-free survival as compared to CVP for some patients with NML. Further prospective study will be needed to answer this question.

Combined modality therapy for stage III and IV disease has been fraught with difficulty. As mentioned previously, the Stanford group treated stage IV patients with split course CVP-TLI-CVP [17]. Complete remissions were achieved in 70% of patients with a median relapse-free survival of 48 months and actuarial survival of >65% at 6 years. These results were not significantly different from CVP or daily single alkylating agent therapy. On the other hand, the combined modality approach often resulted in prolonged bone marrow hypoplasia, making salvage therapy difficult. Similar findings have been reported by the NCI group, comparing combination chemotherapy to whole body irradiation plus the same chemotherapy [19]. Complete response rates (67% vs. 64%), remission durations (60% at 1 year) and actuarial survivals (100% at 2 years) were not significantly different, whereas the combined modality regimen resulted in pronounced hematologic toxicity.

Newer systemic approaches which appear promising include interferon [31] and monoclonal antibody therapy [32]. Thus far, response rates have been high, however follow-up is too short to assess the durability of these remissions.

Gathering both the available prospective and retrospective data, the following conclusions may be drawn: (1) Pathologically documented complete remissions can be achieved in the majority of patients using total lymphoid irradiation for pathologic stage III; and for stages III and IV, with whole body irradiation, single alkylating agent therapy, combination chemotherapy and

---

[3] C-MOPP: cyclophosphamide, vincristine, procabazine and prednisone.

combined modality programs. (2) In spite of the high frequency of complete response, remissions are not durable and a pattern of continuous late relapse is exhibited by all studies to date. (3) Although initially encouraging, the C-MOPP data from the NCI may not be significantly different from that reported by others for other systemic approaches. (4) Since a plateau in the disease-free survival curve has not been achieved by any systemic therapy reported to date, it is unlikely that any of these programs as currently delivered, has curative potential. (5) Newer approaches tested prospectively, are necessary to develop such curative regimens.

5. Treatment deferral

Given that cure remains an elusive goal in patients with advanced indolent lymphomas, then the intent of treatment must be limited to palliation of symptoms and prolongation of survival. Often these patients are clinically well without evidence of threatening disease at diagnosis, making palliative therapy unnecessary. In one prospective study [33], by the Cancer and Leukemia Group B, 43 of 93 patients with NLPD and NML (45%) were judged 'asymptomatic' and potentially eligible for deferral of initial therapy.

To date, there is only one retrospective study [34] which examines the question of deferring initial treatment until required. Forty-four patients with advanced indolent histologies were closely followed without initial therapy. The median observation interval prior to requiring treatment was 31 months for all patients. The median treatment-free interval was significantly different according to histology: 9 months for NML, 32 months for NLPD, and 8+ years for DLWD ($p < 0.02$). In spite of the marked differences in treatment-free interval, no significant differences were noted in actuarial survival according to histologic subtype.

A recent update of this retrospective series [35] continues to show similar trends (see Figs. 3, 4, 5). With 33 additional patients, the median treatment-free interval is 56 months; and histologic subtype remains a significant parameter for the median time to treatment: being significantly shorter for NML (9.5 months) as compared to NLPD (56 months) and DLWD (8+ years) ($p < 0.02$). Median survival is again 10 years without significant differences according to histologic subtype. The survival data reported in this selected retrospective series is comparable to that of other systemic therapies initiated at diagnosis rather than at the time of disease progression (see Table 2).

The potential benefits of deferring initial therapy are listed in Table 3. (1) The patient may experience a prolonged treatment-free interval following diagnosis. This is particularly relevant for patients with NLPD and DLWD in whom this period may measure many years (median of 4.7 and 8+ years,

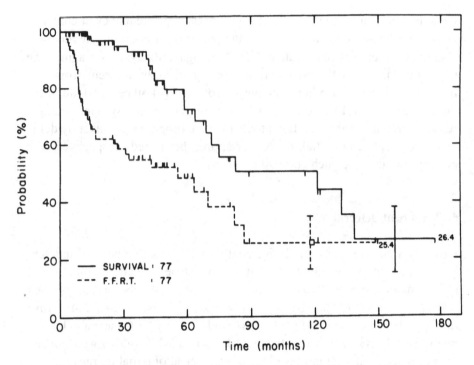

Figure 3. Actuarial survival and freedom from receiving treatment in 77 patients with indolent non-Hodgkin's lymphomas whose initial treatment was deferred (from Portlock [35] by permission).

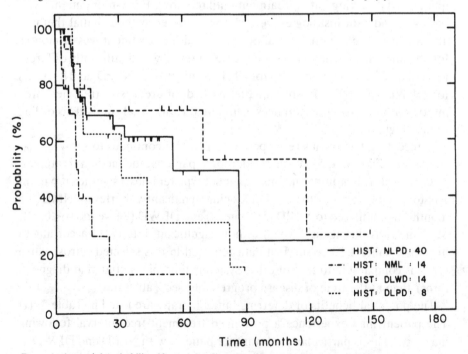

Figure 4. Actuarial probability of remaining free of treatment, for 76 patients whose initial treatment was deferred. One patient with diffuse lymphocytic intermediate differentiation lymphoma is excluded from the analysis (from Portlock [35] by permission).

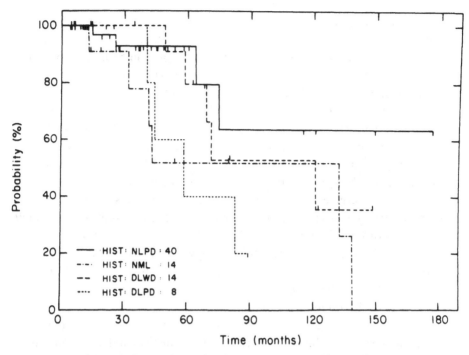

Figure 5. Actuarial survival, according to histology, for 76 patients whose initial treatment was deferred. One patient with diffuse lymphocytic intermediate differentiation lymphoma is excluded from the analysis (from Portlock [35] by permission).

Table 3. Potential benefits of withholding initial therapy.

1. Prolonged treatment-free interval
2. No exposure to agents selecting for drug resistance
3. Spontaneous tumor regression
4. Selection of appropriate therapy
5. Histologic evolution

respectively). For those with NML, only 4 of 14 in the updated Stanford series remain untreated with a median treatment-free interval of 9.5 months. (2) During the treatment-free period, patients will not be exposed to agents which might select for drug resistance. (3) The patient may experience spontaneous tumor regression during the observation period: Gattiker *et al.* [36] have reported an 8% incidence of objective regression in patients with nodular lymphoma. Among the 44 patients reported by Portlock and Rosenberg, 7 have experienced spontaneous regressions: 3 were complete (21+–60+ months duration) and 4 were partial (6–34 months duration). (4) When disease progression occurs, appropriate therapy may be selected (see Table 2). Deferring treatment at diagnosis does not commit the patient to a 'conservative' or 'aggressive' management approach. Decisions regarding therapeutic strategies can be delayed until the patient evidences disease progression. (5) There may be evolution of the indolent histology to an aggressive histologic subtype (NHL, DHL, DUL) with greater likelihood of prolonged disease-free survival. Histologic evolution of the non-Hodgkin's lymphomas is a well-recognized phenomenon, with loss of nodular architecture and the appearance of increasing numbers of large cells. It has been documented in up to 30% of patients at relapse [7, 38], as well as at autopsy [2, 39]. It is not known whether this evolution occurs without treatment. On the other hand, multiple histologic subtypes are present at diagnosis in up to 20% of patients with non-Hodgkin's lymphomas. (6) In previously treated patients with indolent lymphomas, the emergence of an aggressive histology connotes a poor prognosis. Median survival was 11 months following histologic progression at relapse in 19 patients reported by Hubbard *et al.* [36] as compared to a median survival of 77 months for 40 patients whose relapse histology remained nodular. Prospective studies are underway to determine the incidence of histologic evolution prior to treatment and to test whether the emergence of such aggressive histologies can lead to cure with intensive therapy.

The potential hazards of deferring initial therapy are listed in Table 4. (1) The patient must be followed closely at regular intervals and observed expectantly for evidence of disease progression. This approach requires that the patient be reliable and not lost to follow-up. In spite of careful observation, there may be clinically silent disease progression in the retroperitoneum or into such threatening sites as the epidural space. (2) Some patients and even some physicians may be unable to tolerate the added psychological burden of withholding treatment. (3) It is theoretically possible that the results of treatment, when initiated for progressive disease, may be compromised by the advanced extent of untreated lymphoma. For example, at diagnosis, the presence of systemic symptoms or extranodal disease involving sites other than bone marrow or liver have been reported to adversely affect prognosis. It is not known whether these and other prognostic factors become relevant in the patient whose initial therapy is deferred. Median actuarial survival in the Stanford retrospective study was 10 years and not significantly different from the results of protocol studies initiated at diagnosis. However, since patients eligible for a deferred approach have the most indolent disease, is it possible

Table 4. Potential hazards of withholding initial therapy.

1. Close follow-up
2. Clinically silent disease progression in threatening sites
3. Psychological burden of remaining untreated
4. Compromised results of therapy due to disease progression
5. Histologic evolution

that their survival could have been even longer had they received treatment at diagnosis, rather than at the time of disease progression? (4) If histologic evolution to a more aggressive histologic subtype occurs during the observation period, is it possible that such a transformation could decrease survival rather than increase it? As previously discussed, results in relapsing patients with histologic progression and in those with composite lymphoma [40] suggest that this is possible.

Given the relative merits and disadvantages of withholding initial therapy until required, on balance, such a management strategy appears reasonable. Since treatment decisions are only delayed and not modified or forfeited by this approach, nothing may be lost by deferral while a real gain in freedom from treatment may be achieved by some patients. This is particularly true for patients with NLPD and DLWD whose median treatment free period is 55+ months in the Stanford retrospective study. Clearly, prospective trials are necessary to test the utility of treatment deferral as well as to better define its real and potential hazards.

6. Management decisions

Determining an initial plan of management for the patient with advanced indolent lymphoma depends upon a large number of factors (see Table 5). These include some of the following:

1) Histopathology. Deferral of initial therapy in patients with NLPD and DLWD may result in a prolonged treatment-free interval (median of 56 months and 8+ years, respectively) [53]. On the other hand, patients with NML often require treatment within months of diagnosis, even if they initially appear appropriate for treatment deferral (the median time to requiring treatment in the Stanford study was 9.5 months). Secondly, patients with NML may achieve more durable complete remissions with combination chemotherapy (C-MOPP) [30]. If an aggressive histology is detected, either at a separate site or as part of a composite lymphoma, then appropriately intensive combination chemotherapy is indicated.

2) Stage. Deferral of initial treatment is not appropriate for patients with PS

Table 5. Some factors in determining management plan.

1. Histopathology	6. Age
2. Stage	7. General medical health
3. Sites and bulk of disease	8. Potential treatment morbidities
4. Pace of disease	9. Psychological make-up
5. Systemic symptoms	10. Anticipated benefits of treatment

I and II disease since regional irradiation may result in prolonged disease-free survival (>80% at 10 years) with minimal morbidity [9]. For CS I and II disease, regional irradiation may also provide good local control with minimal morbidity, however it is highly probable that undetected intra-abdominal lymphoma is present [11, 12]. Results of total lymphoid irradiation [13, 14] as reported to date for patients with stage III do not appear to be significantly different from the systemic therapies listed in Table 2. Consequently, treatment decisions for stage III patients cannot be based on stage alone.

3) *Sites and bulk of disease.* Since advanced stage alone does not determine the necessity to begin treatment, factors such as local tumor bulk, bone marrow reserve, and involvement of threatening sites may play a more important role. For example, if there is ureteral obstruction secondary to retroperitoneal adenopathy, splenomegaly resulting in hypersplenism, and/or epidural lymphoma, then treatment clearly must be initiated.

4) *Pace of disease.* Even if the lymphoma is not locally bulky or compromising function, it may require therapy if growth is progressive. In particular, if there is rapid progression, then repeat biopsy may be indicated to rule out histologic transformation. On the other hand, if the patient reports a history of slowly progressive or even waxing and waning adenopathy, then a deferred approach may be possible.

5) *Systemic symptoms.* Patients with systemic symptoms usually require therapy in order to palliate their symptoms, regardless of disease extent or other factors.

6) *Age.* Although indolent lymphomas are not common in patients less than 40 years of age, the disease appears to have a similar clinical course to that of middle-aged and elderly patients. Intensive treatment regimens may be better tolerated, but the results of such therapy are not significantly different according to age.

7) *General medical condition.* Treatment deferral or single alkylating agent therapy may be valuable alternatives in the patient with multiple medical problems.

8) *Potential treatment morbidities.* By delaying treatment until it is required, exposure to agents with known toxicities may be minimized. Relative toxicities of the therapies listed in Table 2 will be discussed below.

9) *Psychological make-up.* Deferral of initial treatment may not be possible if the patient or physician is uncomfortable with this management alternative. Close follow-up is mandatory and therefore, the patient must be reliable.

10) *Anticipated benefits of treatment.* If at diagnosis the patient is asymptomatic, clinically well and without threatening disease, then initiation of palliative therapy may be of little value, particularly for those with NLPD and DLWD. On the other hand, for patients with NML, the treatment-free period will probably be short and C-MOPP many offer a prolonged complete remission.

7. Treatment alternatives

Once the decision has been made to initiate therapy, it is important to assess the relative effectiveness of each approach (see Table 2). Deferral of treatment at diagnosis does not dictate a 'conservative' or 'aggressive' treatment strategy with disease progression. However, treatment results and outcome as listed in Table 2 are based on previously untreated patients whose therapy was initiated at diagnosis. Factors to be considered include:

1) Complete response rate. Pathologically documented complete remissions can be obtained in 40–80% of patients. Prospective trials have not demonstrated significant differences between those treatments listed.

2) Duration of therapy required to achieve complete remission. Daily single alkylating agent therapy induces complete responses gradually, sometimes requiring a year or more of continuous therapy [17]. On the other hand, pulse alkylating agent therapy has been reported to yield more rapid responses [41]. Prompt complete responses (2–10 months) are achieved with all other therapies listed in Table 2.

3) Duration of complete response. In prospective trials, [17, 19, 20, 21, 25] significant differences have not been found in disease-free survival among systemic treatment options. In retrospective series, only C-MOPP has been reported to yield superior disease-free survival as compared to CVP in patients with NML. This finding has not been confirmed in prospective testing [25].

4) Survival. Greater than 60–80% of all patients survive 5 years and few 10 year statistics are available. Thus far, significant differences have not been seen, but longer follow-up is necessary.

5) Acute toxicity. Table 6 outlines the relative toxicities of systemic therapy.

Table 6. Relative toxicities of systemic therapy.

	Whole body irradiation	Single alkylating agent therapy	Combination chemotherapy	Combination chemotherapy plus irradiation
Nausea, vomiting	−	−	+ +	+ +
Alopecia	−	−	+ +	+ +
Bacterial infections	+	+	+	+
Herpes zoster	+	+	+	+
Thrombocytopenic hemorrhage	+	+	+	+
Hemorrhagic cystitis	−	+ +	+	+
Chronic bone marrow suppression	+	+	+	+ +

In general, these programs have reproducible, manageable and acceptable toxicity.

6) Chronic or delayed toxicities. Prolonged myelosuppression occurs more frequently with combined modality regimens [17, 19, 22]. Second malignancies have been reported following all systemic therapies [42]. The relative incidence and risk of this complication is not known and will require longer follow-up.

7) Ability to salvage following relapse. Few data are available to answer this important question. Therapies which result in chronic myelosuppression would be expected to limit subsequent therapeutic options.

In summary, the choice of initial systemic therapy cannot be based upon the clear superiority of one treatment over another. The usual parameters of complete response rate, remission duration and survival are of little value since significant differences have not been identified. The need to achieve a rapid response to therapy and the relative acute and chronic toxicities of each regimen play a much greater role in the management decision. Just as there may be no compelling reason to initiate treatment at diagnosis, there may be no clear cut treatment approach which is indicated when disease progression occurs. Table 7 attempts to summarize this difficult management problem and some of the alternative approaches which may be applicable.

Table 7. Alternative approaches to management (adapted from Portlock CS, [35], by permission).

	WBI	SA	CVP	C-MOPP	CM	Deferred RX
Histology						
NLPD	+	+	+	?	±	+ +
NML	+	+	+	+ +	±	±
DLWD	+	+	+	?	±	+ +
Disease sites						
Threatening	+	−	+	+	+	−
Not threatening	+	+	+	+	±	+
Pace of disease						
Rapidly progressive	+	−	+	+	+	−
Stable or						
slowly progressive	+	+	+	+	±	+ +
Systemic symptoms						
Present	+	+	+	+	+	−
Absent	+	+	+	+	±	+ +

WBI: whole body irradiation; SA: single alkylating agent; CVP: cyclophosphamide; C-C-MOPP: cyclophosphamide, vincristine, procarbazine, prednisone; CM: combined modality.

8. Conclusion

A quagmire of data surrounds the management decisions of patients with advanced indolent histology non-Hodgkin's lymphomas. Although highly treatable, these diseases are probably not curable with the several modes of therapy (as currently delivered) discussed above. Management decisions are often based on vague and ill-defined logic since cure is not a realistic therapeutic goal and palliative therapy is often not necessary at diagnosis.

Clearly, new directions are needed in clinical research and patient management. Prospective trials with prolonged follow-up will be necessary to advance toward the goal of cure. New agents, more effective interdigitation of chemotherapy and irradiation, and intensive treatment programs are all being tested.

The role of treatment deferral at diagnosis also requires prospective investigation. As a valid alternative, criteria for selection and reasons for treatment intervention must be regularized. Outcome must also be assessed prospectively in larger patient numbers. Whether treatment deferral will be an important approach in reaching the goal of cure remains to be defined.

References

1. Jones SE, Fuks Z, Bull M, et al.: Non-Hodgkin's lymphomas: IV. Clinicopathologic correlation in 405 cases. Cancer 31:806–823, 1973.
2. Rappaport H, Winter WJ, Hicks EB: Follicular lymphoma – A re-evaluation of its position in the scheme of malignant lymphoma, based on a survey of 253 cases. Cancer 9:792–821, 1956.
3. The non-Hodgkins lymphoma pathologic classification project: National Cancer Institute sponsored study of classifications of non-Hodgkin's lymphomas. Cancer 49:2112–2135, 1982.
4. Sweet D, Golomb H: The treatment of histiocytic lymphoma. Semin Oncol 7:302–309, 1980.
5. Portlock CS: Non-Hodgkin's lymphomas. In: Prognosis, Fries JF, Ehrlich GF (eds), The Charles Press Publishers, 1981, pp. 91–94.
6. Chabner BA, Johnson RE, Young RC, et al.: Sequential nonsurgical and surgical staging of non-Hodgkin's lymphomas. Ann Intern Med 85:149–154, 1976.
7. Goffinet DR, Warnke R, Dunnick NR, et al.: Clinical and surgical (laparotomy) evaluation of patients with non-Hodgkin's lymphomas. Cancer Treat Rep 61:981–992, 1977.
8. Ribas-Mundo M, Rosenberg SA: The value of sequential bone marrow biopsy and laparotomy and splenectomy in a series of 200 consecutive untreated patients with non-Hodgkin's lymphoma. Eur J Cancer 15:941–952, 1979.
9. Rosenberg SA: Is intensive treatment of favorable non-Hodgkin's lymphoma necessary? In: Controversies in Oncology, Wiernik PH (ed), New York: John Wiley & Sons, 1982, pp. 45–60.
10. Monfardini S, Banfi A, Bonadonna G, et al.: Improved five year survival after combined radiotherapy-chemotherapy for stage I–II non-Hodgkin's lymphoma. Int J Rad Oncol Biol Phys 6:125–134, 1980.
11. Jones SE, Fuks Z, Kaplan HS, et al.: Non-Hodgkin's lymphomas: V. Results of radiotherapy. Cancer 32:682–291, 1973.

12. Chen MG, Prosnitz LR, Gonzalez-Serva A, et al.: Results of radiotherapy in control of stage I and II non-Hodgkin's lymphoma. Cancer 43:1245–1254, 1979.
13. Glatstein E, Fuks Z, Goffinet DR, et al.: Non-Hodgkin's lymphomas of stage III extent: Is total lymphoid irradiation appropriate treatment? Cancer 37:2806–2812, 1976.
14. Cox JD, Komaki R, Kun LE, Wilson JF, Greenberg M: Stage III nodular lymphoreticular tumors (non-Hodgkin's lymphoma): Results of central lymphatic irradiation. Cancer 47:2247–2252, 1981.
15. Carabell SC, Chaffey JT, Rosenthal DS, et al.: Results of total body irradiation in the treatment of advanced non-Hodgkin's lymphomas. Cancer 43:994–1000, 1979.
16. Choi NC, Timothy AR, Kaufman SD, et al.: Low dose fractionated whole body irradiation in the treatment of advanced non-Hodgkin's lymphoma. Cancer 43:1636–1642, 1979.
17. Hoppe RT, Kushlan P, Kaplan HS, et al.: The treatment of advanced stage favorable histology non-Hodgkin's lymphoma: A preliminary report of a randomized trial comparing single agent chemotherapy, combination chemotherapy, and whole body irradiation. Blood 58:592–598, 1981.
18. Thar TL, Million RR, Noyes WD: Total body irradiation in non-Hodgkin's lymphoma. Int J Radiot Biol 5:171–176, 1979.
19. Young RC, Johnson RE, Canellos GP, et al.: Advanced lymphocytic lymphoma: Randomized comparisons of chemotherapy and radiotherapy, alone or in combination. Cancer Treat Rep 61:1153–1159, 1977.
20. Kennedy BJ, Bloomfield CD, Kiang DT, et al.: Combination versus successive single agent chemotherapy in lymphocytic lymphoma. Cancer 41:23–28, 1978.
21. Lister TA, Cullen MH, Beard MEJ, et al.: Comparison of combined and single-agent chemotherapy in non-Hodgkin's lymphoma of favourable histological type. Br Med J 1:533–537, 1978.
22. Portlock CS, Rosenberg SA, Glatstein E, et al.: Treatment of advanced non-Hodgkin's lymphomas with favorable histologies: Preliminary results of a prospective trial. Blood 47:747–756, 1976.
23. Anderson T, Bender RA, Fisher RI, et al.: Combination chemotherapy in non-Hodgkin's lymphoma: Results of long-term follow-up. Cancer Treat Rep 61:1057–1066, 1977.
24. Bitran JC, Golomb HM, Ultmann JE, et al.: Non-Hodgkin's lymphoma, poorly differentiated lymphocytic and mixed cell types: Results of sequential staging procedures, response to therapy, and survival of 100 patients. Cancer 42:88–95, 1978.
25. Glick JH, Barnes JM, Ezdinli EZ, et al.: Nodular mixed lymphoma: Results of a randomized trial failing to confirm prolonged disease-free survival with COPP chemotherapy. Blood 58:920–925, 1981.
26. Jones SE, Grozea PN, Metz EN, et al.: Superiority of adriamycin-containing combination chemotherapy in the treatment of diffuse lymphoma: A Southwest Oncology Group study. Cancer 43:417–425, 1979.
27. Portlock CS, Rosenberg SA: Combination chemotherapy with cyclophosphamide, vincristine, and prednisone in advanced non-Hodgkin's lymphomas. Cancer 37:1275–1282, 1976.
28. Rodriquez V, Cabanillas F, Burgess MA, et al.: Combination chemotherapy ('CHOP-Bleo') in advanced (non-Hodgkin) malignant lymphoma. Blood 49:325–333, 1977.
29. Skarin AT, Rosenthal DS, Maloney WC, et al.: Combination chemotherapy of advanced non-Hodgkin lymphoma with bleomycin, adriamycin, cyclophosphamide, vincristine, and prednisone (BACOP). Blood 49:759–568, 1977.
30. Longo D, Hubbard S, Wesley M, et al.: Prolonged initial remission in patients with nodular mixed lymphoma (NML). Proc Am Soc Clin Oncol 22:521, 1981 (abstr).
31. Louie AC, Gallagher JG, Sikora K, Levy R, Rosenberg SA, Merigan TC: Follow-up observa-

tions on the effect of human leukocyte interferon in non-Hodgkin's lymphoma. Blood 58:712–718, 1981.

32. Miller RA, Maloney DG, Warnke R, Levy R: Treatment of B-cell lymphoma with monoclonal anti-idiotype antibody. N Engl J Med 306:517–522, 1982.

33. Peterson BA, Sartiano GP, Frizzera G, Pajak TF, Bloomfield CD, Gottlieb AJ: Symptoms in patients with favorable subtypes of non-Hodgkin's lymphoma. Proc Am Soc Clin Oncol 1:158, 1982.

34. Portlock CS, Rosenberg SA: No initial therapy for stage III and IV non-Hodgkin's lymphomas of favorable histologic types. Ann Intern Med 90:10–13, 1979.

35. Portlock CS: 'Good risk' non-Hodgkin's lymphomas: Approaches to management. Semin Hem (in press), 1983.

36. Gattiker HH, Wiltshaw E, Galton DAG: Spontaneous regression in non-Hodgkin's lymphoma. Cancer 45:2627–2632, 1980.

37. Cullen MH, Lister TA, Brearley RL, et al.: Histological transformation of non-Hodgkin's lymphoma. A prospective study. Cancer 44:645–651, 1979.

38. Hubbard SM, Chabner BA, DeVita VT Jr, Simon R, Berard CW, Jones RB, Garvin AJ, Canellos GP, Osborne CK, Young RC: Histologic progression in non-Hodgkin's lymphoma. Blood 59:258–264, 1982.

39. Risdall R, Hoppe RT, Warnke R: Non-Hodgkin's lymphoma. A study of the evolution of the disease based upon 92 autopsied cases. Cancer 44:529–542, 1979.

40. Kim H, Hendrickson MR, Dorfman RF: Composite lymphoma. Cancer 40:959–976, 1977.

41. Cadman EC, Drislane F, Waldron J, Farber L, Prosnitz L, Bertino JR: High dose pulse chlorambucil is effective therapy for rapid remission induction in nodular lymphocytic poorly differentiated lymphoma. Cancer, 50:1037–1041, 1982.

42. Zarrabi MH: Association of non-Hodgkin's lymphoma (NHL) and second neoplasms. Semin Oncol 7:248–259, 1980.

13. Early intervention with combined modality therapy for 'favorable' non-Hodgkin's lymphomas of advanced stage

TIMOTHY J. KINSELLA

1. Introduction

The non-Hodgkin's lymphomas encompass a heterogenous group of neoplastic diseases of lymph nodes with varying morphologic, immunologic and clinical subtypes. These malignant lymphomas are known not only for their involvement of lymph nodes but also for their ability to spread and involve extralymphatic organs as well, often in a non-contiguous fashion. However, in the vast majority of patients, the dominant clinical features are lymph node involvement and its' secondary manifestations of obstruction, pain and possibly organ failure (e.g. hydronephrosis).

In the last two decades, new advances in cancer treatment, both with chemotherapy and radiation therapy, have had a major impact on the treatment of Hodgkin's disease and malignant lymphomas. The approach to patients with advanced Hodgkin's disease (stage III and IV) has been revolutionized from a palliative approach with involved field irradiation and single agent chemotherapy to a present day highly curative approach with wide-field total lymphoid irradiation, combination chemotherapy, and combined modality therapy [1–3].

For patients with advanced non-Hodgkin's lymphomas, the results of modern treatment are clearly more difficult to interpret. Certainly, the most important development in the management of these diseases has occurred in diffuse histocytic lymphoma (Rappaport classification) where combination chemotherapy has unequivocally resulted in prolonged disease-free survival (? cure) in a significant proportion (40–60%) of patients with advanced disease [4, 5]. However, diffuse histiocytic lymphoma comprises only 15–20% of non-Hodgkin's lymphomas. The curability of other advanced stage adult non-Hodgkin's lymphomas (80–85%) remains generally evasive to combination chemotherapy and/or radiation therapy. This is particularly true for the so-called 'indolent' or 'favorable' histologic subtypes of the Rappaport classification, including nodular lymphocytic poorly differentiated (NLPD), nodular mixed (NM), and diffuse lymphocytic welldifferentiated (DLWD).

Bennett JM (ed), Controversies in the Management of Lymphomas. ISBN 0-89838-586-5.
© *Martinus Nijhoff Publishers, Boston. Printed in the Netherlands.*

The past strategies for treatment of the advanced non-Hodgkin's lymphomas have largely been based on approaches that have been so effective for Hodgkin's disease. However, the natural and treated histories of malignant lymphomas, particularly the 'favorable' histologic subtypes, are clearly different from Hodgkin's disease. In order to interpret the treatment results of the past and to design future treatment strategies for these lymphomas, it is important to clearly define the clinical and pathological differences between Hodgkin's disease and favorable histology malignant lymphomas (Table 1).

2. Comparison of Hodgkin's disease and the favorable histology non-Hodgkin's lymphomas

In general, patients with Hodgkin's disease are younger, and less debilitated. This is particularly true for favorable histology non-Hodgkin's patients who are typically two or three decades older and subject to all of the cardiovascular and pulmonary disease associated with aging and western civilization. Approximately one-third of Hodgkin's disease patients will have the systemic ('B') symptoms defined by the Ann Arbor Staging Classification. In contrast, the vast majority of malignant lymphoma patients will have no systemic symptoms at presentation.

The extent and location of disease at presentation is another major dif-

Table 1. Comparison between Hodgkin's disease and favorable histology non-Hodgkin's lymphomas.

Hodgkin's disease	Favorable histology non-Hodgkin's lymphomas
1. Age: typically young; 2nd and 3rd decade of life.	1. Usually 3–4 decades older and often more debilitated by coexisting chronic diseases.
2. 'B' symptoms: up to 35% with systemic symptoms.	2. Less than 15% with systemic symptoms.
3. 60–70% with loco-regional (stage I and II) disease at presentation.	3. Greater than 75% with advanced disease (stage III and IV) at presentation.
4. Patterns of nodal involvement: up to 40% with mediastinal nodes; less than 5% with Waldeyer's ring and mesenteric nodes.	4. Only 10–15% with mediastinal nodes; up to 70% with mesenteric nodes; up to 15–20% with Waldeyer's nodes.
5. Extra-nodal involvement: bone marrow and liver infrequently involved (<5%).	5. Bone marrow involvement up to 60%; liver involvement up to 20–30%.
6. Accepted histopathologic classification.	6. At least 6 different histopathological classifications.

ference between these diseases. In Hodgkin's disease, at least one-half of patients will have loco-regional disease (stage I and II) whereas patients with malignant lymphomas more commonly present with advanced stage disease, usually involving one or more extralymphatic sites. Following clinical and limited pathological staging, 75–80% of patients with non-Hodgkin's lymphoma will be stage III or IV. This percentage is somewhat lower for patients with diffuse lymphomas and somewhat higher for patients with nodular lymphomas.

The orderly progression of spread from one lymph node site to an adjacent nodal site in patients with Hodgkin's disease has long been recognized [6]. Patients with non-Hodgkin's lymphomas are less likely to fit the concept of contiguity of spread as proposed in Hodgkin's disease. Nevertheless, the majority of stage II and III patients with non-Hodgkin's lymphomas present with lymphomatous involvement of contiguous sites. However, in contrast to patients with Hodgkin's disease, patients who fail treatment of malignant lymphoma are more likely to fail in non-contiguous sites than those with Hodgkin's disease [7].

Approximately 40% of patients with Hodgkin's disease will have mediastinal involvement at presentation and often this is the major site of tumor bulk [8]. For the non-Hodgkin's lymphomas, involvement of the mediastinum at presentation or relapse is uncommon [9]. Typically, the retroperitoneum is the site of bulky lymph node involvement in non-Hodgkin's lymphomas. Additionally mesenteric lymph node involvement is found in approximately 30% of patients with diffuse histologies and in 70% of patients with nodular histologies compared to 5% of patients with Hodgkin's disease [8,9]. Involvement of Waldeyer's ring and peripheral lymph nodes (epitrochlear, femoral, popliteal) are also more common with non-Hodgkin's lymphomas, particularly with favorable histologic subtypes [8, 9].

Extralymphatic involvement of the bone marrow, liver, and gastrointestinal tract further distinguishes the clinical manifestations of these diseases [10]. Bone marrow involvement while uncommon in Hodgkin's disease (5%), occurs in up to 60% of patients with favorable histology non-Hodgkin's lymphoma [11]. Liver involvement is also more common in the non-Hodgkin's lymphomas particularly in patients with NLPD histology [10]. An important reason for the decline in the clinical usefulness of the staging laparotomy for non-Hodgkin's lymphoma is the relatively high yield of the less invasive surgical procedures of bone marrow and percutaneous or laparoscopy directed liver biopsy.

In Hodgkin's disease, the Rye histological classification [12] is both accepted and relatively reproducible from center to center. Indeed, with today's highly effective treatment of Hodgkin's disease, the histological subtype appears to be less important as a prognostic variable [13]. In the non-Hodgkin's lymphomas, there exists six histologic classifications, most of which were proposed during the last decade when new information concerning lymphocyte maturation and function led to some dissatisfaction with the Rappaport classification. This plethora of histologic classifications has been a source of frustration for the clinician with a fragmentation of clinical information and limitation of comparison of treatment results from center to center. Interestingly, a recent NCI sponsored study on the clinical utility of these 6 histologic classifications found that the most reproducible histologic characteristic was the distinction between a nodular or follicular pattern versus a diffuse pattern of lymph node architecture [14].

The pathological interpretation in non-Hodgkin's lymphomas is further complicated by presence of both nodular and diffuse patterns in some lymph nodes. It is now recognized that the prognosis of these patients is similar to patients whose lymph node biopsy shows only a nodular pattern [15]. Additionally, up to 20% of patients may have different histological subtypes based on the Rappaport scheme when at least two separate lymph nodes are biopsied [16].

Finally, the histological presentation of Hodgkin's disease and the favorable histology non-Hodgkin's lymphomas can be distinguished by the relative proportion of neoplastic cells to reactive inflammatory cells evident on lymph node biopsy. In Hodgkin's disease, the Reed–Sternberg (or variant) cell population is considerably smaller than the surrounding inflammatory cell population. By contrast, in non-Hodgkin's lymphomas, the nodal pattern, either nodular or diffuse, is almost completely effaced by neoplastic cells with few inflammatory cells. The relative paucity of neoplastic cells in Hodgkin's disease might in part explain the reason why modern treatments are far more curative for Hodgkin's disease than they are for the favorable histology non-Hodgkin's lymphomas.

3. The great paradox of advanced stage favorable lymphomas

The great paradox of non-Hodgkin's lymphomas is that most patients who present with favorable histology tend to have an advanced stage and yet their survival appears to be relatively good (median survival in excess of 5 years). A clear understanding of this paradox is lacking and this underscores our need for further study of the basic biology of these diseases.

Most clinical studies in the literature report quite high (60–85%) complete response rates for advanced favorable lymphomas with systemic therapy including single agent chemotherapy, combination chemotherapy, whole body irradiation and combined modality therapy. In properly staged III patients, total lymphoid irradiation alone appears highly effective in rendering a majority of patients disease free. However, unlike the complete responders with Hodgkin's disease and diffuse histocytic lymphoma, the complete responders with favorable histology lymphomas generally do not remain in complete remission. Thus, while these lymphomas have been called favorable in comparison to diffuse lymphomas, almost all patients will relapse and die of their disease. A possible exception in the literature is patients with advanced nodular mixed lymphoma treated with C-MOPP at the NCI [17]. Initially, a plateau on the disease-free curve was reported. However, with follow-up beyond 5–6 years in this group of patients, late relapse is occuring [18]. A recent randomized prospective trial of C-MOPP in patients with nodular mixed lymphoma also reports a similar pattern of continuous relapse with time [19].

In the favorable histology lymphomas, the importance of actuarial disease-free data cannot be overstated. Overall survival data simply provide information concerning the natural history of the disease and has led some to conclude that nodular lymphomas are favorable [20]. Disease-free data plotted as a function of time on an actuarial basis will denote the possibility of a relapse. By definition, a cure will be achieved only when a patient remains free of disease far beyond the statistical likelihood of a relapse. To generate these data accurately for advanced stage favorable lymphoma patients, careful follow-up with annual bone marrow evaluation and assessment of the retroperitoneum by repeat lymphangiography and computerized tomographic scanning are necessary. Such follow-up has rarely been done. The lack of routine follow-up studies can only lead to overestimations of disease-free survival. As was found with longer follow-up of nodular mixed patients at the NCI [18], it is difficult to determine when patients with favorable histology lymphomas are disease free long enough to entertain the possibility of cure. Even 10 years of follow-up may be insufficient to judge reliably whether or not curative treatment has been delivered in these patients.

4. Methods of managing advanced favorable lymphoma patients

Precisely because these patients live for long periods of time, there are major controversies concerning their optimal management. Presently, there are at least six major ways to manage a patient with advanced favorable histology lymphoma: (1) initially deferred treatment; (2) single-agent chemotherapy; (3) combination chemotherapy; (4) conventional high-dose radiation therapy (for stage III only); (5) whole or total body radiation therapy; and (6) combined-modality therapy (usually combination chemotherapy and some form of conventional radiation therapy to all lymph nodes or at least those with bulky involvement). The thesis of this chapter is that early intervention with combined modality therapy offers the greatest potential for cure in a patient with advanced stage favorable histology non-Hodgkin's lymphoma. Toward this thesis, I will review the philosophy and treatment results of the various approaches to treatment with emphasis on curative potential.

4.1. Deferral of initial treatment

There has been a recent toward recommending no initial treatment in these patients, based on a report of 44 selected patients seen over a 15-year period at Stanford University Hospital [21]. These patients were selected for deferral of initial treatment since they were asymptomatic, had no impending medical problems related to lymphoma (eg. hydronephrosis, bowel obstruction), and were ineligible for protocol studies. With this 'watch and wait' approach, close careful follow-up (every 2–4 months) is required by the primary physician. Additionally, the patient must understand the rationale for deferral of treatment and the importance of close follow-up. Treatment is initiated only when there is evidence of disease progression as manifested by the development of systemic symptoms or local complications of progressive adenopathy. This approach inherently assumes that the favorable–histology lymphomas are not curable with present-day treatment.

There are at least three reasons to adopt a 'watch and wait' approach in these patients. First, these patients may not require any treatment for a considerable period of time. Secondly, patients may undergo a spontaneous regression which may be associated with prolonged survival [22, 23]. Finally, patients may have a histologic conversion to a diffuse ('unfavorable') histology with disease progression and this patient may then be curable (assuming a conversion to DHL).

Although a 'watch and wait' approach seems reasonable in an asymptomatic patient, hard data to support this approach is quite limited. In a follow-up report on the Stanford study, the median actuarial treatment-free period was 32 months for the whole group, being relatively short for NML patients (10 months) and quite long for the other 2 major favorable histology subtypes (55 months for NLPD; 73+ months for DLWD) [24]. Although the treatment-related morbidity was delayed, most of these patients have progressed and required treatment with single agent chemotherapy, local irradiation or both. To date, no other institution has reported on the feasibility of this approach, although it is under study at the National Cancer Institute. Certainly, a theoretical argument against 'watch and wait' is that, with disease progression, the tumor burden (# logs of tumor cells) may have increased beyond any possibility for cure [25]. Additionally, disease progression may be associated with serious morbidity (eg. epidural cord compression) which may not be reversible with treatment.

The finding of a spontaneous objective regression has been confirmed by another group but it appears to be uncommon ([10%) [22, 23]. Even in the Stanford report on 6 patients with spontaneous regression, two have required treatment for disease recurrence or progression [24]. Although spontaneous objective regression may be associated with prolonged survival, the relative rarity of this occurence hardly argues for adopting a general policy of 'watch and wait'.

Finally, it is not known whether histologic conversion occurs in favorable histology patients whose initial therapy is deferred. It should be re-emphasized that up to 20% of patients with non-Hodgkin's lymphoma may have multiple histologic subtypes even at diagnosis, as has been revealed when more than one lymph node is biopsied [16]. Although the incidence of histologic progression is reported as high as 30% in previously treated patients [26, 27], it appears that this conversion may actually confer a poor prognosis in spite of aggressive combination chemotherapy. In a series from the National Cancer Institute of 21 patients with histologic conversion, only 15 patients (70%) had a diffuse histocytic pattern in the lymph node biopsy at relapse [27]. The other 6 patients 'converted' to diffuse mixed lymphoma. Although one-third of these patients had a complete response to combination chemotherapy, the median survival of the entire group was significantly shorter than that of relapsed favorable histology patients who retained their nodular pattern (46 *versus* 79 months). Only three patients (14%) remain disease-free with a median follow-up of 4 years.

4.2. Early intervention with chemotherapy in advanced favorable lymphoma

Based on the previous arguments, it appears reasonable to institute therapy for advanced favorable histology lymphoma patients at or shortly after their initial presentation. Certainly, a general principle of cancer treatment which appears applicable to these patients is that any improvement in long term survival (? cure) can only be derived from patients achieving a complete response to treatment. However, the definition of a complete response in advanced favorable lymphoma patients requires a meticulous re-evaluation of all prior sites of disease at the completion of treatment. In addition to a repeat physical examination with careful inspection of *all* peripheral nodes, other diagnostic studies need to be repeated including a lymphangiogram, CT scan and contrast studies where indicated. Since there is no reliable non-invasive study to evaluate bone marrow and liver involvement, repeat biopsies are necessary. Additionally, regular (at least yearly) careful follow-up examinations with repeat biopsies (especially bone marrow) and lymphangiogram and/or CT scanning are essential.

Historically, the favorable histology lymphomas represent diseases with a high response rate to a wide variety of chemotherapeutic agents including corticosteroids, alkylating agents, vinca alkaloids, and the antibiotics like adriamycin and bleomycin. For example, treatment with a single alkylating agent can produce a complete response rate of 60–65% in patients with NLPD histology [28]. Combination chemotherapy has also been found to have a high response rate [17, 29]. However, unlike Hodgkin's disease and diffuse histocytic lymphomas, it is not clear whether combination chemotherapy is superior to single-agent treatment in terms of response rate, actuarial disease-free survival and overall survival in favorable histology patients. The results of a recent trial in stage III and IV patients at Stanford failed to reveal any response or survival advantage to cyclophosphamide, vincristine and prednisone (CVP) over single agent cyclophosphamide or chlorambucil [30]. Combining the data from a previous Stanford study [31], the actuarial disease free data favored single agent treatment. These single agent data appear excellent but it must be pointed out that the use of 'disease-free' status to patients receiving single agent chemotherapy in these trials is a misnomer. If patients randomized to receive single agent chemotherapy required no significant change in treatment, then the patient was considered 'disease-free'. In reality some patients achieved a complete response but many did not. Similar to other trials, the main difference between combination chemotherapy such as CVP and single agents like cyclophosphamide and chlorambucil is the duration of treatment time required to achieve a complete response. Patients receiving single agent treatment may require up to 18–24 months to achieve a complete response compared to 3–6 months for CVP [30].

4.3. Early intervention with radiation therapy in advanced favorable lymphoma

There are definite limitations to the use of conventional radiation therapy alone for advanced favorable lymphoma. First, these patients usually present with involvement (often bulky) of multiple lymph node areas, which requires prolonged treatment and assumes that the patient has good overall health. Second, the possibility exists for further tumor progression in one area not actively treated while a different site is being treated. Third, there is the significant probability of occult tumor beyond the radiation portals such as in the bone marrow or other lymph nodes (e.g. popliteal, epitrochlear). Yet, despite these theoretic objections to conventional radiation therapy, initial relapse in irradiated sites is comparatively uncommon [7], which is the converse of the experience with chemotherapy [32].

It is clear that high doses of irradiation (i.e. >3500 rad) are capable of permanently sterilizing lymphomatous masses [7, 33]. If adequate volumes are treated with sufficient doses, then a definite cure rate is achieved for early stage favorable lymphoma patients. The results of high-dose, wide-field total lymphoid irradiation (TLI) in advanced favorable histology patients are quite scant. If there is any curative potential to primary radiation therapy alone, it would have to be restricted to patients with well-documented stage III disease. At best, this represents a minority of advanced favorable histology patients. The radiation technique for these patients must be distinguished carefully from the techniques used for the treatment of Hodgkin's disease. A wide-field approach to the abdomen appears essential if radiation therapy alone is used, because of the high propensity (>70%) for mesenteric nodal involvement [9]. Conversely the infrequent involvement of mediastinum at presentation or relapse argues for an alteration of the supradiaphragmatic radiation technique ('mini-mantle') to limit lung and heart irradiation in this typically middle-aged group of patients.

The results of TLI in patients with stage III nodular lymphoma are quite good. In a group of 51 stage III patients treated at Stanford, the actuarial relapse-free survival was 35% at 10 years [34]. These results compare quite favorably to results reported with combination chemotherapy alone [35]. More importantly, a smaller series reported from another institution rendered even better results with wide field irradiation, with approximately 60% of stage III nodular patients disease-free at 10 years [36]. It needs to be restated, however, that in the natural history of patients with nodular lymphoma, 10 years may be an insufficient period of follow-up to judge reliably whether or not curative treatment has been delivered.

The work of Johnson et al. [37] at the NCI and Chaffey et al. [38] at the Harvard Joint Center for Radiation Therapy established interest in the use of total body irradiation (TBI) in advanced favorable histology lymphoma. The use of TBI as a systemic treatment offers some theoretic advantage over TLI. In general, it appears well tolerated with myelosuppression (especially thrombocytopenia) as the major toxicity. The response rates and overall survival are comparable to those achieved by either single agent or combination chemotherapy [30, 35]. However, long term follow-up shows that virtually all of these patients have relapsed [39]. TBI should be considered a palliative modality with no evidence of curative potential when used either alone [39] or in combination with chemotherapy [30, 35].

4.4. Early intervention with combined modality in advanced favorable lymphomas

Given the relatively modest disease free survival for stage III patients receiving conventional radiation therapy and at least a potential curative role for combination chemotherapy, it is surprising how seldom these two modalities have been combined to treat patients with advanced favorable lymphoma. The reasons for this are not clear but may reflect the initial euphoria concerning the success of combination chemotherapy in treating patients with diffuse histocytic lymphoma (as distinct from other histologies) and the growing awareness of potential leukemogenic consequences of combined modality therapy in Hodgkin's disease [40, 41]. However, a combined modality approach appears attractive when the patterns of failure are analyzed in patients with favorable lymphoma treated with either radiation therapy or combination chemotherapy.

With careful follow-up of stage I, II, and III patients treated by radiation therapy alone, long term local control of involved lymph nodes varied from 92% to 98% in one study [7] (Table 2). Two other interesting findings in the follow-up of these patients were: (1) among patients relapsing in nodal sites, only one-half relapsed in contiguous nodal areas which might have been included in wide-field irradiation; and (2) approximately one-third of relapsing patients failed in extranodal sites with or without lymph node failure. Both of these findings underscore the limitations of conventional high-dose irradiation alone in managing patients with advanced favorable lymphoma. Additionally, since each site of lymph node involvement appears independent of other areas in terms of local control, it is not surprising that the actuarial disease free survival for a heterogenous group of Stage III patients is only 35%.

The typical stage III patient has involvement of multiple lymph node areas on both sides of the diaphragm. The theoretic probability of tumor control or 'cure' (Pc) is a function of local control within each involved lymph node site. Thus,

$$Pc = (1 - R)^n$$

where R = Recurrence rate for a single involved lymph node
and   n = Number of sites involved

Table 2. Local control of lymph node involvement in 'favorable' lymphoma patients treated with radiotherapy (3500 rad or more).*

Histology	Stage			No. of patients	No. of failures in irradiated nodes	% Local control of nodal disease
	I	II	III			
NLPD	11	16	22	49	1	98%
NM	9	16	31	56	3	92%

* Fuks et al. 1975 [7].

Assuming a recurrence rate of 10% for a lymph node site treated to >3500 rad (see Table 2) and five or six involved lymph node sites in a stage III patient, the probability of cure is 30–39%, which is remarkably consistent with the long term disease-free data (35% at 10 years) from Stanford [34].

Using combination chemotherapy with either CVP, C-MOPP or BACOP in advanced favorable histology patients, relapse in previously involved lymph nodes is a more common problem (Table 3) [17]. It can be assumed that those patients who did not achieve a complete response had persistent nodal disease. Also it is reported that 80% of relapses in patients achieving a complete response recurred in nodes only [17]. Thus, in over one-half of patients with favorable histology lymphoma, the involved lymph nodes at presentation were not controlled. The best group appears to be NML patients, where local control of lymph nodes was found in 65% of the 31 patients. Local lymph node control in patients with NLPD or DLWD histology was only 25%. With longer follow-up, a further drop in the disease-free survival curve is reported, presumably with more nodal relapses [18].

Combined modality therapy with high dose TLI and CVP chemotherapy has been used in a prospective trial in patients with stage IV nodular lymphoma at Stanford [42]. The TLI was given after two cycles of CVP chemotherapy and then patients received additional cycles of CVP. The complete response rate, median survival and actuarial disease-free survival did not differ from those of patients who were randomized to receive CVP alone or even single-agent chemotherapy. This study was considered a disappointment for combined modality treatment. However, there was a major flaw in its design which may explain the poor results. The study was limited to stage IV patients, virtually all of whom had bone marrow involvement. Following two cycles of CVP, the bone marrow was not rebiopsied to assess whether the marrow had been 'cleared'. Instead, patients automatically went on to TLI for approximately 4–5 months prior to receiving further systemic therapy. One question whether

Table 3. Local control of lymph node involvement in advanced favorable lymphoma patients treated with CVP, C-MOPP, or BACOP.[a]

Histology	No. of patients	No. of CR	No. of not relapsed	No. of nodal relapses[b]	Total No. of nodal failures
NPDL	49	33	12	17	33 (67%)
NML	31	24	20	3	10 (32%)
DWLD	11	7	2	4	8 (73%)
Total	91	64 (70%)	34 (53%)	24 (27%)	51 (56%)

[a] Anderson *et al.* 1977 [17].
[b] 80% of relapses occurred in lymph nodes only.

286

better results might have been found if a pathologic complete response was required of the chemotherapy prior to the use of TLI. The logic for such an approach is predicated on the observation of a continuous relapse rate following a complete response to combination chemotherapy [32]. This aggressive combined modality approach is being studied at the NCI and is being compared in a random prospective fashion to a 'watch and wait' approach (Fig. 1).

The use of 'consolidation' irradiation following a complete response to combination chemotherapy might be considered as the ultimate in 'non-cross resistance' based on the pattern of lymph node relapse when combination chemotherapy or radiation therapy is used alone. A major issue in a combined modality approach is how combination chemotherapy and irradiation might be integrated to optimize curative potential and minimize morbidity, especially hematologic toxicity. Following clinical and limited pathologic staging (short of laparotomy), patients are started on combination chemotherapy until a complete clinical response has resulted. If the complete response is confirmed by pathologic restaging (bone marrow biopsy, liver biopsy, peritonescopy, etc.), then sequential wide field radiation is begun. An alternative approach after a pathologic complete response would be the repetive alteration of several (2–3) cycles of chemotherapy with large field radiation therapy as described for advanced Hodgkin's disease [43]. However, I would expect that myelosuppression especially thrombocytopenia would severely hamper this latter approach.

The dose and volume of irradiation are two additional variables to be

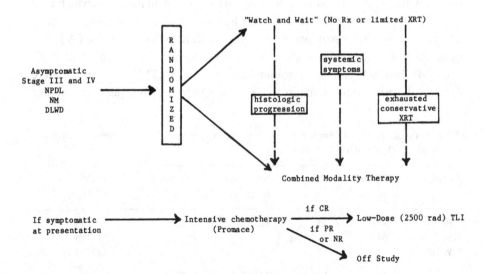

Figure 1. National Cancer Institute study for advanced favorable histology non-Hodgkin's lymphomas.

considered in the optimal design of a combined modality regimen. Since most patients will have involvemen of multiple lymph node areas above and below the diaphragm, sequential wide field irradiation even in a 'consolidative' approach is probably necessary.

Although the radiotherapeutic approach to patients with advanced favorable lymphoma is different thanthat of patients with Hodgkin's disease, the basic principles are the sme. The salient features include the use of a tumoricidal dose, the use of large field radiation via opposed fields to encompass multiple lymphnode areas, and the use of megavoltage beam energy with the ability to treat at an extended source to skin distance. Since many of the lymph node and extra lymphatic sites (e.g. gastrointestinal tract) are midline in crosssectional anatomy, the most efficient treatment plan usually involved equally weighted opposed fields, with both fields being treated daily. The use of a simulator is invaluable to accurate treatment planning to encompass multiple lymph node areas. A linear accelerator (usually 4–6 Mev) is recommended for treatment, with its high dose rate and small penumbra to minimize scatter outside of the designated radiation portals.

There appears to be a rather steep dose-control relationship for the favorable histology lymphomas with conventional fractionated radiation therapy [7]. However, the total dose required to establish long term control in lymph nodes after a complete clinical response to combination chemotherapy is not known. In our combined modality study, TLI to 2500 rad with daily fractionation of 125–175 rad is being used.

An understanding of the tolerance of normal tissues traversed by the radiation beams in treating these advanced lymphoma patients is essential, particularly with combined modality treatment. Typically, the tolerance of several normal tissues must be considered in designing the very large radiation portls to be used. In certain clinical situations, the choice of optimal radiation therapy is limited by the statistical rik of causing significant radiation or combined modality damage to a specific organ. While radiation therapy can result in both acute and late effects, the late effects are the most worrisome. Most acute effects of radiation alone or combined modality therapy are both transient and reversible. Late effects, occurring from several months to a few years following completion of treatment, are often progressive and irreversible, leading to considerable morbidity or even mortality. The mechanism(s) of late injury is not completely understood, although it is speculated to result from damage to the supportive stroma of a normal tissue. The threshold for late radiation injury may be lowered by the concomitant or sequential use of certain chemotherapy drugs like adriamycin, bleomycin, and methotrexate, commonly used in treating the advanced favorable lymphomas.

Since most patients will have involvement above and below the diaphragm, wide field irradiation to these lymph nodes sites seems appropriate. With such extensive irradiation the tolerance of the heart, lung, kidney, bowel and liver as well as bone marrow must be carefully considered. As previously mentioned, the infrequent involvement of the mediastinum and hila at presentation and relapse in these favorable histology patients allows for a modification of supradiaphragmatic irradiation (mini-mantle) to limit heart and lung irradiation. This is especially important if adriamycin and bleomycin are used. With high cervical neck disease or obvious involvement of Waldeyer's ring, large lateral opposed fields to include the involved area are used with the anteroposterior mini-mantle fields blocked back to match below the site of gross nodal involvement.

The high probability of mesenteric lymph node involvement demands whole abdominal pelvic irradiation which will include the liver, kidneys, and bowel as well as the lumbar vertebrae and elvic bone marrow.

Acute bowel damage occurs in most patients and is manifested by diarrhea, colicky abdominal pain and nausea. Damage results from a transient disruption of the normal homeostatic cell renewal system of the intestinal mucosa [44]. Fortunately, it is usually self-limiting and should not be used as criteria for terminating radiation therapy. To improve bowel tolerance to sub-diaphragmatic irradiation, the abdomen and pelvis are treated separately with equally weighted AP-PA fields using a daily fraction of 100–125 rad for the abdominal field and a daily fraction of 150–175 rad for the pelvis. When possible, we attempt to allow a period of 3–4 hours between the abdominal and pelvic fields. The dose to the liver and kidneys is limited to <1500 rad, well below what is felt to represent the threshold for significant radiation injury [45]. With the pelvic field, a midline pelvic block is placed at the level of the pubic symphysis in order to adequately encompass the presacral lymph nodes which may be involved n these favorable histology lymphoma patients.

The potential leukemogenic consequences of combined-modality therapy in these favorable histology patients is of concern in light of the evolving data on combined modality for Hodgkin's disease [40, 41]. However, it should be noted that the chemotherapy usually associated with this uncommon but dreaded late complication includes procarbazine, a drug known for its potential leukemogenicity in animal studies [46]. Procarbazine is not commonly employed in the treatment of the favorable histology patients. An increased incidence of acute non-lymphocytic leukemia has been reported in nodular non-Hodgkin's lymphoma patients receiving intensive radiotherapy [47]. However, it must be pointed out that these patients often received one or more cycles of low dose fractionated total body irradiation as well as prolonged exposure to a single alkylating drug on a daily basis. The combined-modality approach that I have outlined is considerably different and hopefully less leukemogenic.

5. Summary

In summary, a combined-modality approach using combination chemotherapy and high-dose wide-field irradiation appears to have the greatest curative potential for patients with advanced non-Hodgkin's lymphomas of the favorable histologic subtypes. The major argument supporting this approach stems from an analysis of the pattern of relapse following either combination chemotherapy or radiation therapy alone. Since most patients have stage IV disease at presentation, emphasis should be placed on documenting a pathologic complete response to initial chemotherapy (especially in bone marrow) prior to wide field irradiation. The technique of radiation therapy requires a modification in treatment volume and dose. In this setting, long-term control ('cure') of lymph node disease appears possible.

References

1. Kaplan HS: Radiation Therapy. In: Hodgkin's Disease, Harvard University Press, 1980.
2. DeVita VT, Simon RM, Hubbard SM *et al.*: On the curability of advanced Hodgkin's disease with chemotherapy: Long-term follow-up of MOPP treated patients at NCI and the influences of disease variables on prognosis. Ann Intern Med 92:587–595, 1980.
3. Rosenberg SA, Kaplan HS, Hoppe RT, Kushlan P, Horning J: The Stanford randomized trials of the treatment of Hodgkin's disease: 1967–1980. In: Malignant lymphomas, etiology, immunology, pathology, treatment, Rosenberg SA, Kaplan HS (eds), Academic Press, 1982, pp. 513–522.
4. DeVita VT, Canellos GP, Chabner B, *et al.*: Advanced diffuse histocytic lymphoma, a potentially curable disase: Results with combination chemotherapy. Lancet 1:248–250, 1975.
5. Fisher RI, DeVita VT, Johnson RL, Berard CW, Young RC: Prognostic factors for advanced diffuse histiocytic lymphoma following treatment with combination chemotherapy. Am J Med 63:177–182, 1977.
6. Rosenberg SA, Kaplan HS: Evidence for an orderly progression in the spread of Hodgkin's disease. Cancer Res 26:1225–1231, 1966.
7. Fuks Z, Glatstein E, Kaplan HS: Patterns of presentation and relapse in non-Hodgkin's lymphomata. Br J Cancer 31:286–297, 1975.
8. Kaplan HS, Dorfman RF, Nelson TS, *et al.*: Staging laparotomy and splenectomy in Hodgkin's disease: Analysis of indications and patterns of involvement in 285 consecutive unselected patients. Natl Cancer Inst Monogr 36:291–303, 1973.
9. Goffinet DR, Warnke R, Dunnick NR, *et al.*: Clinical and surgical (laparotomy) evaluation of patients with non-Hodgkin's lymphomas. Cancer Treat Rep 61:981–992, 1977.
10. Chabner BA, Johnson RE, Young RC *et al.*: Sequential nonsurgical and surgical staging in non-Hodgkin's lymphoma. Ann Intern Med 85:145–154, 1976.
11. Coller BS, Chabner RA, Gralnick HR: Frequencies and patterns of bone marrow involvement in the non-Hodgkin's lymphomas: Observation on the value of bilateral biopsies. Am J Hematol 3:105–119, 1979.
12. Lukes RJ, Craver LF, Hall TC, Rappaport H, Rubin T: Report of the Nomenclature Committee. Cancer Res 26:1311–1318, 1966.
13. Torti F, Dorfman RF, Rosenberg SA, Kaplan HS: The Changing significance of histology in

Hodgkin's disease. Proc Am Assoc Cancer Res ASCO 20:401, 1979.

14. The non-Hodgkin's lymphoma pathologic classification project: National Cancer Institute sponsored study of classifications of non-Hodgkin's lymphomas: summary and description of a working formulation for clinical usage. Cancer 49:2122–2130, 1982.

15. Warnke RA, Kim H, Fuks Z, Dorfman RF: The coexistence of nodular and diffuse patterns in nodular non-Hodgkin's lymphomas. Significance and clinicopathologic correlation. Cancer 40:1229–1233, 1977.

16. Goffinet DR, Castellino RA, Kim H, Kaplan HS et al.: Staging laparotomies in unselected previously untreated patients with non-Hodgkin's lymphomas. Cancer 32:672–681, 1973.

17. Anderson T, Bender RA, Fisher RI et al.: Combination chemotherapy in non-Hodgkin's lymphomas. Results of long-term follow-up. Cancer Treat Rep 61:1057–1066, 1977.

18. Longo D, Hubbard S, Wesley M, Young RC: Prolonged initial remission in patients with nodular mixed lymphoma (NML). Proc Am Assoc Cancer Res ASCO 22:251, 1981.

19. Glick JH, Barnes JM, Ezoinli EZ et al.: Nodular mixed lymphoma: Results of a randomized trial failing to confirm the prolonged disease-free survival with COPP. Blood, 1981.

20. Jones SE, Fuks Z, Bull M, Rosenberg SA, Kaplan HS: Non-Hodgkin's lymphomas IV. Clinicopathologic correlation in 405 cases. Cancer 31:806–823, 1973.

21. Portlock CS, Rosenberg SA: No initial therapy for stage III and IV non-Hodgkin's lymphomas of favorable histologic type. Ann Intern Med 90:10–13, 1979.

22. Krikorian JG, Portlock CS, Cooney DP et al.: Spontaneous regression of non-Hodgkin's lymphoma: A report of nine cases. Cancer 46:2093–2099, 1980.

23. Gattiker HH, Wiltshaw E, Galton DAG: Spontaneous regression in non-Hodgkin's lymphoma. Cancer 45:2627–2632, 1980.

24. Portlock CS: Deferral of initial therapy for advanced indolent lymphomas. Cancer Treat Rep 66:417–419, 1982.

25. Goldie JH, Coldman AJ: A mathematic model for relating the drug sensitivity of tumors to their spontaneous mutation rate. Cancer Treat Rep 63:1727–1733, 1979.

26. Cullen MH, Lister TH, Brearley RL et al.: Histological transformation of non-Hodgkin's lymphoma: A prospective study. Cancer 44:645–651, 1979.

27. Jones R, Young RC, Berard CW et al.: Histologic progression in non-Hodgkin's lymphoma. Implications for survival and clinical trials. Proc Am Assoc Cancer Res ASCO 20:253, 1979.

28. Jones SE, Rosenberg SA, Kaplan HS, Kadin ME, Dorfman RF: Non-Hodgkin's lymphoma. II. Single-agent chemotherapy. Cancer 30:31–38, 1972.

29. Portlock CS, Rosenberg SA: Chemotherapy of non-Hodgkin's lymphomas: The Stanford experience. Cancer Treat Rep 61–1049–1054, 1977.

30. Hoppe RT, Kushlan P, Kaplan HS et al.: The treatment of advanced stage favorable histology non-Hodgkin's lymphoma: A preliminary report of a randomized trial comparing single agent chemotherapy, combination chemotherapy, and whole body irradiation. Blood 58:592–598, 1981.

31. Glatstein E, Donaldson JS, Rosenberg SA et al.: Combined modality therapy in malignant lymphomas. Cancer Treat Rep 61:1199–1227, 1977.

32. Schein PS, Chabner BA, Canellos GP et al.: Non-Hodgkin's lymphoma: Patterns of relapse from complete remission after combination chemotherapy. Cancer 35:354–357, 1975.

33. Fuks Z, Kaplan HS: Recurrence rates following radiation therapy of nodular and diffuse malignant lymphomas. Radiology 108:675–684, 1973.

34. Glatstein E, Fuks Z, Goffinet DR et al.: Non-Hodgkin's lymphomas of stage III extent: Is total lymphoid irradiation appropriate treatment? Cancer 37:2806–2812, 1976.

35. Young RC, Johnson RE, Canellos GP et al.: Advanced lymphocytic lymphoma: Randomized comparisons of chemotherapy and radiotherapy, alone or in combination. Cancer Treat Rep 61:1153–1159, 1977.

36. Cox JD, Komaki R, Kun LE *et al.*: Stage III nodular lymphoreticular tumors (non-Hodgkin's lymphoma). Results of central lymphatic irradiation. Cancer 47:2247–2252, 1981.
37. Johnson RE: Management of generalized malignant lymphomata with 'systemic' radiotherapy. Br J Cancer (Suppl II) 31:450–455, 1975.
38. Chaffey JT, Hellman S, Rosenthal DS, Maloney WC: Total body irradiation in the treatment of lymphocytic lymphoma. Cancer Treat Rep 61:1149–1154, 1977.
39. Carabell SC, Chaffey JT, Rosenthal DS *et al.*: Results of total body irradiation in the treatment of advanced non-Hodgkin's lymphomas. Cancer 43:994–1000, 1979.
40. Coleman CM, Williams CJ, Flint A *et al.*: Hematologic neoplasia in patients treated for Hodgkin's disease. N Engl J Med 297:1249–1252, 1977.
41. Coleman CN, Burke JS, Varghese A, Rosenberg SA, Kaplan HS: Secondary leukemia and non-Hodgkin's lymphoma in patients treated for Hodgkin's disease. In: Advances in Malignant Lymphomas, Rosenberg SA, Kaplan HS (eds), Academic Press, 1982, p. 259–275.
42. Portlock CS, Rosenberg SA, Glatstein E *et al.*: Treatment of advanced non-Hodgkin's lymphomas. Preliminary results of a prospective trial. Blood 47:747–756, 1976.
43. Hoppe RT, Portlock CS, Rosenberg SA *et al.*: Alternating chemotherapy and irradiation in treatment of advanced Hodgkin's disease. Cancer 43: 472–481, 1979.
44. Kinsella TJ, Bloomer W: Tolerance of the intestine to radiation therapy. Surg Gynecol Obstet 151:273–284, 1980.
45. Kinsella TJ, Fraass BA, Glatstein E: Late effects of radiation therapy in the treatment of Hodgkin's disease. Cancer Treat Rep 66:991–1001, 1982.
46. Sieber SM, Correa P, Dalgard PW *et al.*: Carcinogenic and other adverse effects of procarbazine. Cancer Res 38:2125–2134, 1978.
47. Green MH, Young RC, Glatstein E *et al.*: Acute nonlymphocytic leukemia (ANL) following treatment of non-Hodgkin's lymphoma. Proc Am Assoc Cancer Res ASCO 22:515, 1981.

Subject index

Abdominal involvement, imaging modality
  for staging, 111–125
ABVD chemotherapy, complications with,
  162
Adriamycin
  complications with, 162, 163
  nodular mixed cell lymphomas with,
    251–252
Advanced stage favorable lymphomas,
  278–279
  combined modality therapy in, 283–288
  deferral of initial treatment in, 280–281
  early intervention with chemotherapy in,
    281–282
  management of, 279–288
  radiation therapy alone for, 282–283
Alkeran, see PAVe chemotherapy
Angioimmunoblastic lymphadenopathy
  (AILD), 28, 80, 199
Ann Arbor staging system, 129, 140, 178, 276
Antigens, and Hodgkin cell line, 79
Arteriosclerotic heart disease, and radiation
  therapy, 161
Autopsy findings, 15–16
  clinically unsuspected HD in, 15–16
  progressive among subtypes seen in, 40

BACOP chemotherapy, 233
  nodular mixed cell lymphoma with, 242,
    243
Basal cell skin carcinoma, from radiation
  therapy, 160
Biopsy
  freezing extra tissues for later examination
    in, 49
  HD patients as compromised host in, 48
  relapse, after treatment, 40

Bleomycin
  complications with, 162, 163
  nodular mixed cell lymphomas with,
    251–252, 253
Blood vessel system, and HD, 81
B lymphocyates
  histiocytic lymphoma and, 226
  nodular lymphomas and, 209
  Reed-Sternberg cell origins and, 66–67,
    100, 101, 102, 106
BCNU, in nodular mixed cell lymphoma,
  244–245, 253
BCVP chemotherapy, in nodular mixed cell
  lymphoma, 244–250, 253
Bone
  chemotherapy side effects in, 162, 262
  radiation therapy and growth retardation
    in, 161
Bone marrow biopsy, in staging, 130
Bone marrow involvement, 277
  diagnostic criteria for HD with, 15–16
  granulomatous reaction in HD in, 43
  non-Hodgkin's lymphoma with, 122
  poorly differentiated lymphocytic (PDL)
    lymphomas with, 203
  Reed-Sternberg cells and, 68–72, 80
  staging laparotomy of, 41–42
Breast cancer, and radiation therapy, 160,
  233
Burkitt's lymphoma, in Rappaport
  classification, 185, 193, 204–205

Cancer, and radiation therapy, 160–161
Castleman's disease, 34
Cellular phase of nodular sclerosis, 9, 36–38,
  59
Chemotherapy, 151–164, 227–228

advanced stage favorable lymphomas in, 281–282

anatomic substage in stage III-A disease and, 171–176

complications with, 162

histologic changes after, 45

imaging used in, 121

limited stage disease with, 151–164

nodular mixed cell lymphomas with, 227–228, 230

non-Hodgkin's lymphoma stages I and II and, 260

non-Hodgkin's lymphoma stages II and IV and, 261

radiation therapy combined with, 134; *see also* Combined modality therapy

stage IA and IIA disease in, 154–155

stage IB and IIB disease in, 156–157

stage IIIA disease in, 156, 167–180

toxicity of, 167, 269

see also specific chemotherapeutic regimens

Children, and HD treatment, 155, 161

Chlorambucil

complications with, 233

nodular mixed cell lymphomas with, 227, 235, 250–251

CHOP-BCG chemotherapy, with nodular mixed cell lymphomas, 251–252, 253

Classification systems, 225–226; *see also* specific systems

Clinical stage (CS) of HD, 129

C-MOPP chemotherapy, 279

nodular mixed cell lymphomas with, 234, 235, 242–243, 244–250, 253

non-Hodgkin's lymphoma with, 262

Collagen bands, in nodular sclerosing HD, 59

Combined modality therapy, 134, 151–164

anatomic substages in stage III-A disease with, 171–176

complications of, 163

early intervention with, 275–289

E stage in, 159–160

limited stage disease in, 151–155

mediastinal disease with, 141, 157–158

non-Hodgkin's lymphoma stages III and IV with, 261–262

sites of relapse in, 138

stage I-II disease with, 136, 138

stage IA and IIA disease with, 154–155

stage IB and IIB disease with, 156–157, 159

stage IIIA disease with, 156, 159, 170–176

stage IIIB disease in, 142

stage III and IV disease with, 261–262

Computed tomography (CT)

accuracy of, 116, 118–120

chemotherapy evaluation with, 121

comparative parameters of lymphography and, 115

cost of, 116–117

follow-up treatment after, 279

intravenous contrast agent EOE-13 in, 120

mediastinal masses in stage IA and IIA disease on, 158

non-Hodgkin's lymphoma on, 122–125

residual nodal masses after treatment on, 125

splenic involvement on, 119, 145

staging of HD with, 111, 118–120, 130

strategy in, 120–121

Contraceptives, and chemotherapy, 162

COPP chemotherapy, in nodular mixed cell lymphoma, 232

CP chemotherapy, in nodular mixed cell lymphomas, 244, 246, 247

CT, *see* Computed tomography (CT)

CVP chemotherapy

nodular mixed cell lymphomas with, 242, 243

non-Hodgkin's lymphoma stages III and IV with, 261–262

Cyclophosphamide, 172

nodular mixed cell lymphomas with, 227, 250–251

see also C-MOPP chemotherapy; CP chemotherapy; CVP chemotherapy

Deferred treatment programs

advanced, indolent non-Hodgkin's lymphomas with, 258–261

advanced stage favorable lymphomas with, 280–281

management decisions in, 267–268

nodular mixed cell lymphomas in, 231

potential hazards in, 266–267

Dendritic reticulum cell, and Reed-Sternberg cells, 73–74, 103, 104

Diagnosis of HD, 20–36

cytologic, 48–49

on frozen section, 44

in liver and bone marrow, 15–16
Lukes-Butler classification and, 3
lymphocytic dominance and, 7–9
relapse of HD in, 45
Reed-Sternberg cells in, 4, 20, 80–81, 91, 95
Diffuse Burkitt's lymphoma, 190
Diffuse fibrosis type, lymphocyte depleted HD, 11, 12, 30, 37
Diffuse histiocytic lymphoma, 190–191, 206–207
Diffuse L & H type, HD, 37
Diffuse lymphoblastic lymphoma, 204
Diffuse lymphocytic well-differentiated (DLWD) lymphoma
  chemotherapy for, 250
  combined modality therapy for, 275
  treatment deferral in, 263, 267
Diffuse mixed cell lymphoma, 189–190, 206
Diffuse poorly differentiated lymphocytic (PDL) lymphoma, 188–189
Diffuse lymphomas
  classification comparisons for, 211–214
  diagnosis of, 7
  Rappaport classification of, 194–201
Diffuse undifferentiated non-Burkitt's lymphoma, 193, 194
DTIC, 162

E-lesions, and radiation therapy, 135, 137, 140–141
Eosinophilic granuloma, with HD, 31
E stage disease, in combined modality therapy, 159–160
Extralymphatic involvement, 43–44, 277
  non-Hodgkin's disease in, 277
  radiation therapy for, 140–141

Fertility
  chemotherapy and, 162
  radiation therapy and, 161
Fibroblastic HD, 38
Fibrous histiocytoma, HD resembling, 31–33
Follicle center cell lymphomas, 209
Follicular hyperplasia, in HD differential diagnosis, 22, 30
Follicular lymphomas, 7, 22, 188–189, 226, 229, 235, 241

Gallium scanning, 114

Germ cell neoplasms, in HD differential diagnosis, 44
Germinal centers, giant lymph node hyperplasia resembling, 34
Giant lymph node hyperplasia, in HD differential diagnosis, 34, 44
Graft versus host reaction, 65
Granulocytes, and Reed-Sternberg cells, 104–105
Granulomas
  HD associated with, 31
  Reed-Sternberg cells in, 80
Granulomatous infection
  necrosis in HD resembling, 34
  staging laparotomy of, 42–43
Granulopoiesis, and Hodgkin's cell line, 78
Growth retardation, and radiation therapy, 161

Hematological malignancies, from radiation therapy, 161
Herpes viral infections, 80
Histiocytes
  HD and, 3–4
  Reed-Sternberg cell origins and, 67, 98–100
Histiocytic lymphoma
  B-cell origin of, 209
  classification of, 190–192, 226, 228
  diagnosis of, 9
Histiocytic medullary reticulosis, 67
Histiocytoma, fibrous, HD resembling, 31–33
Histiocytosis, malignant, 25, 67
Hodgkin cell line, 95, 101
  antigen presentation in, 79
  granulopoiesis in, 78
  monokines-fibroblast and lymphocyte growth factors and, 78–79
  spontaneous cell-mediated cytolysis and, 78
Hodgkin's disease (HD)
  differential diagnosis of, 13–15
  extensive necrosis in, 33–34
  at extralymphatic sites, 43–44, 140–141, 277
  histologic background for, 3, 4, 40
  historical aspects of, 91, 92–94
  imaging modalities in, 117–121
  infectious agent in causation of, 92–93
  long-term follow-up and second malignancies in, 232–233
  Lukes-Butler classification definition of,

3–4
non-Hodgkin lymphoma related to, 93, 94
occult, at autopsy, 49
patient as compromised host in, 48
Hoin's disease, 55
Hydantoin-induced lymphadenopathy, 80
Hypothyroidism, from radiation therapy, 161

Imaging
accuracy of modalities in, 111–112
comparison of modalities in, 111–114
Hodgkin's disease and, 117–121
non-Hodgkin's lymphoma on, 121–125
receiver operating characteristic (ROC)
curve in, 113
sensitivity of, 112–113
specificity of, 112
strategy in, 120–121, 123–125
see also Computed tomography (CT);
Lymphography
Immune deficiency in HD, 78, 82
Immunoblastic lymphomas, 102
clinicopathic correlations in, 206–207
immunologic correlations in, 209–210
Rappaport classification of, 187–192,
199–200, 207
Immunoblasts
HD diagnosis and, 13–14
Reed-Sternberg cells similar to, 20, 63, 100
Immunoglobulin G (ImG), and Reed-
Sternberg cells, 66
Immunoglobulin M (ImM), in well-
differentiated lymphocytic lymphoma
(WDL), 196, 206
Infectious agents, and causation of HD,
92–93
Infectious granulomas, necrosis in HD
resembling, 34
Infectious mononucleosis, 63, 80
Interdigitating reticulum cells (IDC), and
Reed-Sternberg cells, 74, 76, 103–104, 106
Interfollicular HD, 30
Interleukin I, 78–79
Intermediated lymphocytic lymphoma (IL),
187
B-cell origin of, 209
Rappaport classification of, 196–197, 206
Inverted Y-field, in radiation therapy,
132–133

Kaposi's sarcoma, HD associated with, 35–36
Kiel classification system, 226, 241
Kiluchi's lymphoma, 210, 211

L & H cells, 5
lymphocyte predominant HD with, 22–23
nodular paragranuloma with, 57–59
L & H type, lymphocyte predominant HD,
57
Lacunar cell predominant nodular sclerosis,
12
Lacunar cells, 59
antigens to, 72
cytologic diagnosis with, 48
interdigitating reticulum cells (IDC) and,
74
L & H cells differentiated from, 5
mixed cellularity HD with, 25
nodular sclerosis with, 9, 10, 23–24, 31
occurrence in sheets or clusters, 24, 31
sarcomatous variant of HD with, 31
Laparotomy, see Staging laparotomy
Large cell follicular center cell lymphoma,
102
Large cell lymphomas
HD differential diagnosis and, 9, 12, 80
non-Hodgkin's lymphoma similar to, 45
Lennert's lymphoma
HD differential diagnosis and, 28, 80
Rappaport classification of, 186, 201, 207
Leukemia
intermediated lymphocytic lymphoma with,
206
radiation therapy and, 161
Limited stage disease, 151–164
chemotherapy alone or combined modality
treatment in, 154–157
complications of treatment in, 160–163
definition of, 151
mediastinal disease in stages IA and IIA
and, 157–158
radiation therapy alone in, 152–154
Lipogranuloma, granulomatous reactions in
HD as form of, 43
Liver involvement, 277
death rates and irradiation of, 146
diagnostic criteria in HD and, 15–16
granulomatous reaction in, HD in, 43
lymphography and computed tomography
(CT) of, 119, 120

in non-Hodgkin's lymphoma, 122, 123
radiation therapy fields and, 133
Reed-Sternberg cells and, 80
splenic involvement related to, 177–178
staging laparotomy of, 41–42
Lukes-Butler classification 1–50, 226, 235, 241
clinical usefulness of, 1, 19–20
definition of HD in, 3–4
diagnosis and, 3
earlier versions of, 212–213
latest version of, 212, 213
modifications of, 1–3
progression in, 13
Rappaport classification compared with,
188–189, 189–190, 191, 193, 194, 196, 197,
199, 200, 201, 207, 210–214
Rye classification modification of, 1–2, 19
Lung carcinoma, from radiation therapy, 160,
232
Lung involvement
nodular sclerosis and, 9
radiation therapy prognosis and, 137
Lymphadenopathies, HD differential
diagnosis with, 80
Lymphangiography, 41
Lymph nodes, 4
granulomatous reaction in HD in, 43
mycosis fungoides in, 35
occult HD in biopsy of, 49
rebiopsy of, after treatment, 6–7
skin involvement in HD and, 15, 43–44
staging laparotomy of, 41
Lymphoblastic leukemia, acute (ALL),
lymphoblastic lymphoma similar to, 187,
197, 207
Lymphoblastic lymphoma, 187
immunologic correlations in, 209
Rappaport classification of, 197–198
Lymphocyte depletion HD (LDHD), 1
antigens to Reed-Sternberg cells in, 72
diagnosis of, 11–13, 80
differential diagnosis of, 12–13, 35
diffuse fibrosis variant of, 12, 30
histologic findings in, 12
progression among subtypes in, 40
reticular variant in, 12, 30
Lymphocyte growth factor, and Hodgkin's
cell line, 78–79
Lymphocyte predominant HD (LPHD)
antigens on Reed-Sternberg cells in, 72

diagnosis of, 7–9
differential diagnosis of, 35
diffuse lymphocyte and histiocyte (L & H)
type, 23
mixed cellularity type differentiated from,
25
nodular lymphocyte and histiocyte (L & H)
form of, 22
nodular paragranuloma type of, 59
progression among subtypes in, 40
Reed-Sternberg (RS) cells in, 8–9
staging laparotomy in, 130
Lymphocytes, 4
diagnosis of HD and, 7–9
nodular sclerosing HD (NSHD) with, 39
Reed-Sternberg cell origins and, 100–103,
106
in relapse biopsies, 40
Lymphocytic leukemia, chronic (CLL)
HD diagnosis and, 23, 34, 35
pseudofollicular proliferation centers
pattern in, 195
well-differentiated lymphocytic lymphoma
similar to, 205
Lymphoepitheloid cell lymphoma, 201
Lymphography
accuracy of, 115, 118, 119–120, 122–123
anatomic substage with, 177
chemotherapy evaluation with, 121
comparative parameters of computed
tomography (CT) and, 115
cost of, 116–117
criteria for nodal involvement in, 116
follow-up in, 115–116, 279
lymphatic cannulation in, 115
lymph node sites covered in, 114–115
mediastinal masses in stage IA and IIA
with, 158
non-Hodgkin's lymphoma in, 122–123, 124
radiation therapy follow-up with, 134
splenic involvement on, 119
stage I-II diseases in radiation therapy on,
141
staging of HD with, 111, 114–116, 117–121,
130
strategy in, 120–121
Lymphoid cells, and Reed-Sternberg cell
origins, 63–77, 99
Lymphoid hyperplasia, mixed cellularity HD
differentiated from, 26–28

298

Lymphoproliferative disorders, HD associated with, 34–36

Macrophages, and Reed-Sternberg cells, 67, 99, 100
Malignant histiocytosis, 25, 67
Malignant lymphoma, 225
Malignant melanoma, in HD differential diagnosis, 25
Malpighian bodies, splenic, in HD, 15
Mantle field, in radiation therapy, 131–132
Mantle zone lymphoma, 196
Mediastinal disease
    radiation therapy for, 45, 140, 141, 142
    stage IA and IIA disease treatment with, 155, 157–158
Mediastinoscopy, 44
Mesenteric nodes, in HD, 117
Metastatic disease
    HD diagnosis and, 14
    lacunar cells and, 24, 31
Mixed cellularity HD (MCHD), 202
    antigens on Reed-Sternberg cells in, 72
    B-cell origin of Reed-Sternberg cells and, 66
    cellular phase of nodular sclerosis as, 9
    diagnosis of, 11, 25–29, 80
    differential diagnosis of, 25–28, 35, 37
    nodular and/or diffuse, 189–190
    progression among subtypes of, 40
    reticular type, lymphocytic depletion HD differentiated from, 12
    T-cell lymphomas and, 28–29
    use of term, in Lukes-Butler classification, 2–3
Monoclonal antibodies, and Reed-Sternberg cells, 72, 77, 103, 104–105
Monoclonal gammopathy, in well-differentiated lymphocytic lymphoma (WDL), 196, 206
Mononuclear variants of Reed-Sternberg cells, 41, 95
MOPP chemotherapy, 234
    complications with, 162
    mediastinal disease with, 141
    radiation therapy combined with, 134
    stage IA and IIA disease with, 155
    stage IIIA disease with, 142, 156, 163, 172
Mummified cells, 20
Murine lymphoid dendritic cells, 75–76

Mycosis fungoides
    HD associated with, 35
    Rappaport classification of, 185, 208
Myocardial infarctions, with radiation therapy, 161
Myeloid cells, and Reed-Sternberg cells, 68–73
Myelomonocytic leukemia, acute (AMML), 72

Nasopharyngeal carcinoma, and HD differential diagnosis, 25
Nitrogen mustard, see MOPP chemotherapy
Nodular Burkitt's lymphoma, 193
Nodular histiocytic lymphoma, 190–192
Nodular L & H form, HD, 7, 37
Nodular lymphomas, 98
    classification comparisons for, 210–211
    clinicopathic correlations in, 201–205
    immunologic correlations in, 208–209
    Rappaport classification of, 188–194
    reproducibility of, 208
    treatment program for, 226–227
Nodular mixed cell lymphoma, 189–190, 202, 228–254
    adriamycin in combination chemotherapy in, 251–252
    biological course of, 233–237
    chemotherapy for, 227–228, 242–254
    classification of, 227
    combined modality treatment of, 275
    deferred initial therapy in, 231
    Eastern Cooperative Oncology Group (ECOG) chemotherapy trials in, 243–250
    lack of consensus in histopathological classification of, 236, 240–242
    National Cancer Institute chemotherapy trials with, 242–243
    non-aggressive therapy for, 230–233
    pathological classification issues in, 228–230
    reproducibility of classification of, 228
    Stanford chemotherapy trials in, 250–251
Nodular paranguloma, 57, 66–67
Nodular poorly differentiated lymphocytic (NPDL) lymphoma, 188–189, 228, 229, 239
    combined modality therapy for, 275
    deferred treatment in, 263, 267
    nodular mixed cell lymphoma

differentiated from, 233–237
Nodular sclerosis HD (NSHD), 1, 4
  antigens to lacunar variants in, 72
  B-cell origin of Reed-Sternberg cells and,
    66
  cellular phase of, 9, 36–38, 59
  collagen bands in, 59
  diagnosis of, 9–10, 23–25, 80
  differential diagnosis in, 25, 37
  fibroblast growth factors in, 78–79
  histologic diagnosis of, 9
  lacunar cells in, 9, 31, 59
  with lymphocyte depletion, 39
  mummified cells in, 21
  necrosis in, 9–10, 24–25
  pleomorphic cells in, 6
  progression among subtypes in, 40
  rebiopsy after treatment for, 7
  Reed-Sternberg cells in diagnosis of, 21
  relapse biopsies in, 40
  staging before radiation therapy in, 176
Nodular undifferentiated non-Burkitt's
  lymphoma, 193–194
Non-Hodgkin's lymphoma (NHL)
  B lymphocytes in, 101
  chemotherapy and, 162, 163
  classification of, 277–278
  composite lymphomas with, 35
  diagnosis of, 45
  with diffuse epitheloid histiocytic reaction,
    201, 207
  HD related to, 93, 94
  imaging examination in, 121–125
  Rappaport classification of, 183–214
  Rye classification of, 1
  stages I and II, 258–260
  stages III and IV, 260–263
  treatment deferral for advanced, indolent,
    257–271
Non-lymphocytic leukemia, acute (ANLL),
  162, 163, 232, 233

Oral contraceptives, and chemotherapy, 162
Ovaries, and radiation therapy, 161

Paracortical hyperplasia, 22
Pathological stage (PS) of HD, 129
PAVe chemotherapy
  radiation therapy combined with, 134
  stage IIIA disease with, 142

Pericarditis, and radiation therapy, 161
Pericardium involvement, and radiation
  therapy prognosis, 137
Periopheral T-cell lymphomas, 209–210, 211
  diffuse mixed cell lymphomas and, 206
  HD differential diagnosis and, 13
  non-Hodgkin's lymphoma and, 186, 192,
    207
Phagocytosis, and Reed-Sternberg cells, 67,
  99
Phenylalanine mustard, complications with,
  233
Pleomorphic cells, 5–6, 59
Pneumonitis, radiation, 161, 163
Poorly differentiated lymphocytic (PDL)
  lymphoma, 188–189, 202–203
Popcorn cells, 7, 22
Prednisolone, see C-MOPP chemotherapy;
  CP
  chemotherapy; CVP chemotherapy;
  MOPP chemotherapy
Procarbazine, see C-MOPP chemotherapy;
  MOPP chemotherapy; PAVe
  chemotherapy
Progressive transformation of germinal
  centers lesion, 22, 59
Proteins, within Reed-Sternbeg cells, 102
Pseudofollicular proliferation centers,
  194–195
Pulmonary infiltrates, acute, 48
Pyknotic giant cells, 6, 7, 9

Radiation pneumonitis, 161, 163
Radiation therapy, 129–148
  advanced favorable lymphomas with,
    282–283
  anatomic substage in stage III-A disease
    and, 171–176
  complications with, 138, 160–161
  computed tomography (CT) with, 125
  E stage disease with, 160
  extralymphatic extension of HD and,
    140–141
  fields used in, 131–133
  histologic changes after, 45
  limited stage disease with, 152–154
  lymphography follow-up after, 140
  nodular mixed cell lymphoma with,
    230–231, 232
  non-Hodgkin's lymphoma stages I and II

with, 260
non-Hodgkin's lymphoma stages III and IV
    with, 260–261
outcome of, 133–148
prognostic factors in, 143–144
sites of relapse in, 138, 145–146
stage I-II disease in, 134–142
stage IIIA disease in, 142–148, 168–169
stage IIIB disease in, 169
staging considerations in, 129–131
techniques in, 131–133
toxicity of, 269
tumoricidal doses in, 131
see also Combined modality therapy
Rappaport classification, 98, 183–214
clinicopathic correlations in, 201–208
description of, 186–210
development of, 183–184
diffuse lymphomas in, 194–201
histiocytic in, 226–228
immunologic correlations in, 208–210
morpholic subtypes in, 188–192
NHL classification (1975) of, 184
NHL classification (1976) of, 186–187
nodular lymphomas in, 188–194, 229
nodular mixed cell lymphomas in, 226, 239,
    240
reproducibility of, 208
terminology used in, 186–187
Reactive follicular hyperplasia, 30
Receiver operating characteristic (ROC)
    curve, in imaging, 113
Reed-Sternberg (RS) cells, 55–107
B-cell origin of, 66–67, 101
biologic activities of, 78–79
bone marrow biopsies with, 41, 42
cellular origin of, 96–106
definition of HD and, 3
dendritic reticulum cells and, 73–74
diagnosis of HD and, 4, 20, 49, 80–81, 91,
    95
diffuse fibrosis form of lymphocyte
    depleted HD with, 30
evidence for, as malignant cell in HD,
    55–57
granulocytes and, 104–105
histiocytes and, 67, 98–100
histologic judgment in recognition, of, 92
immune defects in HD and, 82
immunoblasts similar to, 20

immunoglobulin in, 101–102
interdigitating reticulum cells (IDC) and,
    74, 103–104
lacunuar variants of, 59; see also Lacunar
    cells
liver biopsies with, 41, 42
lymph node on staging laparotomy with, 41
lymphocytes and origin of, 100–103
lymphocytic predominance types, HD,
    with, 8–9
lymphoid origin of, 63–77, 99
macrophage properties of, 67
methods for study of, 62–63
MGP atain in identification of, 5
mixed cellularity HD with, 11, 25, 29
monoclonal antibody immunohistochemical
    studies of, 104–105
mononuclear variants of, 95
murine lymphoid dendritic cell and, 75–76
myeloid cells and, 68–73
necrosis in HD and, 34
nodular L & H form, lymphocyte
    predominant HD with, 22
nodular sclerosis with, 9, 10, 23, 45
phagocytosis and, 67, 99
pleomorphic or sarcomatous variant of, 59
progression among subtypes in
    classification and, 40
proteins in, 102
rarity of, in HD, 93
reticular variant, lymphocyte depleted HD,
    with, 30
reticulum cells and, 96–98
significance of, in future control of HD,
    80–83
single versus multiple disease hypothesis
    in, 82
stromal background for, and diagnosis,
    20–21
thymic or T-cell origin of, 64–65, 103
toxoplasmic lymphadenitis and, 31
unidentified normal cell (UNC) in, 76–77,
    106
variants of, 4–6, 57–62
Reticular type, lymphocytic depletion HD, 4,
    12
diagnosis of, 30
differential diagnosis in, 37
mixed cellularity HD differentiated from,
    25–26

pleomorphic cells in, 6, 59
Reticulum cells, and Reed-Sternberg cells, 96–98, 100
Reticulum cell sarcoma, 101
Rye classification, 1–2, 19, 98, 277

Sarcoidosis, and granulomatous reaction in HD, 43
Sarcomatous variant of HD, 31
Sarcomatous variant of Reed-Sternberg cells, 59
Sclerosis
  fibroblastic proliferation differentiated from, 38
  HD differential diagnosis with, 44
  histologic progression in, 40
  nodular L & H type, lymphocyte depletion HD with, 22
  nodular sclerosing HD (NSHD) with, 23, 25, 36, 37, 38, 40
Sinusoidal large cell lymphoma, 14
Skin carcinoma, from radiation therapy, 160
Skin involvement
  approach to, 43–44
  differential diagnosis of HD and, 35
  lymph node biopsy and, 15
Small lymphocytic lymphoma, in differential diagnosis of HD, 23
Spade field, in radiation therapy, 132–133
Spleen involvement, 177–179
  diagnosis of HD and, 15
  granulomatous reaction in HD and, 43
  liver involvement related to, 178–179
  lymphography and computed tomography (CT) of, 119
  malpighian bodies in HD and, 15
  non-Hodgkin's lymphoma with, 123
  radiation therapy fields and, 133
  Reed-Sternberg cells in, 74, 80
  stage III disease and, 178, 179
  stage IIIA disease and, 142, 144–145, 146
  staging laparotomy of, 40–41
Splenectomy
  stage I-II disease with radiation therapy and, 141
  staging laparotomy with, 130
Stage IA and IIA
  chemotherapy alone or combined modality therapy in, 154–155
  mediastinal masses and treatment in,
      157–158
  radiation therapy alone for, 152–153
Stage IB and IIB disease
  chemotherapy alone or combined modality treatment in, 156–157
  combined modality therapy in, 159
  radiation therapy alone in, 154
Stage IIIA disease, 167–180
  anatomic substage of, 144, 146–147, 171–176
  causes of death in, 146
  chemotherapy alone or combined modality therapy in, 156
  chemotherapy alone as initial therapy in, 167–168
  combined modality therapy in, 159, 170–171
  prognostic factors in, 143–144
  radiation therapy for, 142–148, 153–154, 168–169
  sites of initial relapse in, 145–146
  splenic involvement in, 178–179
Stage IIIB disease, and radiation therapy, 169
Staging
  anatomic substage in, 176–177
  imaging modality in, 111–125
  radiation therapy and, 129–131, 141
  Reed-Sternberg cells in, 80–81
  studies included in, 129–131
Staging laparotomy, 40–43, 117, 130
  in clinical stage IIB disease, 42–43
  granulomatous reaction in, 42–43
  importance of, 20
  infradiaphragmatic involvement in, 117
  liver and bone marrow involvement in, 41–42
  lymph nodes in, 41
  lymphography before, 116
  mediastinal masses in stage IA and IIA with, 158
  nodular sclerosis with, 176–177
  splenectomy with, 130
  splenic involvement on, 40–41, 177
  technique in, 130
  treatment program planning with, 130–131
Subtotal lymphoid irradiation (STLI), 133
Suchi's lymphoma, 210, 211
Superior vena cava syndrome, 45
Syncytial variant, nodular sclerosis, 9

T-cell lymphoma, 63

immunoblastic lymphomas with, 200
mixed cell HD differentiated from, 28–29
Testicular shielding, in radiation therapy, 161
Thoracotomy, 44
Thymoma, in HD differential diagnosis, 44
Thymus, HD originating from, 64–65
T lymphocytes
    interdigitating cells and, 74
    Reed-Sternberg cell origins and, 64–65, 99,
        100, 103, 106
Total lymphoid irradiation (TLI), 133
Toxoplasma, in HD differential diagnosis,
    30–31, 80
Treatment programs, 226–227
    deferred, with advanced, indolent non-
        Hodgkin's lymphomas, 257–271
    histologic changes after, 45
    long-term follow-up and second
        malignancies after, 232–233
    non-Hodgkin's lymphoma evaluation in,
        122
    rebiopsy after, 6–7
    relapse biopsies after, 40
    residual nodal masses after, 125
    staging laparotomy and planning for,
        130–131

Ultrasound, 114, 146

Undifferentiated non-Burkitt's lymphoma, in
    Rappaport classification, 193–194, 204–205
Unidentified normal cell (UNC), and Reed-
    Sternberg cell origins, 76–77, 97, 106
Urography, 114

Vascular system, and HD cells, 81
Vinblastine, 162, 172; see also PAVe
    chemotherapy
Vincristine, see C-MOPP chemotherapy;
    CVP chemotherapy; MOPP chemotherapy

Waldeyer field, in radiation therapy, 132
Waldron's lymphoma, 210, 211
Well-differentiated lymphocytic lymphoma
    (WDL)
    B-cell origin of, 209
    clinicopathic correlations of, 205–206
    differential diagnosis of HD and, 7, 23
    Rappaport classification of, 194–196
WHO classification system, 226
Working Formulation classification nodular
    mixed cell lymphoma in, 241–242
    Rappaport classification comparisons with,
        188, 189, 191, 193, 196, 197, 198–199, 200,
        201, 203, 210–214

Zombie cells, 6, 7